Clinics in Developmental Medicine No. 171
PEOPLE WITH HYPERACTIVITY:
UNDERSTANDING AND MANAGING
THEIR PROBLEMS

© 2007 Mac Keith Press
30 Furnival Street, London EC4A 1JQ

Editor: Hilary M Hart
Managing Editor: Michael Pountney
Sub Editor: Pat Chappelle

First published in this edition 2007

British Library Cataloguing-in-Publication data:
A catalogue record for this book is available from the British Library

ISSN: 0069 4835
ISBN: 978 1 898683 46 9

Printed by The Lavenham Press Ltd, Water Street, Lavenham, Suffolk
Mac Keith Press is supported by Scope

Clinics in Developmental Medicine No. 171

People with Hyperactivity: Understanding and Managing Their Problems

Edited by

ERIC TAYLOR
Institute of Psychiatry
King's College London
London
England

2007
Mac Keith Press

CONTENTS

AUTHORS' APPOINTMENTS

Philip J Asherson
Professor of Molecular Psychiatry, MRC Social Genetic Developmental Psychiatry, Institute of Psychiatry, King's College London, London, England

Gillian Baird
Professor and Consultant Paediatrician, Guy's and St Thomas' Hospital NHS Foundation Trust, Guy's Hospital, London, England

Wai Chen
Research Fellow and Honorary Consultant Child Psychiatrist, MRC Social, Genetic and Developmental Psychiatry Centre, Institute of Psychiatry, King's College London, London, England

Sarah Curran
Senior Lecturer and Honorary Consultant Psychiatrist, Department of Psychological Medicine (Section of Brain Maturation), Institute of Psychiatry, King's College London, London, England

Paul Gringras
Consultant in Paediatric Neurodisability in Sleep Medicine, Paediatric Neurosciences, Evelina Children's Hospital, St Thomas' Hospital, Guy's and St Thomas' Hospital NHS Foundation Trust, London, England

Peter Hill
Consultant Child and Adolescent Psychiatrist, Guy's and St Thomas' Hospital NHS Foundation Trust, Guy's Hospital, London, England

Adam Jaffe
Associate Professor and Staff Specialist, Paediatric Respiratory Medicine, Sydney Children's Hospital, Randwick, NSW, Australia

JJ Sandra Kooij   Consultant Psychiatrist and Head, Department of Psychiatry, ADHD bij volwassenen, Den Haag, the Netherlands

Paramala Janardhanan Santosh   Consultant and Honorary Senior Lecturer, Centre for Interventional Paediatric Psychopharmacology, Department of Child and Adolescent Mental Health, Great Ormond Street Hospital for Children, London, England

Kapil Sayal   Senior Lecturer and Honorary Consultant Child Psychiatrist, Department of Community-Based Medicine, University of Bristol, Bristol, England

Stephen Sheldon   Associate Professor of Pediatrics *and* Director, Sleep Medicine Center, Children's Memorial Hospital, Chicago, USA

Emily Simonoff   Professor and Honorary Consultant Child Psychiatrist, Dept. of Child and Adolescent Psychiatry, Institute of Psychiatry, King's College London, London, England

Maxine Sinclair   Clinical Psychologist, Developmental Neuropsychiatry Service, South London and Maudsley NHS Trust, London, England

Edmund Sonuga-Barke   Professor of Developmental Psychopathology, Developmental Brain-Behaviour Unit, School of Psychology, University of Southampton; Visiting Professor of Developmental Psychopathology, Social, Genetic and Developmental Psychiatry Centre, Institute of Psychiatry, King's College, University of London, England; *and* Adjunct Professor of Child Psychiatry, Child Study Center, New York University, New York, USA

Angie Stevens   Specialist Registrar, Child and Adolescent Psychiatry, South London and Maudsley NHS Trust, Maudsley Hospital, London, England

Eric Taylor

Professor and Honorary Consultant Child Psychiatrist, Department of Child and Adolescent Psychiatry, Institute of Psychiatry, King's College London, London, England

Margaret Thompson

Clinical Reader in Child and Adolescent Psychiatry, University of Southampton; *and* Consultant CAMHS, Ashurst Hospital, Ashurst, Southampton, England

Jody Warner-Rogers

Consultant Clinical Psychologist, Guy's and St Thomas' Hospital NHS Foundation Trust, Guy's Hospital, London, England

PREFACE

The forerunner of this volume, *The Overactive Child*[1], started from a rather European position of scepticism about the neurological theories that gave birth to the idea of hyperactivity. It concluded that much hyperactive behaviour is situationally specific but aetiologically nonspecific; but that a restricted concept of hyperkinetic disorder carried scientific power and clinical value. We did not foresee just how true the scientific prediction would prove. The 20 years since it was published have seen striking advances in the ability to investigate children's brains noninvasively and to measure their genetic constitutions; hyperkinetic disorder and ADHD have yielded a robustness of neuroimaging findings and DNA alterations that has eluded other complex psychiatric disorders; there is a greater richness of psychological theory, and a better understanding of the natural history and the risks that hyperactive behaviour imposes. There has also been a much wider recognition of the problem and a corresponding rise in the numbers recognized and treated: from an estimate of fewer than 0.5 per 1000 children in the UK then, to more than 3 per 1000 now[2]. The rates in the USA have risen too, but from a much higher base; from about 12 per 1000 then to about 50 per 1000 now. The terminology in Europe has also changed, and 'ADHD' has become the preferred diagnostic phrase even when the criteria of hyperkinetic disorder are still applied.

The methods of treatment, however, have not changed greatly. In the UK, stimulants were withdrawn from the market and then reintroduced 10 years ago; their use has increased in many European countries; but only one new drug has been introduced, and that very recently. The behavioural treatments described in the original book are still used; cognitive approaches have still failed to prove their value. The outcome of treated groups of children remains one of considerable developmental risk, in spite of well-established therapies remaining available.

This version of the book therefore has a different focus from the first, as well as a different group of authors. We no longer feel it necessary to deal at length with the concepts and their validity, and some of the lengthy arguments are now things of the past. Rather, we have tried to produce a text that will be useful for what we see as the most pressing current need, the provision of good quality of understanding and service to those affected and their families. There is a rapid expansion in many parts of the world outside North America, often via the establishment of specialist clinics. New groups of professionals are taking on the challenge: child psychiatry and clinical psychology have been joined by paediatricians and nurses enthusiastically, by educational psychology and teaching professions occasionally, and by police and youth justice systems increasingly. Adult services, by contrast, have on

---

[1] Taylor E (1987) *The Overactive Child. Clinics in Developmental Medicine No. 97.* London: Spastics International Medical Publications.

[2] This is an increase in recognition, not necessarily in the numbers affected, as discussed in Chapter 1.

the whole not incorporated the concepts of ADHD into their practice. We have set out to provide a basic framework of understanding, assessing and intervening that can be adapted to varying local circumstances.

Eric Taylor
March 2007

1
CLINICAL AND EPIDEMIOLOGICAL FOUNDATIONS

Eric Taylor

The concepts of hyperactivity and attention deficit are founded on observations of behaviour. The key ideas are those of impulsiveness, overactivity and inattentiveness. They sound easy to recognize, but in practice confusion can arise from their overlap with other common behaviour problems and from uncertainty about what is developmentally appropriate. This chapter will therefore begin by describing the behaviours that clinicians need to recognize, and the extent to which they reflect known disturbances of psychological processes. It will then go on to the epidemiology that is founded upon the behaviours and the corresponding diagnostic constructs. This epidemiological research suggests a developmental model of interacting risks and protective factors, in which variation is determined by a large number of interacting factors, each of small effect, and in which variation in the population is continuous. The boundaries of 'disorder' are therefore somewhat blurred; decisions about what to recognize and when to intervene are often difficult, and controversy has attended them.

Clinicians usually rely on descriptions made by adults who know the child well. Recognition would be easier if an experienced professional could observe every child in detail over representative periods. Teachers can certainly do this, and teacher ratings have been at the heart of research and clinical identification; but ratings can be puzzling and misleading even for an experienced teacher. The words that are used can mean different things to different people.

Inattention

Inattentiveness in behaviour predicts later problems – especially, problems in education. It often accompanies restlessness and impulsiveness, but is not a necessary part of them. If it is not accompanied by overactivity and impulsiveness, then the later outcome is of educational and occupational underachievement rather than the psychiatric complications that attend poor impulse control.

Several concepts are used in describing an inattentive style. Affected children show an apparent lack of focus on tasks, they seem disorganized and fail to attend to details. They are often seen as forgetful, prone to lose things, not taking in instructions, and leaving activities incomplete. They "do not sustain attention" or they are "distracted by external stimuli". These types of problem can be considered separately, but the coexistence of several of them is the hallmark of inattentiveness.

"Lack of focus and attention to detail"
Robert had been referred at the age of 10 years because of increasing parental concern that he was underachieving at school. School had regarded him as a slow learner (and otherwise unproblematic), yet his measured IQ was 110. During a period of observation at school he was initially easy and docile for the teacher to settle to an individual task (a number sheet based on train journeys). He began it swiftly, apparently without realizing what was entailed. He then realized that a pencil and eraser were needed, and bent down to get them from his bag; after prolonged fumbling he found them and went back to the paper sheet. The teacher had emphasized the written instruction that he should do the first three first; but a later exercise was set out more prominently, with attractive pictures to follow, and he began on that. He realized at once he could not do it, and put up his hand; the teacher resettled him to the first questions, about speed of movement. He wrote an answer about distance, not speed, looked pleased and began to draw a picture of the train. The time for that part of the class then expired, and he went off to a corner with models set out, leaving the paper behind on the table. The teacher called him back to bring her the paper, which he did cheerfully.

At no point had he been disruptive, or engaged in unrelated activity, or been distracted by external stimuli, and the task was quite easy by the standards of the class; yet he had made no headway and presumably learned nothing from it. Further neuropsychological analysis looked for a working memory deficit, but did not find one. The structure provided by the psychologist administering the tests enabled him to achieve well when he did not do so spontaneously.

Forgetfulness and 'losing things' are often responsible in themselves for an appearance of muddle and disorganization. They can be due to a memory impairment, so psychological testing of short-term memory is particularly useful. If a memory loss is the only cognitive problem, it has rather different implications for advice about learning than would be the case for an attention problem.

'Not sustaining attention' and 'distractibility' are frequent descriptions, yet experimental analyses of attention have indicated clearly that neither actually applies to children with ADHD (see next section). This apparent paradox emphasizes what a gulf there is between descriptions at behavioural and cognitive levels. Clinicians should therefore be careful about applying theoretical explanations derived from cognitive psychology.

'Distractibility', for instance, is the application of a theory to describe the behaviours, and the theory has not worked well. What is actually seen is a sequence of activities each of short duration, and correspondingly a high rate of change in activities. Observation schemes and the formulation of interview questions take account of this and define behaviours in terms of what is seen rather than inferences about their cause.

COGNITIVE ANALYSES OF INATTENTION
The behaviours of inattention do not map on to the cognitive changes in a simple way. The phrase 'attention deficit' has been seductive in implying that the task of cognitive analysis is to find the component of the attentional process that is impaired in children with ADHD.

TABLE 1.1
Cognitive changes in ADHD

Executive function tests (e.g. working memory, planning)
Variable reaction times
Inhibitory function (e.g. in 'Stop' tests – see text)
Motivational changes (delay aversion)
Visuospatial understanding
Perception of time
Flexibility of attention (e.g. switching tests)
Poor error correction

Much research has focused on the search, and much of it is distinguished. So far, however, the conceptualization has not worked very well in either research or clinical terms.

In research terms, a large body of literature has addressed the puzzles, and the interested reader can consult several scientific reviews (e.g. Sergeant et al. 2003). I would like to summarize it further into some provisional conclusions:

• There are indeed cognitive changes that distinguish groups of children with ADHD from ordinary children. The most widely used test is probably the Continuous Performance Test, of which there are several commercially available forms including the TOVA and the Conners (for references, see Taylor et al. 1998). This requires detection and quick response to some signals but not to others. Errors can be either missing responses to signals or making 'errors of commission' – responding to a stimulus that did not call for a response. Reaction times are more variable than in controls. The mistakes can be due to off-task behaviour, such as simply not looking at the computer screen. Mistakes, however, are common in people with ADHD even when they are overtly concentrating on the signal.

• The changes are not in the abilities traditionally called 'attention'. If it were an inability to sustain attention over time, then mistakes would cluster towards the end. In fact, however, children with ADHD make more mistakes even at the very beginning. Similarly, if it were due to distractibility then the performance of children with ADHD would be affected by adding irrelevant information more than that of ordinary children. This turns out not to be the case.

• The relationship between test scores and behaviour has not yet been shown to be due to a shared genetic basis. With the exception of variability in response speed, there is little evidence for genes in common (Kuntsi and Stevenson 2001) (Table 1.1).

• There is no single deficit. The various cognitive associations of ADHD cannot all be reduced to one underlying problem or group of problems (Solanto et al. 2001).

'Executive function' changes include poor performance on tests of working memory, planning and foresight, and flexibility in switching from one aspect of the world to another. They involve brain systems using networks extending from frontal cortex to basal ganglia (Swanson et al. 2004). They are an important part of higher function, and tests show impairment not only in ADHD but also in autism, learning difficulties and other neurodevelopmental problems. Particular mention should be made of 'error detection and correction', which are affected in ADHD, and may be more specific to this disorder (Sergeant et al. 2003). There is less of the usual reaction to making a mistake – which should be to notice it and learn from it. This is reflected in a smaller neurophysiological response when an error has been made (Rubia et al. 2005).

'Dual task' tests, in which people have to combine two simultaneous activities effectively, are often performed in a disorganized way. Such tests are included in convenient test batteries such as the Tests of Everyday Attention for Children (TEA-ch) (see Chapter 4). Switching attention from one aspect of a stimulus array to another also seems to be less effective in children with diagnosed ADHD than in normal controls.

Impulsiveness is also an important aspect of the cognitive changes. It is usually measured by tests in which a response has to be given to most stimuli but suppressed for others ('Go–No Go'), or in which some signals require the suppression of a response that has already been started ('Stop' tests). Behavioural impulsiveness is considered in the next section, together with the idea that impulsiveness may be more a motivational change than a cognitive deficit. The important points to raise here are that there is considerable variation between individuals with ADHD in the abilities that are impaired, and that the cognitive abilities do not all have a single brain basis. Functional neuroimaging has been able to identify localized activation during the performance of several cognitive tests (Rubia et al. 2003), and different networks are involved. Error detection and response activate a left-sided inferofrontal system, in contrast to the right-sided inferofrontal and striatal activity during the inhibition of response in a 'Stop' test. There are more posterior patterns of neuroactivation in attention switching and in timing tasks. Yet all these systems show underactivation in children and adolescents with ADHD by comparison with typical young people. The suggestion therefore is that the cognitive changes in ADHD are heterogeneous. We are some way from a diagnostic set of cognitive tests, and their value may prove to be in analysing an individual child's strengths and weaknesses even more than in contributing to a diagnosis.

CLINICAL IMPLICATIONS
At the clinical level, one is analysing individual children rather than groups. It is then apparent that most – but not all – children with ADHD have a weakness on at least one of the 'attention' tests, few have weaknesses on all of them, and there is no single pattern of impairment. The type of problem that is shown is often a characteristic of the individual; that is, it may well be persistent over repeated testing and not just a random fluctuation of performance on different tests. The aim of clinical testing is therefore to analyse the individual's strengths and weaknesses rather than to detect a characteristic and diagnostic clustering of tests. Chapter 4 will take further the issues of how to do this.

In summary, 'attention deficit' is not a single deficit, and not an explanatory concept. Rather, it is descriptive of a set of changes in behaviour that carry adverse consequences for later development.

Impulsivity
Again, one needs to get behind the word and distinguish what one can see from theories about it. In ordinary English usage, an impulse is not only "a sudden inclination to act

without premeditation" (which corresponds to definitions of hyperactivity), but also an "incitement arising from some state of mind or feeling" (*Oxford English Dictionary*). The second meaning is closer to the professional idea of being 'impulse-ridden' than to that of impulsiveness: a chronically resentful child, for example, may be seen as bursting out in rage because of the strength of the impulse rather than any deficiency in its control. The difficulty with this second meaning in professional discourse is that it is wholly circular: the only evidence for the state of mind is the behaviour that it is supposed to explain.

A corresponding diagnostic trap is for disobedient behaviour to be rated as impulsive. Much hyperactive behaviour is rule-breaking; but much rule-breaking behaviour is not hyperactive.

CASE STUDY

"Oppositional behaviour"

Declan was referred at the age of 11 for evaluation of possible ADHD by his school nurse, with particular concern about a diet consisting largely of junk food. Teachers were aware of great variety in his behaviour in different lessons, which was sometimes highly disruptive to the work of the class. Observation clarified strong contingencies related to the behaviour of other children in the class. Misbehaviour, such as throwing books at neighbouring desks and shouting jokes across the class to other children, was followed by attention and sometimes laughter from them, which he clearly relished. In classes with a clearer work ethic, he was rather subdued and took little part. Outside the classroom he was a high-status and controversial figure in the peer group. In the setting of a detention class, with authoritative control from the supervising teacher over the whole group, he worked very effectively and attentively, and used these 'punishment' sessions to maintain a good academic output.

The motivated and oppositional quality of his misbehaviour did not in itself rule out ADHD; poor impulse control could have contributed to his poor conduct; but the behaviour was not evidence in itself for impulsiveness since there was evidence of planned and intended rule violations rather than lack of control.

It would be useful if objective tests could identify a generalized tendency towards *action without reflection*, and interpret specific behaviour problems in this light. Cognitive analyses of impulsiveness have been fruitful, but the present state of knowledge emphasizes a variety of pathways rather than one underlying problem.

Barkley (1997) has argued that a lack of inhibition is the common pathology for all cases of ADHD and underlies the various 'surface' manifestations. People behave impulsively in this view because they lack the ability to suppress unwanted actions, and their actions are correspondingly erratic and ill-considered.

Sonuga-Barke (2004) proposed an account based not on disability but on motivation. In effect, the children are able to restrain themselves, but are in a situation where they choose to reduce delay, because it is unusually unpleasant for them ('delay aversion'). They therefore tend to adopt a strategy of making fast guesses and responses, and moving on to another if the first does not work out. People with ADHD are then seen as able to slow themselves down and wait if essential, but as being chiefly motivated by the need to avoid delay rather than to win reward.

Van der Meere et al. (1992) suggested a basic deficit in 'state regulation'. The idea comes from the now-you-see-it-now-you-don't quality of children's cognitive performance. For example, in the continuous performance test mentioned above, children with ADHD are disproportionately sensitive to the speed with which stimuli are presented. At some speeds (e.g. one response every 4 seconds or so), they perform as well as other children, but if the presentation is either quicker or slower, their responses become slower and more variable. This leads to the notion that the speed of presentation affects the physiological state of the brain's control mechanisms, and people without ADHD can maintain an optimal state more effectively than those with the disorder.

Sagvolden et al. (2005) have tied the phenomenon of ADHD in humans together with some states seen in animals with dopamine abnormalities. In both, there is a "rapid delay-of-reward gradient" – i.e. a reward has to follow a correct response unusually quickly if it is to be effective in encouraging learning. This notion is often applied in behaviour therapy, with an emphasis on rewarding desired behaviours much more quickly and consistently than would be natural.

Each theory can be formulated in a way that predicts the others. Perhaps they should be seen not as alternative and unique explanations, but as descriptions of coexistent processes. These theories are all expanded by their originators in much more rigorous ways than here, and I have deliberately simplified to the point of being inaccurate. I have done this because clinicians have found this a very complex literature to grasp, yet can take some useful points from it.

In particular, it is helpful to think of several possible ways in which a child might become impulsive (prone to action without reflection), and therefore might be helped:
- Decision to respond quickly (to avoid the unpleasantness of waiting)
- Inaccurate time perception (so that insufficient time is taken for an activity)
- Inability to plan actions (so the simplest is chosen)
- Inability to inhibit response.

All these have to overcome an apparent paradox: the reaction times of children with ADHD are not too rapid, but slower than the average and more variable. This is not truly a contradiction, but a caution against thinking in over-simple terms. A response may be both slow and premature; and a response may be slow because it has not been sufficiently prepared.

Overactivity

Overactivity refers to an excess of movements, especially in situations that expect calm. The best way to identify a child with restless overactivity is not on the football field: in situations expecting high activity, a child with hyperkinetic disorder will not stand out from other children in this respect, although they may well stand out for other reasons, such as the disorganization and diffuseness of their activity). Rather, situations such as the classroom, family visits, or mealtimes – when children can ordinarily modulate their activity to a calmer level – will distinguish the hyperactive child from others.

'Restlessness' is perhaps a better word to use than overactivity. Lay understanding is often confused by the idea that being active is a problem, and fears that energy and vigour are being turned into pathologies by an intolerant society. Many active children, after all, are engaged in positive and desirable activities rather than unfortunate ones. Nevertheless, a locomotor excess remains a useful concept for understanding children with hyperactivity. Excessive movement can still be detected even when the child is asleep, so overactivity cannot be reduced to inattentiveness or lack of compliance, but is a feature of ADHD in its own right.

Subjective experiences

The definitions of hyperactivity have all been based on observable behaviour. By comparison with many psychiatric disorders, at least those seen in adults, there is little emphasis on the subjective sensations of those affected. Nevertheless, subjective accounts are often helpful. They play a greater part in the identification of adults, but even in children they can be helpful to elicit so as to help the children's understanding of themselves.

Some of the accounts of children are descriptions of the reactions of others. "Everybody is against me", "I'm in trouble but it's not my fault", and "I'd like to have friends" are all based on their perceptions of how other people behave, and can be easier for children than the introspection of their own state.

Other accounts are about the subjective experience of impulsiveness, and many will recognize that they do not stop and think ahead or that they commit actions that they would not do if they put time into thinking about it. It can be helpful to work through a checklist such as those of the DSM (*Diagnostic and Statistical Manual of Mental Disorders*; APA 1994) and ICD (*International Statistical Classification of Diseases and Related Health Problems*; WHO 1992) – not so much for the diagnosis, since these self-ratings are not very reliable, but as explanation of what others see. Beyond this, some children will develop explanations of their impulsive actions in terms of influences they cannot control (which can include the sensation of a voice instructing wrong actions or the sensation of "a bad boy in me").

Adults will often describe sensations of craving activity, or of thoughts "whirling" in their head, and being confused with other thoughts, or not carried through to their conclusion. Younger children may not have the concepts for this, but often will describe it in retrospect, when it changes. For example, the experience of starting on medication can be one of relief from disconnected and restless thinking, and the relief allows the patient to recognize and describe what it was like before.

Associated features

It is worth adding a short list of some complaints by teachers or parents that do not by themselves suggest hyperactivity, although they may be associated with it:
• sleep disturbance
• noncompliant behaviour
• aggression
• temper tantrums
• clumsiness
• literacy problems
• emotional outbursts.

These can all occur in children with a diagnosis of ADHD; they can sometimes result from ADHD: indeed, they may be the most important things needing intervention for an individual child. But they are not in themselves grounds for diagnosis, because they can result from many different causes. These different causes need to be sought in assessment even if ADHD is present and has been diagnosed.

The diagnostic schemes

ICD-10 CRITERIA (WHO 1992)

The ICD-10 definition of 'hyperkinetic disorder' (HKD) is based upon the simultaneous presence of attention deficit, overactivity and impulsiveness (see Chapter 3). The Research Diagnostic Criteria are algorithmic, with the rule that all three cardinal problems need to be present in more than one situation – for instance, at school as well as at home, or in observation at the clinic as well as at school. They need to be at a level that is out of keeping with the child's development – not just chronological age, but cognitive development as well. The problems also need to have been present from an early age – before the age of 7 years by definition, and in practice usually even earlier. There are also a number of exclusion criteria – in particular, the presence of other disorders that could themselves be causes of hyperactive behaviour.

The Clinical Guidelines of ICD-10 are not couched in the same format of specific rules. Rather, they provide descriptions of the conditions for clinicians to compare with presenting cases. The concept of the disorder is very similar, but the scheme seems to reflect a different conceptualization of the nature of psychiatric diagnosis, in which cases are matched to a prototype rather than built up from specific symptoms. This may well be closer to what happens in most diagnostic encounters, but provides less explicit guidance on handling the common problems of boundaries with normality and with other conditions.

The ICD-10 is formulated as a single-diagnosis system, especially in the Clinical Guidelines format. It is not impossible to have multiple diagnoses, but most cases are expected to fit one pattern. This can make for difficulties when several other types of problems are present as well as hyperactivity, as is usually the case. There are therefore several rules to cope with this, with mixed categories and exclusion criteria. For instance, the coexistence of hyperactivity and conduct problems is tackled by a separate definition of 'hyperkinetic conduct disorder', which is a subcategory of hyperkinesis. By contrast, the coexistence of hyperactivity with autism is dealt with by diagnosing only the latter. By way of further contrast, the coexistence of hyperactivity with Tourette syndrome is unspecified, with the implication that one should diagnose both.

DSM-IV CRITERIA (APA 1994)

The DSM-IV category is called Attention Deficit/Hyperactivity Disorder (ADHD) and this terminology has gained universal currency. The category is based on very much the same list of behaviours as those that characterize the ICD-10 definition of HKD (Table 1.2). There are a few slight differences in wording of the items, but they are clearly intended to refer to the same general pattern. The rules for making a diagnosis from these items are, however, quite different.

TABLE 1.2
Symptom domains for ADHD/HKD in ICD-10 and DSM-IV

Inattention (IN)	Hyperactivity (H)	Impulsivity (IMP)
Fails to attend to details	Fidgets with hands or feet	Talks excessively (ICD-10)
Difficulty sustaining attention	Leaves seat in classroom	Blurts out answers to questions
Does not seem to listen	Runs about or climbs	Difficulty waiting turn
Fails to finish	Difficulty playing quietly	Interrupts or intrudes on others
Difficulty organizing tasks	Motor excess	
Avoids sustained effort	("on the go" in DSM-IV)	
Loses things	Talks excessively (DSM-IV)	
Distracted by extraneous stimuli		
Forgetful		

- DSM-IV does not require that all three of the cardinal problems should be present. Rather, impulsiveness/overactivity or inattentiveness can be grounds for the diagnosis even in the absence of the other. The subdivisions within ADHD are 'inattentive', 'impulsive/overactive' and 'combined'. The ICD-10 criteria are therefore not met unless cases fall within the 'combined' category of DSM-IV.
- The requirements for pervasiveness across situations in the DSM-IV are less stringent. Rather than criteria having to be met in more than one situation, there is only the requirement that some impairment should be present in more than one situation – and the impairment may be based on a subset of symptoms.
- The exclusion criteria applying to the coexistent presence of other disorders are less stringent. Instead of the requirement that problems such as autism and affective disorders should be absent, the criterion is that the symptomatology should not be better explained by another syndrome. This often leads to multiple diagnoses in DSM-IV terminology.

HKD DIAGNOSIS AND ADHD DIAGNOSTIC SUBTYPES
HKD (ICD-10)
Six or more from the IN domain, plus three or more from the H domain, plus one or more from the IMP domain.

ADHD subtypes (DSM-IV)
Combined: six or more from the IN domain and six or more from the H/IMP domain.
Inattentive: six or more from the IN domain and less than six from H/IMP domain.
Hyperactive/Impulsive: six or more from H/IMP domain and less than six from the IN domain.

HKD subtypes based on comorbid disorder diagnosis
- Disturbance of activity and attention (without conduct disorder).
- Hyperkinetic conduct disorder (with conduct disorder).
- Diagnosis of HKD if there are anxiety and mixed disorders is not recommended.

The consequences of these differences in criteria are considered further in Chapter 3.

Epidemiology

Several studies converge on a point prevalence in the primary school-age population of about 1.5% for hyperkinetic disorder; and about 5% for ADHD.

The two main surveys in the UK have been the Newham studies, starting in the mid-1980s (Taylor et al. 1991), and a National Morbidity Survey carried out some 20 years later (Meltzer et al. 2000). The Newham studies were based on a two-stage population survey of all children aged 6 to 8 years on school rolls in one London borough, comprising more than 5000 children. An initial questionnaire survey (based on Rutter's parent and teacher rating scales) identified about 9% of boys as at-risk (i.e. scoring above the cut-off – 3 out of 6 – on both teacher and parent scales). A random sample of those children, and of control groups, were studied more closely with parent and teacher interviews, examinations and psychological tests; a research diagnosis was made, and by weighting the rates in each of the stratified groups an estimate could be made of the rates of diagnosable disorders in the child population. The rate for hyperkinetic disorder was about 17 per 1000 in boys (rather lower in girls – see below). The point prevalence rate for 'ADDH' (which was the DSM-III diagnosis in use at the time) was about 40 per 1000. The administrative prevalence – the rate with which the diagnosis was made in practice – was too low for a robust estimate, but a case register from that time, in another London borough, had indicated only about 1 in 2000 being diagnosed.

The National Morbidity Survey used a different methodology. A nationally representative sample of more than 10,000 children was studied with rating scales and structured interviews given by non-clinical researchers, after which clinicians made diagnoses on the basis of the information gathered. The rate for HKD was about 14 per 1000 children, and again the rate was substantially lower in girls. By this time the use of health services was quite high, with nearly half of the children being referred to child mental health services. Most of the referred children, however, were probably not diagnosed by their local services as showing the HKD that the research study had identified.

This pattern of underdiagnosis in the UK is confirmed by national data on the use of stimulant medication: in 1999, only about 3 per 1000 were being treated (Lord and Paisley 2000). Furthermore, a recent epidemiological study in yet another London borough (Croydon) found it still to be the case that only about 1 child in 10, out of those identified by high scores on rating scales from teacher and parent, were in practice receiving the diagnosis (Sayal et al. 2002).

A child whose behaviour is hyperactive has a complex journey to becoming a diagnosed case. In this Croydon survey, the first stage was for the behaviour to be perceived by parents as a problem; teachers played a smaller part in identification. The second stage was the presentation of the child to primary health care, and the third was the recognition by health care professionals that hyperactivity (rather than some other kind of behaviour disturbance) was the diagnosable problem. This third stage of professional recognition was the limiting step for most children, and it was at this point that the journey towards a diagnosis usually stopped. When it was recognized in primary care, there was little further filtering, and virtually all the recognized children were referred on to specialist child mental health or paediatric services. The crucial stage of professional recognition was determined largely by parental knowledge and beliefs: when the parents themselves suggested the possibility of ADHD, the primary care teams were responsive in making specialist referral.*

Internationally, there is some consensus that ADHD is a problem and a risk for development, and affects a significant minority of children. Widely different rates for ADHD are reported from different countries, varying from 2% to 19%, but most of this difference is due to the methods of assessment that are used (Swanson et al. 1998). The usual figures adopted are those from studies that have included a research interview with parents and the DSM-III, -III(R), or -IV criteria. On this basis, ADHD estimates cluster around 5–10% and HKD estimates around 1–2%; screening questionnaire ratings of those at risk are around 10–20% (Schachar and Tannock 2002). Attention deficit without hyperactivity has received less research attention, but is troublesome for something like another 1% of the school age population.

It is doubtful whether there are any major differences between nations. The question is not easy to answer, because hyperactive behaviour is distributed continuously (see below), the exact cut-off taken is somewhat arbitrary, and it is not clear whether the cut-off should be universal or locally defined. In some populations – for instance, the Chinese population in Hong Kong – careful diagnostic measures have suggested that there may be a lower prevalence of disorder than in Europe (Leung et al. 1996). Interestingly, however, the apparent prevalence taken from rating scales was higher in Hong Kong than in Western populations (Ho et al. 1996a), illustrating the extent to which the disorder is socially defined and influenced by the concern that adults feel for these behaviours in different cultural settings.

In ordinary practice, the rates of clinically diagnosed cases differ enormously between societies, indicating a powerful part played by culture in determining the concepts of disorder. Many reviewers have described the enormous differences between the USA on the one hand and European and Asian countries on the other. The frequency of the diagnosis in practice is at least 10 times as great in the USA as in the UK. Furthermore, the rate is increasing: surveys in the 1980s suggested that a little under 1% of American youth were being diagnosed and treated; 10 years later the rate had risen to 3.4%, and it continues to rise (Olfson et al. 2003).

Is the rate increasing?
The administrative prevalence – the rate at which the disorders are in practice recognized – is rising sharply in the UK, and stands at about 3 per 1000. It is not likely that this massive rise (nearly tenfold over 20 years) reflects an epidemic of the disorder. The rates found in the Newham and National Morbidity surveys (see above) are too similar to allow for so great an increase in prevalence. More persuasively, the analysis of successive birth cohorts has made it possible to study directly the changes in behaviour problems over a time span of some 25 years (Collishaw et al. 2004). Some of the mental health problems of young

---

*This crucial role of parents in determining whether a child becomes a case will not apply everywhere. In many places, teachers are the identifiers of the problem. This is likely to alter the case mix presented to specialist services.

people are indeed rising over time in this country: conduct and emotional disorders are, disappointingly, on the increase. Hyperactive behaviour, however, has remained rather stable. This makes it less probable that social factors are responsible for ADHD: the rise of television viewing and eating processed food have both been suggested as causes, but are not supported by historical changes in prevalence. The changes in recognition, however, clearly do reflect social attitudes.

COMPLETING THE CLINICAL PICTURE

Category or dimension?
The behaviour of hyperactivity has a graded distribution in the population. There are progressively fewer children at increasing levels of hyperactivity. The cut-offs taken are not arbitrary. The number of symptoms required for an ADHD diagnosis in the DSM system was set in field trials in the USA, examining the best cut-off that would predict current social impairment. Admittedly, it does not follow that this will generalize to other parts of world, nor that it is the best criterion. The number of symptoms required for the ICD diagnosis of HKD was less systematically investigated, but based on a level that predicted evidence of neurodevelopmental abnormality and a large response to stimulant medication.

Though not arbitrary, the cut-offs have a weaker empirical base than would be desirable. For clinical purposes, the key level should probably be that which predicts that, if untreated, there is a substantial risk of persisting impairment. This would be helpful because it would also set the level at which intervention should be provided. Although some evidence exists, it is complex to interpret because it suggests that the risk itself is graded, with successively higher levels of hyperactivity carrying progressively higher risks of a mental disorder later (Taylor et al. 1996).

At present, therefore, the grounds for the diagnosis include not only the symptoms of the disorder but the requirement that they should impose a significant impairment – for instance, in school progress or the development of peer relationships. This is out of line with most other ICD-10 diagnoses: the general philosophy of the scheme is that one should recognize disease by its signs, and that to define by impairment confuses research and discourages early and preventive intervention. In the case of HKD, however, social impairment still needs to be part of the clinical definition.

Situation specificity
Hyperactive behaviour is not a fixed property of a child, but varies with the context. Variability and unpredictability from day to day are often emphasized in parent and teacher accounts. Some children pose diagnostic puzzles because the information from different sources conflicts. School may see a very stressed child who cannot cope with ordinary expectations for concentration; parents may see a cheerful, happy child at home without apparent problems. Conversely, parents may feel overtaxed by the demands of a disruptive child who, at school, is no less compliant than his or her peers.

In these situations each side may blame the other for inability to cope. This can, of course, be the case. A few parents are unable to cope with ordinary childish misbehaviour and falsely present it as a problem in the child. Some school classes are overwhelmed by problem behaviour, and some teachers cannot keep order. These are, however, unusual reasons for hyperactivity or inattentiveness being confined to one situation. More commonly there are other reasons that need analysis:

- *The child's behaviour is in fact the same across situations, but raters differ.*
  Agreement between raters in different situations is modest at best. Parents and teachers are more likely to agree about whether a child has a problem than about what problem it is (Mota and Schachar 2000).
- *The behaviour is the same across situations, but the impact is different.*
  A short duration of attention could be a problem at school, but inapparent at home if there are no demands for sustaining attention over time.
- *One situation is affecting the other.*
  A restrictive regime at school may keep a child in order, but at the expense of a great outpouring of frustration at home after school.
- *There is an interaction between the child and the situation.*
  Some genetic twin studies have examined separately the influences on home and school behaviour (Nadder et al. 2002). They suggest that there may be specific effects. Some of the genetic influences on behaviour at home do not affect behaviour at school, and vice versa; other genetic influences raise the likelihood of hyperactive behaviour in both situations.

We do not yet know all the genes involved, or the way they work. Some epidemiological evidence, however, gives clues. Ho et al. (1996b) surveyed a school population with parent and teacher questionnaires, and selected those who showed hyperactive behaviour at home only, at school only, or pervasively across both situations. The school-specific group showed more evidence of academic learning difficulties; perhaps some of their off-task behaviour was due to inability to cope with the lessons. The home-specific group showed more evidence of family conflict and adversity; perhaps they reacted with misbehaviour that in turn was poorly controlled. The pervasive group did not, as might be expected on a simple additive model, show the combination of both kinds of problem. Rather, they showed a pattern of neurodevelopmental delays, in language and motor coordination, that is most typically an association of HKD.

Sex ratios

Studies in the general population have suggested that hyperactive behaviour is commoner in boys than in girls, with a ratio of about 3:1 (Schachar and Tannock 2002). In clinical populations, however, the sex ratio is much greater, and figures of 4:1 are common in ADHD clinics, with some reporting sex ratios as high as 9:1. It seems probable both that girls have some protection against the development of hyperkinetic disorders, and that when disorders do develop girls are less likely than boys to be referred for help.

In the studies carried out in the borough of Newham, the male excess for hyperactivity was of the order of 2.5:1. We need to understand the reasons for the sex difference, and especially whether it suggests that the problem is different in males and females, so some details of the measures taken on the girls will be described (Heptinstall and Taylor 2002, Young et al. 2005)

First, the reason could be rater bias, if raters are less likely to identify hyperactive behaviour in girls than in boys. This predicts identified girls will be more deviant than boys on objective measures and implies that girls should be identified by female norms. This, however, turned out not to be the case: when males and females were compared on mechanical measures of movement (actometers) and direct observation of movements in structured situations, then the hyperactive girls were somewhat less active than the hyperactive boys.

Second, it could be that there are different forms of disorder in males and females. This predicts that affected girls will have different symptoms (perhaps more inattentiveness and less hyperactivity) or worse outcomes. This turned out to have some truth in it: the hyperactive girls were not only somewhat less active than the boys but tended to be even more impaired on psychological test measures. The differences were not great, however, and the key measure, of outcome at 10 years, suggested that their course was similar to that of the hyperactive males.

Third, the difference might come from an unbalanced comorbidity – if, for instance, affected girls have less of other patterns of disturbance such as conduct disorder; but there was no sign of this. If anything, the opposite held: the hyperactive girls were at risk for overt emotional disturbance as well as oppositional behaviours, while the boys were at risk for conduct rather than emotional problems.

Finally, the lack of force in the above possibilities suggests that the difference arises from a differential in risk factors – either in the sexes' exposure to risk (in which case risk factors should be less common in girls generally but equal in affected girls and boys), or in the sexes' vulnerability to risk factors (predicting that they should be equal in girls and boys in the general population but greater in girls when considering only the children affected by ADHD). The high rate of neurocognitive abnormalities, mentioned above and reported in some other investigations (e.g. James and Taylor 1990), would be in keeping with the idea that a larger amount of neurological risk needs to be present in girls to overcome the protection against hyperactivity that their sex enjoys. The story here is far from clear, and research is needed. But the implications are that the same criteria should be applied to both genders, that the 2 or 3 to 1 ratio of males to females is likely to be correct, and correspondingly that a more effective recognition of affected girls needs to be developed.

GENETIC AND ENVIRONMENTAL CONTRIBUTIONS

It is now clear that genetic factors contribute strongly to ADHD. Comparisons of monozygotic with dizygotic twins, and of the biological and adoptive relatives of adopted children, give high values for 'heritability'. Chapter 2 will review the genetic and molecular mechanisms that may be responsible. Sometimes this is taken to contradict environmental influences – to suggest for instance that heritability estimates in excess of 90% leave little room for environmental influences. This need not be the case. Genetic–environmental interactions and correlations need to be reckoned with. Many genes will act by modifying the organism's response to particular environmental influences. A weak risk factor for disorder in the population (e.g. physically harsh treatment) may be stronger on a specific outcome (e.g. aggression) and a very strong influence in a vulnerable subgroup (e.g. with a variant of the gene for monamine oxidase A) (Caspi et al. 2002). The ability to define a specific genetic constitution may allow environmental influences to become clearer.

The understanding of effects of early stress has been modified by an increased realization that early damage entails different consequences from late, and its results are sometimes rather nonspecific. A lateralized brain injury such as a stroke in the first year of life may have a direct effect on power in contralateral limbs, but it does not necessarily have the specific psychological consequences that would follow later injury. A left-sided brain lesion does not lead to the predicted language dysfunction but rather to impairment of visuospatial information processing (Frampton et al. 1998). Even a left-sided hemispherectomy is compatible with a satisfactory development of language (though there may still be subtle deficiencies). The young brain when damaged is not so much resilient as plastic: it compensates for functional alteration, and that compensation can bring different sorts of dysfunction (Taylor 1991a). Left- and right-sided lesions are both associated with the development of inattentiveness and impulsiveness.

Specific environmental stresses
• *Alcohol.* The incidence of fetal alcohol syndrome (FAS) is about 1.9 per 1000 live births (Abel 1990). Children with the physical signs of FAS are at risk for hyperactive behaviour as well as generalized learning disability

• *Smoking* during pregnancy has been associated epidemiologically with changes in the offspring. Linnet et al. (2003) review associations with ADHD and find a probable effect; though methodological flaws are marked in this literature (Ramsay and Reynolds 2000). Social confounders are hard to allow for. Nevertheless, a case–control study of 280 cases of ADHD and their controls found a twofold increase in rates of maternal smoking for the controls, even after adjusting for familial psychopathology, social adversity and comorbid conduct disorder (Mick et al. 2002).

• *Maternal use of cocaine* is well known to produce a neonatal abstinence syndrome; in addition its use is associated with a high rate of spontaneous abortions, fetal growth retardation and mental problems including hyperactivity (Chasnoff et al. 1985, Bingol et al. 1987).

• *Medicines* in pregnancy have been reviewed by Altshuler et al. (1996). Better knowledge is urgently needed, but it is already clear that benzodiazepines and anticonvulsants are associated with later behavioural problems including ADHD-like patterns of behaviour (Steinhausen et al. 1994).

• *Low birthweight.* A very low birthweight (e.g. <1.5 kg) is associated with hyperactivity and a low IQ in later life and a higher than average rate of behavioural problems – for example, survivors still had a disadvantage of 9 IQ points at the age of 8 years by comparison with children randomly selected from the same birth cohort (Anderson et al. 2003). A meta-analysis by Bhutta et al. (2002) commented that the relative risk for ADHD was more than doubled, and that the loss of IQ points was greater the lower the birthweight.

Lesser degrees of low birthweight and the presence of obstetric complications have been reported in case–control studies to be more frequent than expected in people with ADHD (and in people with other kinds of developmental disorder). The association, however, is not usually because of a direct cause–effect relationship. Low birthweight is often associated with other kinds of social disadvantage: it may for instance reflect low quality of antenatal care. There may also be a reverse causality. A fetus with an abnormal brain may be more likely to encounter problems of delivery (see below); it not only has greater vulnerability to the risks of prematurity, but also a greater exposure to the risks.

• *Lead exposure.* There is an epidemiological association between behavioural hyperactivity and high body lead (Taylor 1991b). The research has not been able to allow for psychosocial confounders. Nevertheless, there is a known effect of lead on IQ even allowing for other kinds of disadvantage, so it is reasonable to suppose that some of the association with hyperactivity is indeed due to toxic effects on the brain.

• *Selective deficiencies* of iron, zinc and essential fatty acids are often canvassed but the evidence (e.g. from supplementation trials in children with ADHD) is not compelling. Thyroid deficiency is indeed a cause of attentional problems if not corrected. Neonatal screening is desirable, and iodine supplementation in deficient parts of the world should be supported. Deficiency in fetal life as a consequence of maternal hypothyroidism is also an influence on later mental development.

• *Child neglect* represents a failure of the environment to provide the minimum of care, stimulation and supervision. Children who are reared in environments of extreme deprivation and neglect can exhibit marked speech and socialization deficits; yet, they can show great improvements once removed to a more reasonable environment, as long as they do not suffer from other genetic or congenital problems. The question has been, whether the adversity has enduring effects after the environment has been improved.

Recent studies of children who have been adopted into ordinary families in the UK after periods spent in depriving orphanages in Romania have indicated that signs of inattention and impulsiveness are one of the important sequelae (Rutter et al. 2001). Many of the effects can be reversible – children with developmental delays and low body weight after periods of less than a year in the institution appear to recover to normality. However, longer periods of deprivation can be followed by persisting abnormalities of mental development. Hyperactivity in particular is associated with the time spent in the depriving environment, not with the degree of malnutrition evident when they were rescued.

Diagnostic validity
There is plenty of evidence that people with high levels of inattentiveness, overactivity and impulsiveness are different from other people in ways that put them at risk. Faraone (2005) reviews the diagnosis of ADHD and defends it against those who would regard it as a non-illness. Following standard criteria for validity, ADHD has:

- Well-defined clinical correlates distinguishing it from good health: notably, poor school achievement, poor peer relationships, high rates of delinquency and substance abuse, and more injuries.
- Separation from other disorders: though coexistence with other problems is common, those other disorders do not give a complete explanation of hyperactivity. Children with ADHD still keep that diagnosis even when the features that overlap with other conditions are given no weight.
- Characteristic course and outcome: it is a chronic condition and often persists into adult life.
- Evidence for heritability – which is strong, as detailed in Chapter 2.
- Neurobiological characteristics in laboratory studies, also detailed in Chapter 2.
- Characteristic response to treatment: the good response to stimulants (and to other drugs) has historically been a major reason for and support of the diagnosis (see Chapter 8).

LIMITATIONS TO VALIDITY

It is also important to recognize the limitations of knowledge and the possible abuse of diagnostic thinking.

The biological findings characterize groups, not individuals. It is helpful for clinicians to know that when they have diagnosed a case, they can draw on the knowledge amassed from scientific studies. This knowledge, however, does not extend to asserting a single aetiology. Not all individuals show a biological variant (such as an altered dopamine transporter gene or a small caudate nucleus); not all individuals with a biological variant show ADHD. The associations are real, but probabilistic, not defining.

There are environmental as well as genetic contributions, and some of these, such as postnatal neglect, reflect the social environment.

What is inherited is probably not ADHD or HKD, but a continuously distributed trait, or set of traits.

There is no absolute point along the trait at which the cut-off is set. Rather, committees set the level of symptoms required according to that which predicts referral for problems and social impairment (in DSM) or that which is thought to predict neurodevelopmental impairments and treatment response (in ICD-10).

The extent to which high levels of the trait are impairing, or regarded as a problem, depends upon the culture (see 'Epidemiology' above).

The diagnosis is easy only if it is done badly. ADHD is only one of the patterns of disruptive behaviour. If it is invoked merely because of the presence of disruptive behaviour then many of the other causes will be missed. Overmeyer et al. (1999), for instance, showed that raters who were blind to the diagnosis of ADHD detected much more by way of social and family problems than did raters who knew that the features of ADHD were present.

None of this contradicts the validity of disorder, or even tells against it. However, it does caution against simplistic approaches, such as the common practice of telling parents that, because their child shows the behaviour of ADHD, therefore he or she has a genetically determined illness of chemical imbalance. Appendix 1.1 gives a suggested factsheet for parents; many will want to go more deeply into the science of the problem, even to read this book.

The controversies

Most scientific clinicians now accept that the differences that underlie extreme levels of hyperactive behaviour have quite strong genetic and physical environmental influences, and can legitimately be regarded as reflections of brain function. Many, however, will think, "that is all very well, but biological determination does not in itself mean that this is an illness." This is correct. Genetic influences upon height are also strong, but that does not mean that short stature is an illness, nor that there is any absolute level of height below which medical intervention is called for. Rather, there is an interaction between the fact of short stature and the surrounding social context, to which a growth clinic will be sensitive. In the same way, symptoms of hyperactivity and inattentiveness can be more or less impairing according to the demands of the social environment, and clinical management will take that into account.

Some will also protest, "given that ADHD is a valid kind of diagnosis, have we gone too far?" Present knowledge does not allow an absolute judgement about the point at which a cut-off should be placed, so there is a good deal of local variation. Many people in education are troubled by the rise in those being recognized and the extent to which parents regard ADHD as an explanatory diagnosis. Sophisticated clinicians may well recognize that ADHD is not an explanation but a description of behaviour. They know that, in order to achieve reliability in classification, we have had, for the time being, to stop basing our taxonomy on supposedly causative explanations.[*] Nevertheless, in the minds of many parents, the recognition of inattentive and impulsive behaviour implies strong physical causality – and, correspondingly, the welcome lifting of psychological explanations that impose the burden of responsibility or guilt. This sometimes offends teachers who would prefer the parents to recognize aspects of their family life that are problems for their children. All the same, the studies comparing mono- and dizygotic twins (see Chapter 2) indicate that the shared environment – which should include aspects of family life that impinge on all the children – plays little part in the development of hyperactive behaviour. ADHD is a valid category of disorder, even if its boundaries are sometimes unclear.

Public doubts and reservations also come at other levels. "Given that ADHD is worth recognizing, where should we draw the boundaries of disorder?" Chapter 6 will take further the issues of its overlaps with other kinds of disturbance. "Who should receive medication?" is considered further in Chapter 11. Neither expert authority nor scientific consensus go unchallenged, which no doubt is all to the good. Clinicians should recognize the doubts, and refrain from exaggerating the level of confidence with which all the implications of a disease model can be defended. But they should also feel confidence in presenting the idea that hyperkinetic disorder is a valid way of describing the predicament of some children, that the strongest influences on its origin stem from genetic inheritance and the early

---

[*]There is no intention that psychiatric classification will always remain at this rather unsatisfying level of mere description. I very much hope that reliable descriptions are one step on the journey towards an understanding that will be truly medical in that the physiological pathways leading to disorder are clarified. Indeed, ADHD has advanced as far as any condition in mental health in the discovery of the pathways through which genes lead to behaviour. But there is still a long way to go.

physical environment, that a good deal is known already of its neurobiological and psychological roots, and that evidence-based interventions are available.

REFERENCES

Abel EL (1990) *Fetal Alcohol Syndrome*. Oradell, NJ: Medical Economics.

Altshuler L, Cohen L, Szuba M, Burt V, Gitlin M, Mintz J (1996) Pharmacologic management of psychiatric illness during pregnancy: dilemmas and guidelines. *Am J Psychiatry* **153**: 592–606.

Anderson P, Doyle LW, and the Victorian Infant Collaborative Study Group (2003) Neurobehavioral outcomes of school-age children born extremely low birth weight or very preterm in the 1990s. *JAMA* **289**: 3264–3272.

APA (1994) *Diagnostic and Statistical Manual of Mental Disorders, 4th edn (DSM-IV)*. Washington, DC: American Psychiatric Association.

Barkley RA (1997) Behavioral inhibition, sustained attention, and executive functions: constructing a unifying theory of ADHD. *Psychol Bull* **21**: 65–94.

Bhutta AT, Cleves MA, Casey PH, Cradock MM, Anand KJ (2002) Cognitive and behavioral outcomes of school-aged children who were born preterm: a meta-analysis. *JAMA* **288**: 728–737.

Bingol N, Fuchs M, Diaz V, Stone RK, Gromish DS (1987) Teratogenicity of cocaine in humans. *J Pediatr* **110**: 93–96.

Caspi A, McClay J, Moffitt TE, Mill J, Martin J, Craig IW, Taylor A, Poulton R (2002) Role of genotype in the cycle of violence in maltreated children. *Science* **297**: 851–854.

Chasnoff IJ, Burns WJ, Schnoll SH, Burns KA (1985) Cocaine use in pregnancy. *N Engl J Med* **313**: 666–669.

Collishaw S, Maughan B, Goodman R, Pickles A (2004) Time trends in adolescent mental health. *J Child Psychol Psychiatry* **45**: 1350–1362.

Faraone SV (2005) The scientific foundation for understanding attention–deficit/hyperactivity disorder as a valid psychiatric disorder. *Eur Child Adolesc Psychiatry* **14**: 1–10.

Frampton I, Yude C, Goodman R (1998) The prevalence and correlates of specific learning difficulties in a representative sample of children with hemiplegia. *Br J Educ Psychol* **68**: 39–51.

Heptinstall E, Taylor E (2002) Sex differences and their significance. In: Sandberg S, ed. *Hyperactivity and Attention Disorders of Childhood*. Cambridge: Cambridge University Press, pp. 99–125.

Ho TP, Leung PWL, Luk SL, Taylor E (1996a) Establishing the constructs of childhood behavioral disturbances in a Chinese population: a questionnaire study. *J Abnorm Child Psychol* **24**: 417–431.

Ho TP, Luk ESL, Leung PWL, Taylor E, Lieh-Mak F, Bacon-Shone J (1996b) Situational versus pervasive hyperactivity in a community sample. *Psychol Med* **26**: 309–321.

James A, Taylor E (1990) Sex differences in the hyperkinetic syndrome of childhood. *J Child Psychol Psychiatry* **31**: 437–446.

Kuntsi J, Stevenson J (2001) Psychological mechanisms in hyperactivity: II. The role of genetic factors. *J Child Psychol Psychiatry* **42**: 211–219.

Leung PWL, Luk SL, Ho TP, Taylor E (1996) The diagnosis and prevalence of hyperactivity in Chinese schoolboys. *Br J Psychiatry* **168**: 486–496.

Linnet KM, Dalsgaard S, Obel C, Wisborg K, Henriksen TB, Rodriguez A, Kotimaa A, Moilanen I, Thomsen PH, Olsen J, Jarvelin MR (2003) Maternal lifestyle factors in pregnancy risk of attention deficit hyperactivity disorder and associated behaviors: Review of the current evidence. *Am J Psychiatry* **160**: 1028–1040.

Lord J, Paisley S (2000) The clinical effectiveness and cost-effectiveness of methylphenidate for hyperactivity in childhood. Version 2 – for consultation. London: National Institute for Clinical Excellense (online at www.nice.org.uk/download.aspx?o=11655).

Meltzer H, Gatward R, Goodman R, Ford T (2000) *The Mental Health of Children and Adolescents in Great Britain*. London: The Stationery Office.

Mick E, Biederman J, Faraone SV, Sayer J, Kleinman S (2002) Case–control study of attention-deficit hyperactivity disorder and maternal smoking, alcohol use, and drug use during pregnancy. *J Am Acad Child Adolesc Psychiatry* **41**: 378–385.

Mota VL, Schachar RJ (2000) Reformulating attention-deficit/hyperactivity disorder according to signal detection theory. *J Am Acad Child Adolesc Psychiatry* **39**: 1144–1151.

Nadder TS, Rutter M, Silberg JL, Maes HH, Eaves LJ (2002) Genetic effects on the variation and covariation of attention deficit–hyperactivity disorder (ADHD) and oppositional–defiant disorder/conduct disorder (Odd/CD) symptomatologies across informant and occasion of measurement. *Psychol Med* **32**: 39–53.

19

Olfson M, Gameroff M, Marcus S, Jensen P (2003) National trends in the treatment of attention deficit hyperactivity disorder. *Am J Psychiatry* **160**: 1071–1077.

Overmeyer S, Taylor E, Blanz B, Schmidt MH (1999) Psychosocial adversities underestimated in hyperkinetic children. *J Child Psychol Psychiatry* **40**: 259–263.

Ramsay MC, Reynolds CR (2000) Does smoking by pregnant women influence IQ, birth weight, and developmental disabilities in their infants? A methodological review and multivariate analysis. *Neuropsychol Rev* **10**: 1–40.

Rubia K, Smith AB, Brammer MJ, Taylor E (2003) Right inferior prefrontal cortex mediates response inhibition while mesial prefrontal cortex is responsible for error detection. *Neuroimage* **1**: 351–358.

Rubia K, Smith AB, Brammer MJ, Toone B, Taylor E (2005) Abnormal brain activation during inhibition and error detection in medication-naive adolescents with ADHD. *Am J Psychiatry* **162**: 1067–1075.

Rutter ML, Kreppner JM, O'Connor TG, and the English and Romanian Adoptees (ERA) Study Team. (2001) Specificity and heterogeneity in children's responses to profound institutional privation. *Br J Psychiatry* **179**: 97–103; erratum in: *Br J Psychiatry* **179**: 371.

Sagvolden T, Johansen EB, Aase H, Russell VA (2005) A dynamic developmental theory of attention-deficit/ hyperactivity disorder (ADHD) predominantly hyperactive/impulsive and combined subtypes. *Behav Brain Sci* **28**: 397–419.

Sayal K, Taylor E, Beecham J, Byrne P (2002) Pathways to care in children at risk of attention-deficit hyperactivity disorder. *Br J Psychiatry* **181**: 43–48.

Schachar R, Tannock R (2002) Syndromes of hyperactivity and attention deficit. In: Rutter M, Taylor E eds. *Syndromes of Hyperactivity and Attention Deficit In Child and Adolescent Psychiatry: 4th edn.* Oxford: Blackwell Scientific, pp. 399–418.

Sergeant JA, Geurts H, Huijbregts S, Scheres A, Oosterlaan J (2003) The top and the bottom of ADHD: a neuropsychological perspective. *Neurosci Biobehav Rev* **27**: 583–592.

Solanto MV, Abikoff H, Sonuga-Barke E, Schachar R, Logan GD, Wigal T, Hechtman L, Hinshaw S, Turkel E (2001) The ecological validity of delay aversion and response inhibition as measures of impulsivity in AD/HD: a supplement to the NIMH multimodal treatment study of AD/HD. *J Abnorm Child Psychol* **29**: 215–228.

Sonuga-Barke EJ (2004) On the reorganization of incentive structure to promote delay tolerance: a therapeutic possibility for AD/HD? *Neural Plast* **11**: 23–28.

Steinhausen HC, Losche G, Koch S, Helge H (1994) The psychological development of children of epileptic parents. I. Study design and comparative findings. *Acta Paediatr* **83**: 955–960.

Swanson JM, Sergeant JA, Taylor E, Sonuga-Barke EJ, Jensen PS, Cantwell DP (1998) Attention-deficit hyperactivity disorder and hyperkinetic disorder. *Lancet* **351**: 429–433.

Swanson JM, Casey BJ, Nigg J, Castellanos FX, Volkow ND, Taylor E (2004) Clinical and cognitive definitions of attention deficits in children with attention-deficit/hyperactivity disorder. In: Posner MI, ed. *Cognitive Neuroscience of Attention.* New York: Guilford Press, pp. 430–446.

Taylor E (1991a) Developmental neuropsychiatry. *J Child Psychol Psychiatry* **32**: 3–47.

Taylor E (1991b) Toxins and allergens. In: Rutter M, Casaer P, eds. *Biological Risk Factors for Psychosocial Disorders.* Cambridge: Cambridge University Press, pp. 199–232.

Taylor E (1999) Developmental neuropsychopathology of attention deficit and impulsiveness. *Dev Psychopathol* **11**: 607–628.

Taylor E, Sandberg S, Thorley G, Giles S (1991) *The Epidemiology of Childhood Hyperactivity. Maudsley Monographs 33.* Oxford: Oxford University Press.

Taylor E, Chadwick O, Heptinstall E, Danckaerts M (1996) Hyperactivity and conduct problems as risk factors for adolescent development. *J Am Acad Child Adolesc Psychiatry* **35**: 1213–1226.

Taylor E, Sergeant J, Döpfner M, Gunning B, Overmeyer S, Mobins HJ, Eisert HG (1998) Clinical guidelines for hyperkinetic disorder. *Eur Child Adolesc Psychiatry* **7**: 184–200.

van der Meere J, Vreeling HJ, Sergeant J (1992) A motor presetting study in hyperactive, learning disabled and control children. *J Child Psychol Psychiatry* **33**: 1347–1354.

WHO (1992) *International Statistical Classification of Diseases and Related Health Problems. 10th edn (ICD-10).* Geneva: World Health Organization.

Young S, Heptinstall E, Sonuga-Barke EJS, Chadwick O, Taylor E (2005) The adolescent outcome of hyperactive girls: Self-report of psychosocial status. *J Child Psychol Psychiatry* **46**: 255–262.

What is Attention Deficit Hyperactivity Disorder?

Attention Deficit Hyperactivity Disorder (ADHD) is a term used to describe the condition of children who are inattentive, impulsive, and active at levels higher than expected for their mental and chronological age.

How is ADHD diagnosed?

The three core symptoms used to diagnose ADHD are:

• Attention problems: Inattention and distractibility, difficulties in sustaining attention and apparently not listening. Difficulties in organizing and following through instructions. Losing things and forgetfulness.
• Impulsivity: Difficulties in waiting for his/her turn, often blurting out answers before questions are completed. Butting into conversations or games.
• Hyperactivity (restless overactivity): Running about or climbing excessively, always on the go, fidgeting with hands or feet or unable to sit still.

It is important to stress that an ADHD diagnosis is made on the basis of a recognizable behaviour pattern. The cause of the behaviour may be complex. But children with the condition can be helped though good parenting, good management at school and the controlled use of medication.

The symptoms of ADHD will often begin to diminish as the child or adolescent grows up. It is less common for adults to have ADHD.

Children with ADHD are difficult to bring up. They are liable to develop educational, behavioural and conduct problems or emotional difficulties, and to suffer from low self-esteem.

What is the cause?

In the past, professionals tended to blame parents for the behaviour of a child with ADHD. Others have said the condition was due to additives in the food. However, research has not supported the popular view that ADHD is due to eating food additives, preservatives or sugar. Although the symptoms of some children get worse with certain foodstuffs, this is not the main cause of ADHD.

It is now known that ADHD is associated with subtle changes in the structure and function of the brain. It is commonly genetic, and many children with ADHD have a parent or close relative with a similar condition.

In rare cases ADHD is associated with pregnancy or birth complications. In a few cases it arises as a direct result of disease or trauma to the central nervous system.

Poor parental management is not thought to be a primary cause of ADHD but can make the symptoms worse.

What is involved in the assessment?

Parents may be asked to fill in a checklist of symptoms if ADHD is suspected. A similar checklist will also be given to the child's schoolteacher.

In the checklist, parents are asked detailed questions about the child's behaviour in a range of situations. The child will also be observed directly and may undergo tests to clarify ability and attainment.

The evaluation may take time – one to two hours per week over the course of three weeks. This is necessary as a diagnosis in an individual child needs to consider the level of development that the child has reached and rule out other causes, such as deafness or learning disability.

It is also important to find out whether your child has additional problems sometimes found with ADHD. These include learning difficulties, dyspraxias (clumsiness), speech and language problems, and broad spectrum autistic problems.

What is involved in treatment?

Treatment programmes aim to support development in learning and behaviour. The first lines of treatment are usually through non-medication measures such as those in Items 1–5 below, particularly in younger children.

1. Behavioural therapy: The aim is to modify the child's behaviour. Good behaviour is encouraged by a reward and inappropriate behaviour is ignored or something enjoyable is removed.

2. Attention training for young children: The child's ability to attend is gradually developed using structured play activities in a one-to-one situation with an adult, generally the parent.
3. Cognitive behavioural therapy: Includes training in problem-solving and social skills. For older children who are anxious or whose self-esteem is low, helping them correct their distortions in thinking and developing more positive self-talk can be helpful.
4. Educational measures: Children with ADHD have been demonstrated to respond to behavioural programmes at school. They may also have associated problems such as specific learning difficulties or clumsiness that may need special help.
5. Special diets: These are often well known to parents but are difficult to follow. Their general effectiveness has not been proven in research trials. Occasionally a diet may be tried in a child with known allergies under the supervision of a dietician. A food diary will often clarify the situation.
6. Medication: Using stimulant medication should not be regarded as controversial. There is overwhelming evidence over the years for its effectiveness, most recently supported by a large multicentre trial in the USA.

A combination of cognitive–behavioural and educational methods with medication has been found to be the most successful form of treatment. When behavioural methods are used, the dose of medication can be lower.

Finally . . .
Children with ADHD are difficult to rear. Even with medication and treatment we cannot cure ADHD. Our aim is to help parents to bring the child's behaviour under control. This will help the child as well as the parent. Treatment and care can help to improve the child's attention span and encourage his or her enthusiasm to learn and build self-esteem.

APPENDIX 1.2
FURTHER READING AND INFORMATION FOR FAMILIES

Literature
Of the numerous titles available for parents of children with ADHD, some of the best are:

Taking Charge of ADHD: The Complete, Authoritative Guide for Parents. Revised edn.
Russell A Barkley. 2000. New York: Guilford Press.
This is a thick American-style compendium by a respected American expert and researcher in the ADHD field. It is optimistic in tone – problems are for solving – and very sympathetic to the difficulties experienced by children and parents. It covers a very broad range of topics, challenging many myths, correcting misconceptions and giving useful information on strategies of coping at home and at school.

Hyperactivity: Why Won't My Child Pay Attention?
Sam Goldstein and Michael Goldstein. 1992. New York: John Wiley.
Well-balanced and readable account of ADHD. This has a good section on parent behavioural management but the section on medication is now somewhat dated.

1–2–3 Magic: Effective Discipline for Children 2–12.
Thomas W Phelan. 2003. Illinois: Child Management.
Written in an easy, jokey, colloquial style. This book describes a management system that is clear and makes sense to parents. Not surprisingly, it is probably the most popular book for parents, presenting behavioural management in an easy to follow format. This is particularly useful for help in managing the oppositional and non-compliant child. A video illustrating the techniques described in the book is also available (see below).

Put Yourself in Their Shoes: Understanding Teenagers with Attention Deficit Hyperactivity Disorder.
Harvey C Parker. 1998. Plantation, FL: Specialty Press.
Sympathetic view of the teenager with ADHD. Useful strategies for improving communication, problem-solving, study and social skills.

The AD/HD Handbook – A Guide for Parents and Professionals on Attention Deficit/Hyperactivity Disorder.
Alison Munden and Jon Arcelus. 1999. London and Philadelphia: Jessica Kingsley.
Easy to read book giving a well-balanced picture of ADHD, the diagnosis, the causes, the effects in adolescence and adult life. It includes helpful information on interagency support from health, education and social services, as well as useful contacts in the UK and abroad. Compared with the books listed above it is low in advice on behavioural management.

How to Talk So Kids Will Listen and Listen So Kids Will Talk.
Adele Faber and Elaine Mazlish. 2004. New York: Perennial Currents.
Not specifically for children with ADHD, but an excellent book on improving communication between parents and children. Particularly effective at raising self-esteem and supporting problem-solving.

The Incredible Years: a Trouble-Shooting Guide for Parents of Children Aged 3–8.
Carolyn Webster-Stratton. 2006. Seattle, WA: Seth Enterprises.
Outstandingly good book on helping parents understand and cope with children's problem behaviour. Carolyn Webster-Stratton is the pioneer of using videotape to train parents in the most effective approaches to parenting. There is excellent advice on how to cope with a range of problematic situations. What is particularly helpful is the attention to detail in describing the suggested strategies, the sound research base from which the book is written, and the overall frame of sympathy and understanding for parents.

Parenting the ADD Child: Can't Do? Won't Do? Practical Strategies for Managing Behaviour Problems in Children with ADD and ADHD.
David Pentecost. 2000. London: Jessica Kingsley.
Sound and readable book on parenting strategies for children with ADHD.
Well set out and well presented.

Learning to Slow Down and Pay Attention. A Book for Kids About ADHD. 3rd edn.
Kathleen Nadeau and Ellen Dixon. 2004. Washington, DC: Magination Press.
Excellent book aimed at children and adolescents.

Don't Rant and Rave on Wednesdays! The Children's Anger-Control Book. 6th edn.
Adolph Moser. 1994. Kansas City: Landmark Editions.
Picture book for children around 7–11 years old.

Video
1–2–3 Magic: Managing Difficult Behavior in Children 2–12.
Thomas W Phelan. 2004. Illinois: Child Management Inc.
A well illustrated account of the methods described in his book (see above).

Useful contacts (UK)
ADDISS – ADD Information Services
ADDISS provide an excellent source of support and information for parents of children with ADHD. Individuals can visit the office at 10 Station Road, Mill Hill, London NW7 2JU, England. ADDISS distribute an extensive catalogue of books, videos and audio-tapes, including all those listed above.
PO Box 340, Edgware, Middlesex HA8 9HL, England.
Tel: 020 8906 9068
Fax: 020 8959 0727
e-mail: info@addiss.co.uk
Website: see below.

ADDers is another non-profit support group with useful links.
Thanet ADDers, 45 Vincent Close, Broadstairs, Kent CT10 2ND, England.
Tel: 0870 950 3693
Website: see below.

Milton Keynes ADHD Support Group also provides useful information and contacts.
31 Ramsons Avenue, Conniburrow, Milton Keynes MK14 7BB, England.
Tel: 01908 676779
Website: see below.

Benefits Enquiry Line
Freephone: 0800 882200
This gives advice on the benefit situation for children with disabilities.

The Advisory Centre for Education
Tel: 020 7354 8321
They give free telephone advice on issues related to education.

Contact a Family
Tel: 020 7383 3555
This is a charity which puts parents of children with medical or psychiatric problems in touch with others with similar problems.

The Royal College of Psychiatrists
The Royal College of Psychiatrists produces a 'Mental Health and Growing Up' series of 36 factsheets on a range of common mental health problems. They can be ordered through Book Sales at:
The Royal College of Psychiatrists, 17 Belgrave Square, London SW1X 8PG, England.
Tel: 020 7235 2351 ext 146
Fax: 020 7245 1231
e-mail: booksales@rcpsych.ac.uk
The factsheets on ADHD are:
Factsheet 5: Attention deficit disorder and hyperactivity
Factsheet 6: Stimulant medication for hyperkinetic disorder and attention deficit hyperactivity disorder
They can be accessed through the college website at: http://www.rcpsych.ac.uk/info/mhgu/newmhgu5.htm
and http://www.rcpsych.ac.uk/info/mhgu/newmhgu6.htm respectively.

Useful contacts (international)

In the USA the National Resource Center on AD/HD provides an information line:

Tel: 800 233 4050

It is supported by CHADD (Children and Adults with Attention Deficit/Hyperactivity Disorder), which runs many other activities:

CHADD National Office, 8181 Professional Place – Suite 150, Landover, MD 20785.

Tel: 301 306 7070

Fax: 301 306 7090

Many local groups are affiliated (see website below).

There is also a CHADD national organization in Canada:

PO Box 43021, Edmonton, Alberta T5J 4M8.

Tel: 866 434 9004

The ADDers.org website (see below) provides extensive information on support groups around the world.

Websites

Websites change frequently, and some are better maintained than others. Some are frankly fictional and dangerous in their alarmist information. Some useful sites are:

UK:
- http://www.addiss.co.uk (ADDISS)

This site has recently been updated and much improved. The aim is to be accurate and evidence-based. It contains articles by experts and factsheets on ADHD. There are details on conferences, training and support groups, plus the book and video catalogue mentioned above
- http://www.rcpsych.ac.uk (Royal College of Psychiatrists – see above)
- http://adders.org (includes useful international contacts)
- http://www.mkadhd.org.uk (Milton Keynes ADHD Support Group)

Argentina:
- http://www.tdah.org.ar (La Fundacion Trastorno por Deficit de Atencion e Hiperactividad)

Australia:
- http://www.addaq.org.au (Attention Deficit Disorder Association Queensland)
- http://www.ladswa.com.au (Learning and Attentional Disorders Society of Western Australia)

Belgium:
- http://tdah.be
- http://www.zitstil.be

Brazil:
- http://www.tdah.org.br (Associação Brasileira do Déficit de Atenção – ABDA)

Canada:
- http://www.adhdcanada.com

Denmark:
- http://www.adhd.dk

Finland:
- http://www.adhd-liitto.fi

France:
- http://www.tdah-france.fr

Germany:
- http://www.ads-ev.de
- http://www.bv-ah.de

Iceland:
- http://www.adhd.is

Ireland:
- http://www.thechildrensclinic.ie

Italy:
- http://www.aifa.it (Associazione Italiana Famiglie ADHD)
- http://www.aidai.org (Associazione Italiana per i Disturbi di Attenzione e Iperattività)

Japan:
- http://www.e-club.jp

Mexico:
- http://www.deficitdeatencion.org (Asociación Mexicana por el Déficit de Atención, Hiperactividad y Trastornos Asociado)
- http://www.tdah.org

Netherlands:
- http://www.adhd.nl

New Zealand:
- http://www.adhd.org.nz

Singapore:
- http://www.spark.org.sg

Spain:
- http://www.f-adana.org
- http://www.anshda.org (Asociación de Padres de Niños con Síndrome de Hiperactividad y Déficit de Atención)

Switzerland:
- http://www.aspedah.ch (Association Suisse de Parents d'Enfants avec Deficit d'Attention et/ou Hyperactivité)

USA:
- http://www.accap.org (American Academy of Child and Adolescent Psychiatry)

Contains sound research and conference information. There is also a Facts for Families series. The brief sheet on ADHD is accessed on: http://www.aacap.org/publications/factsfam/noattent.htm
- http://www.chadd.org (CHADD – Children and Adults with Attention Deficit Disorders)

CHADD is an American non-profit organization representing children and adults with ADD/ADHD
- http://www.add.org
- http://www.help4adhd.org

2
BIOLOGICAL FOUNDATIONS

Sarah Curran

In current practice, the diagnosis of ADHD is based on clinical history and observation, not on psychological or biological markers. Nevertheless, much of the public and professional understanding of ADHD supposes that it is based on physical aetiology and a demonstrable change of brain function. This chapter therefore goes into more detail and examines more of the primary scientific literature than do other parts of the book, to review the strength of the evidence on which the notion is based.

A widely accepted hypothesis is that ADHD represents dysfunction of the prefrontal cerebral cortex of unknown cause (Faraone and Biederman 1998, Arnsten 2000). Supporting evidence for this hypothesis includes similarities of the clinical features of ADHD patients and patients with injuries or diseases of the frontal lobes, as well as ADHD-like behavioural and neurocognitive deficits in animals with lesions of frontal cortex (Deutch and Roth 1990; Hynd et al. 1990; Shue and Douglas 1992; Arnsten 1997, 2001; Barkley 1997). Neurochemical theories about the biological basis of ADHD have focused on monoamine neurotransmitter pathways, dysregulation in which results in neuropsychological dysfunction (Lou 1996, Castellanos 1997). The striking and consistent beneficial clinical effects of stimulant drugs in patients with ADHD, and evidence that such drugs facilitate monoaminergic synaptic neurotransmission, particularly of dopamine, have strongly encouraged speculation that aberrant, and particularly deficient, cerebral monoamine neurotransmission may contribute to the pathophysiology of ADHD (Pliszka et al. 1996, Seeman and Madras 2002).

Impairments on tasks of executive function, especially inhibition of inappropriate responses, are key neuropsychological associations of ADHD (Tannock 1998). A change in the child's constitution (genetic/inherited, or environmental/acquired) that leads to the symptoms of ADHD is therefore likely to be associated with an alteration in the brain structures and functions that subserve the control of impulse and attention.

Knowledge of parallel circuits in the brain that functionally link prefrontal cortex to basal ganglia, from basal ganglia to thalamus and from thalamus to cortex, has been the single most useful organizing principle in the study of neuropsychiatric disorders (Castellanos 2001). These cortico-striatal-thalamo-cortical (CSTC) circuits have been implicated in ADHD (as well as in Tourette syndrome and obsessive–compulsive disorder). CSTC circuits provide both positive and negative feedback to other cortical regions and have been studied intensively in rodents, nonhuman primates and humans. Cortical, thalamic and subthalamic nucleus (STN) efferents are glutaminergic and excitatory, while striatal (caudate nucleus, putamen and nucleus accumbens) and pallidal efferents are GABAergic and inhibitory. Ventral tegmental area (VTA) and substantia nigra pars compacta (SNc) neurons can be excitatory or inhibitory depending on whether they activate D1 or D2 dopamine receptors, respectively.

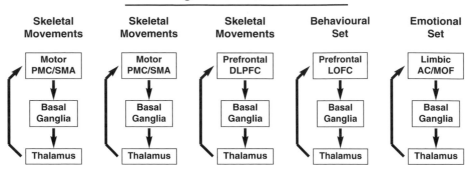

Basal Ganglia Thalamocortical Circuits

Skeletal Movements	Skeletal Movements	Skeletal Movements	Behavioural Set	Emotional Set
Motor PMC/SMA	Motor PMC/SMA	Prefrontal DLPFC	Prefrontal LOFC	Limbic AC/MOF
Basal Ganglia	Basal Ganglia	Basal Ganglia	Basal Ganglia	Basal Ganglia
Thalamus	Thalamus	Thalamus	Thalamus	Thalamus

Fig. 2.1. Simplified diagram of five parallel basal ganglia thalamocortical circuits including (1) the motor circuit with primary projection zones in the premotor cortex (PMC), supplementary motor areas (SMA), and primary motor cortex; (2) the oculomotor circuit with primary projection zones in the supplementary eye fields (SEF) and frontal eye fields (FEF); (3) dorsolateral prefrontal circuit (DLPFC); (4) lateral orbital frontalcircuit (LOFC); (5) the limbic circuit with primary projection zones in the anterior cingulate (AC) and medial orbitofrontal cortex (MOF).

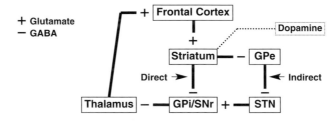

Fig. 2.2. Direct and indirect pathways of the basal ganglia and relevant neurotransmitters.

The 'indirect pathway' maintains a tonic level of inhibition. It involves signals that travel from the striatum to the external segment of the globus pallidus (GPe) and switch off the inhibition on the STN (also being activated by prefrontal efferents), which in turn 'activates' the inhibitory output of the internal segment of the globus pallidus (GPi). The 'direct pathway' extends from the prefrontal cortex (PFC) through the internal segment of the GPi through the thalamus, feeding back to exert a net amplification (via disinhibition) of the original cortical output, resulting in an overall positive feedback to the cortex. The identification of functionally segregated direct and indirect circuits facilitating complex regulation of inhibitory and excitatory influences at thalamic and cortical levels has been one of the principal achievements of the past decade.

CSTC circuits implicated in ADHD (Figs. 2.1, 2.2)
While involvement of the prefrontal CSTC circuits in ADHD were imputed primarily from clinical observations, testing hypotheses and understanding more fully the biological

aetiology has been made possible through advances in neuroimaging techniques. Recent evidence from functional and structural imaging supports the view that ADHD involves a predominantly right hemispheric frontostriatal abnormality (Overmeyer et al. 2001).

Neuroimaging studies

Early studies using computerized tomography (CT) failed to distinguish controls from ADHD patients (Shaywitz et al. 1983). In the last two decades, new methods of brain imaging, along with the neuropsychological ability to break down human behaviours into simpler components that can be studied more easily, have advanced the study of neuro-behavioural disorders such as ADHD. Neuroimaging techniques include magnetic resonance imaging (MRI), positron emission tomography (PET), single-photon emission computed tomography (SPECT), functional MRI (fMRI) and magnetic resonance spectroscopy (MRS). Frank and Pavlakis (2001) provide a good review of the principles of these techniques.

ANATOMICAL MRI (aMRI)

The quantitative study of brain development during childhood and adolescence was not feasible until MRI became available in the late 1980s. Routine brain MRI has not been informative in differentiating the ADHD population from controls; however, the development of volumetric techniques has enabled researchers to consider regional brain variations in the ADHD population. In addition, there have been sufficient numbers of aMRI studies of the developing human brain that the normal developmental trajectory is understood (for a review, see Durston et al. 2001). The most noteworthy findings from these studies are: (1) the total brain volume does not increase significantly after age 5 years; (2) white matter volume increases significantly across the life span and does not stop growth at the end of childhood; (3) cortical grey matter increases during childhood, then decreases during adolescence (probably due to synaptic pruning) before stabilizing in adulthood; (4) subcortical grey matter shows a similar but more prominent pattern of decrease of volume with age, taking place at an earlier age. With the creation of age and sex norms, we have begun to understand the relevance of between-group volumetric differences to clinical symptoms of ADHD.

A large, longitudinal study (Castellanos et al. 2002) examined regional brain volume changes prospectively as a function of increasing age. Comparing a sample of 152 cases diagnosed with ADHD and 139 age- and sex-matched controls, ranging in age from 5 to 18 years, initial volumes and prospective age-related changes of total cerebrum, cerebellum, grey and white matter for the four major lobes, and caudate nucleus of the brain were examined. On initial scan, patients with ADHD had significantly smaller brain volumes in all regions, even after adjustments for covariates. Cerebellar volumes were reduced to an even greater degree than cerebral volume in ADHD. Anterior cortical grey matter, caudate nucleus and cerebellar volumes correlated with parent-derived and clinician-derived ratings of the severity of the diagnostic behaviours of ADHD. Unmedicated children with ADHD also exhibited strikingly smaller total white matter volumes compared with controls and with medicated children with ADHD, providing a certain reassurance that medication does not appear to be structurally harmful. Volumetric differences in total and regional cerebral measures and in the cerebellum persisted with age. Caudate nucleus volumes were initially reduced in patients with ADHD, but diagnostic differences disappeared at follow-up as caudate volumes decreased for controls during adolescence. Results were comparable for male and female patients on all measures. Frontal and temporal grey matter, caudate, and cerebellar volumes correlated significantly with parent- and clinician-rated severity measures within the ADHD sample. It was concluded that developmental trajectories for all structures, except caudate, remain roughly parallel for patients and controls during childhood and adolescence, suggesting that genetic and/or early environmental influences on brain development in ADHD are fixed, non-progressive, and unrelated to stimulant treatment.

Studies using cross-sectional designs are largely supportive of the findings from this longitudinal study. Hill et al. (2003) reported smaller total brain volume, superior prefrontal and right superior prefrontal volumes, as well as significantly smaller areas for cerebellar lobules I–V and VIII–X, corpus callosum and splenium. No group differences were observed for the inferior prefrontal, caudate or cerebellar volumes, or for the area of cerebellar lobules VI–VII. In the ADHD group but not in the control group, greater right superior prefrontal volume predicted poorer performance on a test of sustained attention. Patterns of brain abnormality did not differ in male and female children with ADHD. Mostofsky et al. (2003) found that boys with ADHD had (on average) 8.3% smaller total cerebral volumes. Significant reductions in lobar volumes were seen only for the frontal lobes. Within the frontal lobes, a reduction was seen in both grey and white matter volumes, with some evidence suggesting lateralization of these findings: reduction in frontal white matter volume was specific to the left hemisphere, and there was a bilateral reduction in frontal grey matter volume but more so in the right hemisphere. Subparcellation of the frontal lobe revealed smaller prefrontal, premotor and deep white matter volumes. Findings suggest that ADHD is associated with decreased frontal lobe grey and white matter volumes. More than one subdivision of the frontal lobes appear to be reduced in volume, suggesting that the clinical picture of ADHD encompasses dysfunctions attributable to anomalous development of both premotor and prefrontal cortices. Hesslinger et al. (2003) reported fronto orbital volume reductions in adult patients with ADHD. It remains unknown whether small volumes are a primary deficit or a result of dysfunctional activation during childhood in terms of a residual deficit or a specific type of adult outcome of the disease. Overmeyer et al. 2001 found that children with ADHD had significant grey matter deficits in right superior frontal gyrus [Brodmann area (BA) 8/9], right posterior cingulate gyrus (BA 30) and the basal ganglia bilaterally (especially right globus pallidus and putamen). They also demonstrated significant central white matter deficits in the left hemisphere anterior to the pyramidal tracts and superior to the basal ganglia. Other cross-sectional studies have found abnormalities of the cerebellar vermis (Castellanos et al. 1996, 2001; Berquin et al. 1998) in individuals with ADHD.

Perhaps more relevant for ADHD are studies that relate anatomical changes with cognitive tasks, especially of attention and inhibition. Studies using this design are beginning to emerge (Durston et al. 2001). In a normative study, Casey et al. (1997) first tested 26 children between 5 and 16 years old on a stimulus selection task and measured regions of the prefrontal cortex (e.g. anterior cingulate region). There was a correlation between area of the right, but not the left, anterior cingulate cortex and performance of the stimulus selection task, which remained even after partialing out the effects of age, IQ and total cerebrum. Performance was faster and more accurate on the inhibitory trials for children with larger right anterior cingulate measures, providing evidence for the importance of this region in cognitive control. In a second study of 26 children with and 26 children without ADHD, they tested children on three attention tasks and showed significant correlations between performance on these tasks and asymmetry and size of the basal ganglia (caudate nucleus and globus pallidus) and prefrontal cortex. The behavioural data from the normal volunteers typically correlated with anatomical measures. In contrast, behavioural data from the ADHD children typically was in the opposite direction or did not correlate. These results imply that deficits in cognitive control observed in ADHD may be due to abnormalities of the prefrontal cortex and basal ganglia, and that variations in these structures in healthy individuals relate to performance on cognitive control tasks.

FUNCTIONAL MAGNETIC RESONANCE IMAGING (fMRI)
One of the most important aspects of fMRI is its utility in studying human brain development, because of its non-invasive nature and lack of ionizing radiation. This methodology is central to work on the involvement of prefrontal and basal ganglia circuitry in cognitive control. Of relevance to ADHD is the examination of blood flow patterns during tasks designed to measure the neuropsychological deficits in executive function, in particular response inhibition and selective attention, which have been redesigned for use in the scanner environment. For a review of neuropsychological deficits in ADHD, see Chapter 4.

A number of fMRI studies have been completed with healthy children (Casey et al. 1997, Thomas et al. 1999, Durston et al. 2001). Again as with aMRI, establishing normal patterns of brain activity in children is a critical first step in evaluating the degree of abnormality in patterns of brain activity in children with ADHD. The most relevant developmental fMRI study that has been completed to date, examined brain activity in children using a version of the previously described response inhibition task (i.e. the go/no-go task) (Casey et al. 1997). Based on the results from 18 subjects aged between 7 and 24 years (9 adults and 9 children), prefrontal activity was demonstrated during this task for all subjects, but only activity in the orbitofrontal cortex and right anterior cingulate cortex correlated with behavioural performance. Subjects with the most activity in orbitofrontal cortex performed best on this task, while those who performed worst (more errors) had increased activity of the anterior cingulate cortex. Of significance were the developmental differences observed in patterns of brain activity in children relative to adults. Overall, children had greater volumes of activity with a significant difference in dorsolateral prefrontal regions. There were no significant differences in movement or variance in MR signal between groups to explain this result. It appears that children recruit both dorsal and ventral prefrontal regions while adults recruit predominantly ventral prefrontal regions that correlate with task performance. This finding may suggest a refinement in the organization or efficiency in prefrontal cortex, particularly within the dorsolateral prefrontal cortex, with age. Further work by the group using a cognitive control task that manipulates the preceding context of trials has supported the importance of the prefrontal cortex, anterior cingulate cortex and basal ganglia in overriding repetitive or salient responses with relevant ones (Durston et al. 2001).

Barkley's hypothesis (see Chapter 1) of a core deficit of inhibition in ADHD has influenced many of the early studies using fMRI to address the frontal localisation of 'response inhibition'. Response inhibition refers to the suppression of extraneous unwanted movements in a given behavioural context. Response inhibition is considered critical in the preparation and selection of motor responses and includes the processes involved in selective attention, also considered 'executive attention', which is dependent upon the ability to inhibit responses to 'surrounding' or 'interfering' stimuli. fMRI was used to investigate the hypothesis that ADHD is associated with a dysfunction of prefrontal brain regions during motor response inhibition and motor timing (Rubia et al. 1999). Brain activation of 7 adolescent boys with ADHD was compared to that of 9 comparison boys equivalent in age and IQ while they were performing a stop task, requiring inhibition of a planned motor response, and a motor timing task, requiring timing of a motor response to a sensory cue. The ADHD group showed lower power of response in the right mesial prefrontal cortex during both tasks and in the right inferior prefrontal cortex and left caudate during the stop task.

This study was followed by an investigation of whether this hypofrontality in adolescents with ADHD could be attributed to delayed maturation of frontal cortex (Rubia et al. 2000). Brain activation of 17 healthy subjects (9 adolescents and 8 young adults) during performance of a motor response inhibition task and a motor timing task was measured using fMRI. The effect of age on brain activation was estimated, using the analysis of variance and regression, at both voxel and regional levels. In the delay task, superior performance in adults was paralleled by a significantly increased power of response in a network comprising prefrontal and parietal cortical regions and putamen. In the stop task, alternative neuronal routes – left hemispheric prefrontal regions in adults and right hemispheric opercular frontal cortex and caudate in adolescents – seem to have been recruited by the two groups for achieving comparable performances. A significant age effect was found for the prefrontal activation in both tasks, confirming the hypothesis of a dysmaturational pathogenesis for the hypo-frontality in ADHD. The group went on to show that adolescents with ADHD, compared with controls with other psychiatric conditions, were impaired on tests of response inhibition but not on tasks of motor timing (Rubia et al. 2000, 2001). Reduced right prefrontal activation was observed in hyperactive adolescents during higher level inhibition and delay management, but not during simple sensorimotor coordination. In an fMRI study of 18 medication-naive adolescents with ADHD, abnormal brain activation was observed during several executive functions in task-specific brain regions, including frontal, parietal and striatal brain areas (Rubia 2002).

One study of fMRI effects of methylphenidate administration in 10 male children with ADHD and 6 healthy male controls reported differences in frontal-striatal function and its modulation by methylphenidate during response inhibition tasks (Vaidya et al. 1998). Children performed two go/no-go tasks with and without drug. ADHD children had impaired inhibitory control on both tasks. Off-drug frontal–striatal activation during response inhibition differed between ADHD and healthy children: ADHD children had greater frontal activation on one task and reduced striatal activation on the other task. Drug effects differed between ADHD and healthy children: the drug improved response inhibition in both groups on one task and only in ADHD children on the other task. The drug modulated brain activation during response inhibition on only one task: it increased frontal activation to an equal extent in both groups. In contrast, it increased striatal activation in ADHD children but reduced it in healthy children. These results suggest that ADHD is characterized by atypical frontal–striatal function and that methylphenidate affects striatal activation differently in ADHD than in healthy children.

Another study (Anderson et al. 2002) examined the effects of methylphenidate on fMRI relaxometry of the midline vermis of the cerebellum in boys with ADHD. This region was selected as it has been observed to be significantly smaller in children with ADHD. Also, in preclinical studies, the vermis has been shown to modulate forebrain dopamine (DA) systems, to influence locomotor activity, and to contain a significant density of DA transporters. T2 relaxometry was used to assess blood volume in the cerebellum (hemispheres and midline vermis) of 10 boys with ADHD who were administered placebo or one of three different doses of methylphenidate continuously for 1 week. T2 relaxation time values are inversely proportional to local cerebral blood volume. After each week of treatment, and within 1–3 hours of the boys' afternoon dose, testing for drug efficacy was performed by using objective measures of activity. Moderate and high doses of methylphenidate increased T2 relaxation time in a rate-dependent manner – increasing T2 relaxation time in the most active children with ADHD and reducing T2 relaxation time in children with ADHD who were not objectively hyperactive. This preliminary study supports a role for the vermis in ADHD and suggests that further research is needed to clarify the relationship between vermal size, vermal blood flow, stimulant response, and the developmental pathophysiology of ADHD.

The putamen has also been implicated. In a study measuring resting state basal ganglia and thalamus activation in boys with ADHD using T2 relaxometry, longer relaxation times were found bilaterally in the putamen (which could be normalized by methylphenidate), and these strongly correlated with measures of increased motor activity and decreased sustained attention (Teicher et al. 2000). This supports the link between DA-mediated motor activity and impulsivity/inattention and the view that a common underlying deficit accounts for the different dimensions of ADHD (Rubia et al. 2001).

MRS STUDIES

MR spectroscopy (MRS) allows for noninvasive, in vivo visualization and examination of brain metabolism. MRS offers an advantage over radionucleide neuroimaging techniques (PET and SPECT) for the study of children and adolescents because of its lack of ionizing radiation, which allows repeated examination of a single study subject. MRS can be used to quantify neuronal integrity. Phosphate 31-labeled MRS quantifies phosphate-containing compounds that reflect high-energy phosphate and membrane phospholipid metabolism. In contrast, proton (^{1}H)-MRS provides spectra that can be used to measure N-acetylaspartate (NAA), creatine and phosphocreatine (Cr + PCr), and choline (Cho) containing substances. NAA is present in high concentration in gray matter and neurons, and its synthesis is closely correlated with mitochondrial energy metabolism. Therefore, NAA is often used as a measure of neuronal density and/or mitochondrial function. In contrast, Cr + PCr and Cho concentrations are used as measures of phosphate metabolism and membrane turnover, respectively (Murphy et al. 2002).

Jin et al. (2001) examined 12 previously untreated boys with ADHD ^{1}H-MRS before and after one dose (10 mg) of methylphenidate. Pre- and post-methylphenidate spectra were acquired bilaterally in the globus pallidus. Peaks of NAA, Cho, Cr, myo-inositol and glutamate were measured, and the ratios of the peaks were calculated and compared with data from 10 matched controls. In children having ADHD, the NAA/Cr ratio decreased significantly in the bilateral striatum while the Cho/Cr ratio showed a mild unilateral increase. One oral dose of methylphenidate did not affect the ratios significantly. These findings suggest that the striatum is bilaterally involved in children with ADHD. Approximately 20–25% of neurons may have died or may be severely dysfunctional. There seems to be a mild hyperactivity of the cholinergic system. However, the evidence for these metabolic differences may apply only to ADHD-C (the hyperactive/impulsive and inattentive combined subtype) and not to ADHD-I (inattentive subtype) (Sun et al. 2005).

Carrey et al. (2003) used ^{1}H-MRS to examine metabolite levels in the prefrontal cortex of children with ADHD. Nine age- and sex-matched case–control pairs were examined, aged 7–16 years. A long-echo ^{1}H-MRS scan was acquired from the right prefrontal cortex and left striatum in all subjects. Compounds that can be visualized with ^{1}H-MRS include NAA, glutamate/glutamine/gamma-aminobutyric acid (Glx), Cr/PCr and Cho. Frontal–striatal glutamatergic resonances were elevated in the children with ADHD as compared to healthy control subjects. No differences were noted in NAA, Cho or Cr metabolite ratios. These findings suggest that frontal–striatal Glx resonances may be increased in children with ADHD in comparison with healthy control children. This group went on to examine the effect of treatment on metabolite concentrations. Fourteen children with ADHD were investigated medication-free and after treatment, using ^{1}H-MRS. In the prefrontal cortex and striatum, metabolite peaks of NAA, Glx, Cr/PCr and choline compounds were measured, and ratios of the peaks were calculated and compared before and after treatment. The Glx to Cr/PCr ratio decreased significantly in the striatum. No other metabolites demonstrated any change in response to medication. These findings suggest that glutamate may be involved in treatment response in ADHD, especially in the striatum.

MRS has the potential to measure in vivo neurochemical changes to different medication treatments. Carrey et al. (2003) examined pre- and post-treatment ^{1}H-MRS in two children with ADHD responsive to treatment with methylphenidate and two responsive to treatment with atomoxetine. In the striatum, a striking decrease in the Glu/Cr ratio (mean change 56.1%) was observed between 14 and 18 weeks of therapy in all four children. In the prefrontal cortex, however, changes in the Glu/Cr ratio were noted only in subjects receiving atomoxetine, not in those receiving methylphenidate. These data suggest that in vivo MRS measurement has the potential to assess response to psychopharmacological treatment in children with ADHD.

SPECT AND PET STUDIES

Positron emission tomography (PET) is a nuclear medicine technique for performing physiological measurements in vivo. The PET scanner provides tomographic images of the distribution of positron-emitting radiopharmaceuticals in the body. From these images measurements can be obtained of regional cerebral blood flow (rCBF) and blood volume; glucose, oxygen and protein metabolism; blood–brain barrier permeability; neuroreceptor–neurotransmitter systems; tissue pH; and the concentration of radiolabelled drugs in the brain. Single-photon emission computed tomography (SPECT) is simpler than PET because it uses radiopharmaceuticals labelled with conventional radionucleotides such as technetium-99m (^{99m}Tc).

The limits of radiation dosimetry are such that only a small number of PET/SPECT studies of the brain may be performed during development.

A recent study examined SPECT scans before and after an 8 week course of methylphenidate in 32 right-handed boys aged 7–14 years who had DSM-IV ADHD, had never been medicated, and were free of all comorbid psychiatric conditions including learning disorders (Kim et al. 2001). Drug response was compared to rCBF changes. Clinical responders showed that most (64%) had robust perfusion increases in the caudate nuclei and frontal lobes. Thalamus and temporal lobe perfusion also increased in many responders. Perfusion increases were greater in the right hemisphere than in the left (28 vs 10).

Additional SPECT studies have compared adult ADHD patients and normal controls by labelling the dopamine transporter (DAT) protein (a specific marker for dopaminergic neurons, with nonhydrolysable phenyltropane analogue of cocaine (Dougherty et al. 1999, Dresel et al. 2000, Krause et al. 2000, van Dyck et al. 2002). All but the last of these studies found *increased* binding to DAT in the DA-rich basal ganglia of ADHD subjects. However, the correct interpretation of these observations is far from clear. They may reflect increased abundance or tissue density of DA nerve terminals, or an increase in DAT-per-neuron, perhaps with a net reduction of synaptic availability of DA, and artefacts due to previous treatment are not entirely excluded. In addition, improvement in clinical symptoms with D,L-methylphenidate was associated with decreased DAT binding (Dresel et al. 2000, Krause et al. 2000). This effect evidently reflects the ability of this stimulant, and perhaps of released DA, to compete for DAT binding sites with the radioligands employed, and not necessarily evidence that stimulants alleviate ADHD symptoms by correcting an underlying abnormality in DA neurotransmission.

Additional complex findings that are not readily interpreted derive from PET studies of the brain. This functional imaging technique has demonstrated *increased* uptake of the labelled DA precursor [^{18}F]-L-dopa in the midbrain of some adolescents with ADHD (Ernst et al. 1999), but *decreased* uptake in the prefrontal cortex (PFC) of adult ADHD patients (Ernst et al. 1998).

Volkow et al. (1997) used PET and radiolabelled raclopride – a dopamine (2) receptor (D2R) radioligand – to index changes in the availability of the D2R in the striatum of normal adults, before and after a clinically relevant oral dose of methylphenidate. The authors found that methylphenidate significantly increased extracellular DA concentration, as evidenced by a significant reduction in D2R availability.

Another SPECT study indicates that in non-drug-treated children with ADHD, higher D2R availability is observed at baseline, which is downregulated back to reported near-normal values after methylphenidate therapy (Ilgin et al. 2001). Initially, higher values of D2R availability seem to indicate better response to methylphenidate therapy in ADHD.

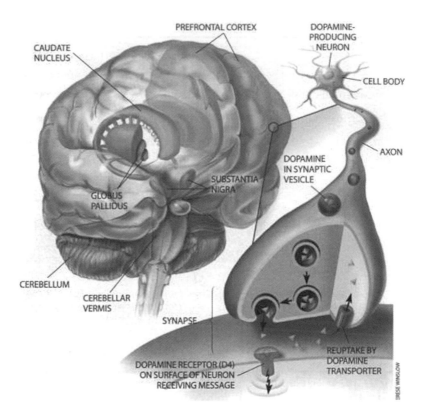

PREFRONTAL CORTEX

DOPAMINE-
PRODUCING
NEURON

CAUDATE
NUCLEUS

CELL BODY

AXON

DOPAMINE
IN SYNAPTIC
VESICLE

SUBSTANTIA
NIGRA

GLOBUS
PALLIDUS

CEREBELLUM

CEREBELLAR
VERMIS

SYNAPSE

DOPAMINE RECEPTOR (D4)
ON SURFACE OF NEURON
RECEIVING MESSAGE

REUPTAKE BY
DOPAMINE
TRANSPORTER

Fig. 2.3. Regions of the brain implicated in ADHD. Picture reproduced by courtesy of Xavier Castellanos.

Brain regions where abnormalities have been noted in people with ADHD are summarized in Figure 2.3.

DIFFUSION TENSOR IMAGING
Diffusion tensor imaging is based on the MR signal being made sensitive to the movement of water molecules at the micron level; it provides a new method for estimating myelination in vivo (Mascalchi et al. 2005).

Animal models of ADHD
Animal models of ADHD include several genetic mutants, either naturally occurring or artificially produced, as well as animals prepared by brain lesioning or exposure to neuro-toxins, typically early in development (Solanto 2002). With relatively homogeneous subjects, these models allow considerable experimental control of factors that may be involved in the pathophysiology of ADHD. They also avoid complex effects of comorbidity, previous drug exposure, family interactions, and other social factors encountered in human ADHD patients.

In general, animal models should resemble a clinical disorder in as many details as possible, including symptomatic expression, treatment responses, pathophysiology, and ideally, aetiology. More specifically, an adequate ADHD model should: (a) mimic the fundamental behavioural deficits found in ADHD patients (*face validity*); (b) conform to a theoretical rationale, such as the proposed pathophysiology or known therapeutics of ADHD (*construct validity*); and (c) predict unknown aspects of ADHD, such as its genetics, neurobiology, or novel therapeutics (*predictive validity*). Construct validity is particularly important in view of a number of recent advances in understanding the genetics and pathophysiology of ADHD. (For a review of the literature on animal models, see Davids et al. 2003.)

MONOAMINE FUNCTIONS IN ANIMAL MODELS OF ADHD
Dopamine
In the spontaneously hypertensive rat (SHR), behavioural deficits analogous to ADHD symptoms are usually considered to be mediated by an impaired DA reward mechanism that consists mainly of dysregulation of DA release, although changes in postsynaptic responses to DA also have been detected. Rats with neonatal 6-hydroxydopamine (6-OHDA) lesions represent another model with decreased DA transmission. Despite losses of DA that are similar to those found in bradykinetic rats with adult 6-OHDA lesions, neonatally lesioned rats display a robust motor hyperactivity that is inhibited by stimulant drugs, but not by selective inhibitors of DA transport. Behavioural deficits in coloboma mutant mice are caused by a mutation of the *SNAP-25* gene, with a resulting deficiency in DA transmission. However, the DAT knockout mouse (DAT-KO) demonstrates persistent hyperdopaminergic function, in striking contrast to the SHR rats with neonatal 6-OHDA lesions, and coloboma mice.

The similarity of behavioural and pharmacological profiles of animal models of ADHD based on deficient DA transmission to those with increased DA transmission is paradoxical. Perhaps, a generalized underactivity of the dopaminergic system in ADHD is rather simplistic and, as proposed by Castellanos (2001), different abnormalities may exist in two DA regions: underactivity in a cortical region (i.e. anterior cingulate) resulting in cognitive deficits, and overactivity in a subcortical region (i.e. caudate nucleus) resulting in motor overactivity. Animal models with decreased DA transmission, such as SHR and the neonatally 6-OHDA lesioned rat, and those with increased DA transmission, such as the DAT-KO mouse, represent deviations from an optimal level, albeit in opposite directions. In models with diminished DA transmission, stimulants may be beneficial by enhancing release of DA. In models with excessive DA function, activation of presynaptic D_2-like autoreceptors and the consequent reduction in DA neurotransmission may contribute to the beneficial effects of stimulants.

Noradrenaline
Stimulants potentiate noradrenaline (NA) as well as DA; and other NA-potentiating agents, including tricyclic antidepressants and more selective NA uptake inhibitors such as atomoxetine are effective in treating ADHD (Biederman and Spencer 2000). These findings suggest that the central noradrenergic system may be involved in the disorder. NA neurons arise

in the locus coeruleus of the brainstem and project widely throughout the CNS. They are sensitive to novelty, which suggests that they are involved in maintaining vigilance and directing attention to relevant stimuli, while reduced central noradrenergic tone may impair these functions (Pliszka et al. 1996). Consistent with this hypothesis, selective and extensive depletion of NA in neonatal rat, which can be achieved with 6-OHDA in the presence of a selective DAT-inhibitor (Teicher et al. 1986), leads to motor hyperactivity and learning deficits (Raskin et al. 1983), and distractibility in a rodent model that selectively assesses sustained attention (Carli et al. 1983). Behavioural effects of drugs that potentiate NA transmission in laboratory models also are consistent with the effectiveness of such agents in the treatment of clinical ADHD.

However, analyses of NA neurotransmission in animal models of ADHD have indicated normal or increased NA transmission. Studies of NA transporter knockout mice did not show altered spontaneous activity or unusual responses to stimulants, although their motor responses to D_2-agonist quinpirole and D_3/D_2-agonist 7-hydroxydipropylaminotetralin (7-OH-DPAT) were increased (Xu et al. 2000). The disparity between the pathophysiology of animal models of ADHD and the beneficial effects of NA-potentiating agents in both animal models and in patients with ADHD, are not easily understood, and further investigation of the role of the NA system in ADHD will help to elucidate the situation.

Serotonin

Serotonergic neurons execute slow, regular discharges that change across the sleep–wake cycle and become virtually silent during rapid eye movement (REM) sleep (Jacobs et al. 1981). These neurons coordinate autonomic and neuroendocrine functions with changing motor output, and regulate sensory information processing, as well as exerting motor-facilitating effects at the lateral horn motoneurons (Gerson and Baldessarini 1980). When the serotonin (5-HT) system is suppressed, such as with orientation to salient stimuli and in REM sleep, motor function is inhibited, and sensory information processing is activated.

Serotonin has been studied closely in only a minority of the animal models of ADHD. Rats that have been poisoned in the neonatal period with 6-hydroxydopamine develop not only hyperactivity but also a prominent hyperinnervation of the neostriatum with serotonergic fibres. Serotonin-potentiating agents can have inhibiting effects on motor hyperactivity (Bishop et al. 2003). In mice that have been genetically altered to knock out the dopamine transporter gene, serotonin may be critically involved in mediating the behaviour-inhibiting effects of stimulants (Gainetdinov et al.1999). All these suggest that serotonin may play a role in pathogenesis in some circumstances, but do not establish serotonin-enhancing drugs as useful treatment.

Most of the experimental models of ADHD rely on behavioural hyperactivity as a primary index to assess effects of clinically proven treatments for ADHD, such as stimulants and tricyclic antidepressants. Much less is known about the effects of these treatments on attention and impulsivity in these models. Animal modelling of ADHD is also limited by the still-evolving understanding of the clinical disorder. Despite the many advances in developing and analysing animal models of ADHD, an ideal laboratory model for ADHD has yet to be established (Solanto 2002).

Genetic studies in ADHD

Current developments in molecular genetics have led to a rapid increase in research aimed at the identification of genetic variation that influences complex human phenotypes (see reviews by Smalley 1997, Asherson and Curran 2001). There has been great interest in ADHD. The driving force behind the molecular genetic research in this area is the overwhelming evidence from quantitative genetic studies that show high heritability ($h^2 = 0.7$–0.9) for the behaviours characterizing the diagnosis of ADHD, whether the disorder is viewed as a categorical entity or a continuous trait. However, the pattern of inheritance is complex and it is likely there are many genes of small effect size contributing to the risk for the disorder.

Molecular genetic research in ADHD has generally focused on candidate gene association studies, and two groups have published completed systematic sib-pair linkage scan data (Fisher et al. 2002, Bakker et al. 2003, Ogdie et al. 2003), although several sib-pair collections are underway.

The linkage results have not implicated a gene or genes of large effect size in ADHD. In the study by Fisher et al. (2002), 126 affected sib pairs were investigated using an approximately 10 cM grid of microsatellite markers. Allele-sharing linkage methods excluded any loci with lambda values ≥ 3 from 96% of the genome and those with lambdas ≥ 2.5 from 91%, indicating that there is unlikely to be a major gene involved in ADHD susceptibility. Under a strict diagnostic scheme they could exclude all screened regions of the X chromosome for locus-specific lambdas ≥ 2 in brother–brother pairs, demonstrating that the excess of affected males with ADHD is probably not attributable to a major X-linked effect.

Qualitative trait maximum lod score analyses have pointed to a number of chromosomal sites that may contain genetic risk factors of moderate effect. None exceeded genomewide significance thresholds, but lod scores were >1.5 for regions on 5p12, 10q26, 12q23, and 16p13. Quantitative-trait analysis of ADHD symptom counts implicated a region on 12p13 (maximum lod 2.6) that also yielded a lod >1 when qualitative methods were used. In summary of work by Ogdie et al. (2002), two regions have emerged as highly likely to harbour risk genes for ADHD: 16p13 and 17p11. Interestingly, both regions, as well as 5p13, have been highlighted in genome-wide scans for autism.

In an independent study (Bakker et al. 2003), a genome scan was performed on 164 Dutch affected sibling pairs (ASPs) with ADHD. Initially, a narrow phenotype was defined, in which all the sib pairs met the full ADHD criteria (117 ASPs). In a broad phenotype, additional sibling pairs were included, in which one child had an autistic spectrum disorder but also met the full ADHD criteria (164 ASPs). This genome scan indicated several regions of interest, two of which showed suggestive evidence for linkage. The most promising chromosome region was located at 15q, with a multiple lod score (MLS) of 3.54 under the broad phenotype definition. This region was previously implicated in reading disability and autism. In addition, MLSs of 3.04 and 2.05 were found for chromosome regions 7p and 9q, respectively, in the narrow phenotype. Except for a region on chromosome 5, no overlap was found with regions mentioned and the other genome scans (Fisher et al. 2002, Ogdie et al. 2003).

Candidate gene association studies have been underway since 1996 and have focused primarily on genes involved in the monoamine pathway as outlined in Figure 2.4. A com-

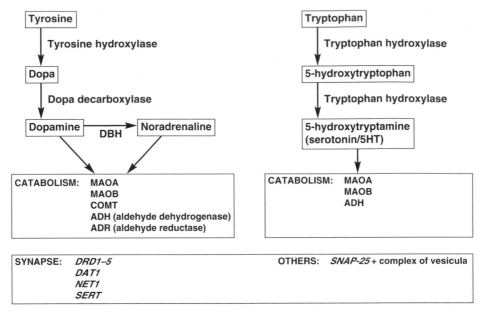

Fig. 2.4. Candidate neurotransmitter genes and their metabolic pathways.

prehensive review and meta-analysis has been published by Bobb et al. (2004). They found that evidence for association exists for four genes in ADHD: the dopamine D4 and D5 receptor genes (*DRD4* and *DRD5* respectively), and the dopamine and serotonin transporter genes (*DAT1* and *SLC6A4*). While other genes were promising, they concluded that they need further replication, and they stressed the fact that all candidate gene approaches continue to face the problem of relatively low power, given modest odds ratios for even the best replicated genes.

D4 RECEPTOR GENE (*DRD4*)
DRD4 is located in the short (p) arm of human chromosome 11, at position 11p15.5. The greatest variance in peptide sequence from other DA receptors occurs in the third intracellular sequence of this peptide, which is required for interaction with G proteins and second-messenger signaling (Van Tol et al. 1992). The 48 base pair sequence is commonly repeated 2, 3, 4 or 7 times, and it is the long 7-repeat that appears to confer the risk of ADHD (Faraone et al. 1999). Failure to replicate by some centres may reflect differences in case identification, genetic stratification in studies using case–control designs, or the fact that effect sizes have been generally small (1–2%).

An interesting feature of the data reported so far has been the wide range of sampling procedures, which give rise to similar positive findings, including both case–control and within-family forms of association analysis, over a broad range of phenotypic criteria. Swanson et al. (1998) used a highly selected group of children who had all responded to methylphenidate and had the combined subtype of ADHD without significant comorbidity. This contrasts greatly with Rowe et al. (1998) who applied diagnostic criteria following completion of DSM-IV rating scales, and Smalley et al. (1998) who applied broader DSM-IIIR and DSM-IV criteria. Meta-analyses have confirmed that the studies taken as a whole give clear evidence of a statistically significant association between ADHD and the 7-repeat variant of the gene ($DRD4\rightarrow$) (Faraone et al. 2001). The odds ratio is modest, at about 1.4. The same $DRD_{4.7}$ genotype has also associated with adult personality traits related to ADHD, including novelty seeking and impulsivity (Benjamin et al. 1996, Ebstein et al. 1996).

The functional significance of the $DRD4$ polymorphism is still uncertain (Watts et al. 1999, Kazmi et al. 2000). It remains possible that the 7-repeat is in linkage disequilibrium with a functional variant, which may confound association studies and lead to discrepant association findings.

D₅ RECEPTOR GENE ($DRD5$)

Initial reports of association between ADHD and the common 148-bp allele of a microsatellite marker located 18.5 kb from the $DRD5$ gene (Daly et al. 1999, Tahir et al. 2000) have been followed by several studies showing nonsignificant trends toward association with the same allele (Barr et al. 2000b, Payton et al. 2001). A recent meta-analysis of genotypic information from 14 independent samples of probands and their parents, found association with the $DRD5$ locus (p=0.00005; odds ratio 1.24; 95% confidence interval 1.12–1.38) (Lowe et al. 2004). This association appears to be confined to the predominantly inattentive and combined clinical subtypes, rather than the hyperactive–impulsive subtype.

DOPAMINE TRANSPORTER GENE ($DAT1$)

The dopamine transporter (DAT) sequesters extracellular dopamine into neurons, is an important regulator of extracellular dopamine and is a principal target of standard anti-hyperactivity medications (e.g. methylphenidate, D-amphetamine) in brain (Giros et al. 1996, Seeman and Madras 1998, Volkow et al. 1998). DAT is the principal regulator of synaptic dopamine concentration and of the duration of dopamine activity, and thus plays a critical role in the regulation of dopaminergic transmission. The gene for this neurotransmitter ($DAT1$) has been mapped to chromosome 5p15.3 (Giros et al. 1992), and its entire sequence, spanning nearly 60 kb, has recently been elucidated (Vandenbergh et al. 2000). At a molecular level, the 3′-untranslated region of the dopamine transporter gene varies in length due to a polymorphic variable number tandem repeat (VNTR) polymorphism (Vandenbergh et al. 1992). The repeat region varies from 3 to 11 copies (Kang et al. 1999, Mitchell et al. 2000), but only alleles with 10 copies of the 40-bp repeat unit have been associated with ADHD.

Replicated associations with ADHD have been reported for a polymorphism of the 480-bp VNTR at the 3′ untranslated region of $DAT1$ (Cook et al. 1995, Levy et al. 1997, Curran et al. 2001). In addition, Barr et al. (2001b) used family trios in a haplotype study of three polymorphisms at the dopamine transporter locus, one of which included the 480-bp VNTR. While they did not find a significant association for any of the alleles examined individually, they found significant evidence for biased transmission of one of the haplotypes containing the 480-bp VNTR, thus providing further evidence that this marker is in linkage disequilibrium with a risk gene for ADHD. There have been several negative studies using both clinical ADHD and epidemiological samples assessed by rating scale measures (Palmer et al. 1999, Holmes et al. 2000, Swanson 2000, Todd et al. 2001). There is evidence that the associated 10 allele may be particularly effective in transporting DA into nerve terminals (Heinz et al. 2000, Michelhaugh et al. 2001, Miller and Madras 2002), and also that expression of *DAT1* is regulated by the 3' UTR VNTR (Fuke et al. 2001, Inoue-Murayama et al. 2002, Mill et al. 2002a).

SEROTONERGIC TRANSPORTER GENE (*SLC6A4*)
The efficiency of serotonergic signalling relates to the concentration of the neurotransmitter in the synaptic cleft and is controlled by the serotonin transporter (5-HTT), which selectively removes serotonin out of the synaptic cleft. The activity of 5-HTT is controlled by a common 44-bp deletion in the promoter region of transporter protein levels. According to a recent meta-analysis of molecular genetic studies in ADHD, the association between a length variation of a repeat in the transcriptional control region of the *5-HTT* gene and ADHD is the third most replicated finding (Bobb et al. 2004). The *5-HTT* gene has also been found to be associated with a dimensional composite rating scale score of ADHD behaviours in a UK population sample (Curran et al. 2005).

OTHER POLYMORPHISMS IN THE SEROTONIN SYSTEM
There has been a replicated association between a polymorphism in the *5HTR 1B* receptor gene and clinical ADHD (Hawi et al. 2002, Quist et al. 2003). An association was reported between a promoter polymorphism in the serotonin transporter (5-HHTTLPR) and clinical ADHD (Manor et al. 2001), and there is a single report of an association for a variant in the *5HTR2A* gene (Quist et al. 2000).

The tryptophan hydroxylase-2 gene (*TPH2*) is the rate-limiting enzyme of serotonin (5-HT) synthesis in the brain. Preferential transmissions were detected for the two single nucleotide polymorphisms (SNPs) in *TPH2*'s regulatory region (rs4570625, p=0.049; rs11178997, p=0.034). Haplotype analysis revealed a strong trend of association between the regulatory region SNPs (rs4570625, rs11178997) and ADHD (p=0.064) (Walitza et al. 2005).

POLYMORPHISMS IN THE NORADRENERGIC SYSTEM
Candidate genes of the noradrenergic (NA) neurotransmission system have also been considered in ADHD. Barr and coworkers (Barr et al. 2001a, Xu et al. 2001) tested genes encoding two α-adrenoceptors, α_{1C} (*ADRA1C*; located in the short arm of human chromosome 8, at 8p11.2) and α_{2C} (*ADRA2C*; at 4p16). With transmission dysequilibrium analysis, they found no biased transmission of any known allele of these genes, and concluded that the alleles considered were not linked to ADHD in the families tested.

Dopamine beta hydroxylase (DBH)
DBH is the enzyme that catalyzes the conversion of dopamine to noradrenaline. This

enzyme is expressed within the secretory vesicles of NA- and adrenaline-producing neurons and neurosecretory cells. Recent data show associations between allelic variation at the DBH locus and plasma DBH activity in three distinct human populations (Zabetian et al. 2001). Several polymorphisms have been described in this locus, all of which are correlated with the levels of DBH activity (Wei et al. 1997). Comings et al. (1999) found a positive association between this polymorphism and continuous ADHD scores in a sample of probands with Tourette syndrome. Daly et al. (1999) found an association between this polymorphism and a sample of children with clinically diagnosed ADHD, and this association was stronger for families where at least one parent was retrospectively diagnosed as having ADHD. Roman et al. (2002) replicated this result in a sample of 88 nuclear families who had a child with clinical ADHD.

SYNAPTOSOMAL-ASSOCIATED PROTEIN (SNAP-25)
A little work has been done on the human homologue of the *Snap* gene, *SNAP-25*. Hess et al. (1995) looked at several markers on chromosome 20 in the region syntenic to mouse chromosome 2, but found no evidence of linkage in five family pedigrees using an autosomal dominant model. Several limitations to this study were raised by Barr et al. (2000a), who carried out an association study of the 3′ untranslated region of the human *SNAP-25* gene and observed biased transmission using the transmission disequilibrium test on haplotypes derived from two SNPs. Mill et al. (2002b) identified a novel microsatellite repeat in *SNAP-25* located between the 5′ UTR and the first coding exon, and tested for association with ADHD. Case–control analyses suggest there may be a role of this polymorphism in ADHD, with one allele over-represented in controls and another over-represented in probands. Within-family tests of linkage and association, however, were not significant, although transmissions of the nominated alleles were in the predicted direction. Further work by Mill et al. (2004), in which they screened the *SNAP-25* gene using denaturing high-performance liquid chromatography (DHPLC) and sequencing, resulted in them genotyping six polymorphic SNPs and two microsatellites in a clinically ascertained sample of 188 probands. Several markers were found to show association with ADHD, both individually and in combination with other markers to form multimarker haplotypes. Analyses of transmission by parental sex demonstrated that the association of *SNAP-25* with ADHD is largely due to transmission of alleles from paternal chromosomes to affected probands, suggesting that this locus may be subject to genomic imprinting. This group have reported evidence supporting the relationship between *SNAP-25* and dimensonal ratings of ADHD in a general population sample of children (Mill et al. 2005). Further work is required to ascertain the role of *SNAP-25* in ADHD and to assess the functional significance of this polymorphism.

NICOTINIC RECEPTORS
Encouraged by findings that nicotinic acetylcholine (ACh) receptor agonists can improve attention, learning and memory in ADHD patients, the α_4 nicotinic receptor gene (*CHRNA4*) has been studied. There are several lines of evidence suggesting that the nicotinic system may be functionally significant in ADHD: (a) nicotine promotes the release of dopamine

and has been shown to improve attention in adults with ADHD, both in smokers and non-smokers (Levin and Simon 1998); (b) ADHD is a significant risk factor for early initiation of cigarette smoking in children (Milberger et al. 1997); (c) maternal cigarette smoking appears to be a risk factor for ADHD (Milberger et al. 1996); (d) nicotine has been shown to stimulate the release of DA in vitro and in vivo in rats (O'Neill et al. 1991); (e) rats demonstrate changes in locomotor activity after nicotine exposure, and prenatal nicotine exposure in rats causes a reduction in a number of nonspecific striatal dopaminergic binding sites (Fung and Lau 1989); and (f) a central nicotinic agonist, ABT-418, improves attention in both monkeys and ADHD adults (Wilens et al. 1999, Fox et al. 2002). Nicotinic acetylcholine receptors are pentameric protein complexes that form a central core for ion movement. Though many subunit genes are expressed in brain, the two primary subunit complexes appear to be an alpha 7 homomeric complex and an alpha4–beta2 heteromeric complex. The nicotinic system has previously been studied in schizophrenia where the neuronal nicotinic acetylcholine receptor alpha 7 subunit gene (*CHRNA7*) has been implicated in decreased P50 inhibition and attentional disturbances in patients with schizophrenia and in many of their nonschizophrenic relatives. Three known microsatellites near *CHRNA7* were studied in 206 ADHD parent-proband trios (Kent et al. 2001), but no evidence for association with ADHD was found. However, another study examined sequence variation at the nicotinic acetylcholine receptor alpha 4 subunit gene (*CHRNA4*) in two independent familial subtypes of ADHD defined by latent class analysis and found a significant association with a 5' intron 2 SNP and severe inattention problems (p=0.007, effect size=4, 95% CI 1.3–4.1). Further investigation is required.

Nicotine agonists may have a functional significance. As stated, maternal smoking is a risk factor for ADHD, and conversely, ADHD is a reported risk factor for early cigarette smoking in children. A central acetylcholinergic system may be involved in ADHD. A role of cholinergic transmission in ADHD is also generally consistent with evidence of the critical importance of this neurotransmission system in cognitive functions (Berger-Sweeney 2003), and is specifically supported by clinical trials finding that treatment with both nicotine and the nicotinic agonist ABT-418 improved attention and arousal in ADHD subjects (Wilens et al. 1999).

Chromosome 6
Warren et al. (1995) reported an association between ADHD and a null (absent) allele of the C4B complement locus in the *MHC* gene region of chromosome 6. This region has been linked with reading disability (Cardon et al. 1995, Grigorenko et al. 1997), raising the possibility that a common susceptibility gene may explain the recognized comorbidity between ADHD and reading disability.

X chromosome
Jiang et al. (2000, 2001) found evidence for association and linkage between two polymorphisms in genes on the X chromosome and ADHD (in the monoaminoxidase A [*MAOA*] gene and the nearby DXS7 locus). *MAOA* and *MAOB* genes code for important enzymes involved in the catabolism of dopamine, noradrenaline and serotonin.

Toxicological/environmental influences

Studies of hypothesized dietary factors, including excessive ingestion of sucrose, have yielded mainly negative results, but other environmental toxins have been implicated in ADHD. Lead exposure during development can produce various nonspecific neurobehavioural abnormalities, including hyperactivity, restlessness, distractibility and impaired cognition. However, lead contamination is not found in most cases of ADHD (Needleman 1990). Parents of ADHD children may consume more alcohol and tobacco than parents of normal controls, and exposure to alcohol or tobacco smoke during early development may be a risk factor for ADHD (Milberger et al. 1997). One might argue that embryological and perinatal insults can selectively damage striatal neurons and affect developing frontal lobe basal ganglia neural networks. Environmental influences are described from a more epidemiological standpoint in Chapter 1.

Discussion

ADHD, as currently defined, is a syndrome or group of syndromes with early onset characterized by problems with attention span, distractibility, impulsivity, and/or the presence of hyperactivity. Genetic influences are strong.

A variety of recent pharmacological, imaging and neuropsychological studies have suggested that the attention problems manifested in ADHD are due to dysfunctions of ventral catecholaminergic pathways projecting to prefrontal and frontal cortex. However, a simple hypofunction is unlikely to be the full story. The precise nature of the abnormalities is complex and likely to vary with particular symptom profiles. More than 30 structural and functional neuroimaging studies of the brain in patients diagnosed with ADHD have been reported, and most of these studies implicate the prefrontal cerebral cortex and its innervation of subcortical regions such as caudate–putamen, nucleus accumbens and amygdaloid complex in the pathophysiology of ADHD. Reduced size of the corpus callosum, particularly in its rostral or splenial portion, has been detected in some children diagnosed with ADHD, and the typically larger corpus callosum in the human female brain may be protective against ADHD. However, a direct link between ADHD and defective transfer of information between the cerebral hemispheres has not been demonstrated in ADHD. Moreover, substantial callosal hypoplasia usually is associated with other major neurodevelopmental disorders that are not specifically associated with ADHD. Recently, the cerebellum has been implicated in cognition and emotion, in addition to its traditional role in coordinating movement and maintaining body posture during ambulation, suggesting a possible contribution to ADHD that is consistent with reports of deficits in fine motor control in some ADHD patients. As the primary site for memory consolidation, the hippocampal formation is also of potential interest in ADHD. Structural brain imaging has not revealed evidence of structural abnormality of the hippocampus, but functional imaging has found reduced cerebral glucose metabolism in this brain region in adolescent girls with ADHD.

With regards to molecular genetic mechanisms in ADHD, it is likely that there are many susceptibility genes, each of small effect size, contributing to the symptoms. There is likely to be a complex interaction between neurotransmitters, and the balance of activity may be more important than absolute amounts. From a molecular viewpoint, therefore, systems/

45

pathway analysis is likely to be needed. Pharmacogenetic studies are now underway and will be important in finding genetic variation predicting therapeutic response to already available medications and are also likely to influence further development of treatments.

We can expect to learn how quantitative variation in the phenotype will be reflected in functional imaging studies and neurotransmitter expression studies, and how specific these brain abnormalities are to the behaviours/syndrome of ADHD. The research so far has provided a partial biological validation for the concept of ADHD. It has not indicated that genetic inheritance and the physical environment are the sole causes, nor indeed that they are necessary, but does suggest that they contribute to most cases. The validation is at a group level, not individual: it is not yet possible to confirm or exclude ADHD by any biological test. But with continuing developments in neuroimaging techniques and molecular genetics, the future looks promising in relation to bridging the gap between clinical and basic research relevant to ADHD.

REFERENCES

Anderson CM, Polcari A, Lowen SB, Renshaw PF, Teicher MH (2002) Effects of methylphenidate on functional magnetic resonance relaxometry of the cerebellar vermis in boys with ADHD. *Am J Psychiatry* **159**: 1322–1328.

Arnsten AF (1997) Catecholamine regulation of the prefrontal cortex. *J Psychopharmacol* **11**: 151–162.

Arnsten AF (2000) Genetics of childhood disorders: XVIII. ADHD, Part. 2: Norepinephrine has a critical modulatory influence on prefrontal cortical function. *J Am Acad Child Adolesc Psychiatry* **39**: 1201–1203.

Arnsten AF (2001) Modulation of prefrontal cortical–striatal circuits: relevance to therapeutic treatments for Tourette syndrome and attention-deficit hyperactivity disorder. *Adv Neurol* **85**: 333–341.

Asherson PJ, Curran S (2001) Approaches to gene mapping in complex disorders and their application in child psychiatry and psychology. *Br J Psychiatry* **179**: 122–128.

Bakker SC, van der Meulen EM, Buitelaar JK, Sandkuijl LA, Pauls DL, Monsuur AJ, van't SR, Minderaa RB, Gunning WB, Pearson PL, Sinke RJ (2003) A whole-genome scan in 164 Dutch sib pairs with attention-deficit/hyperactivity disorder: suggestive evidence for linkage on chromosomes 7p and 15q. *Am J Hum Genet* **72**: 1251–1260.

Barkley RA (1997) Behavioral inhibition, sustained attention, and executive functions: constructing a unifying theory of ADHD. *Psychol Bull* **121**: 65–94.

Barr CL, Feng Y, Wigg K, Bloom S, Roberts W, Malone M, Schachar R, Tannock R, Kennedy JL (2000a) Identification of DNA variants in the SNAP-25 gene and linkage study of these polymorphisms and attention-deficit hyperactivity disorder. *Mol Psychiatry* **5**: 405–409.

Barr CL, Wigg KG, Feng Y, Zai G, Malone M, Roberts W, Schachar R, Tannock R, Kennedy JL (2000b) Attention-deficit hyperactivity disorder and the gene for the dopamine D5 receptor. *Mol Psychiatry* **5**: 548–551.

Barr CL, Wigg K, Zai G, Roberts W, Malone M, Schachar R, Tannock R, Kennedy JL (2001a) Attention-deficit hyperactivity disorder and the adrenergic receptors alpha 1C and alpha 2C. *Mol Psychiatry* **6**: 334–337.

Barr CL, Xu C, Kroft J, Feng Y, Wigg K, Zai G, Tannock R, Schachar R, Malone M, Roberts W, Nothen MM, Grunhage F, Vandenbergh DJ, Uhl G, Sunohara G, King N, Kennedy JL (2001b) Haplotype study of three polymorphisms at the dopamine transporter locus confirm linkage to attention-deficit/hyperactivity disorder. *Biol Psychiatry* **49**: 333–339.

Benjamin J, Li L, Patterson C, Greenberg BD, Murphy DL, Hamer DH (1996) Population and familial association between the D4 dopamine receptor gene and measures of Novelty Seeking. *Nat Genet* **12**: 81–84.

Berger-Sweeney J (2003) The cholinergic basal forebrain system during development and its influence on cognitive processes: important questions and potential answers. *Neurosci Biobehav Rev* **27**: 401–411.

Berquin PC, Giedd JN, Jacobsen LK, Hamburger SD, Krain AL, Rapoport JL, Castellanos FX (1998) Cerebellum in attention-deficit hyperactivity disorder: a morphometric MRI study. *Neurology* **50**: 1087–1093.

Biederman J, Spencer TJ (2000) Genetics of childhood disorders: XIX. ADHD, Part 3: Is ADHD a noradrenergic disorder? *J Am Acad Child Adolesc Psychiatry* **39**: 1330–1333.

Bishop C, Kamdar DP, Walker PD (2003) Intrastriatal serotonin 5-HT2 receptors mediate dopamine D1-induced hyperlocomotion in 6-hydroxydopamine-lesioned rats. *Synapse* **50**: 164–170.

Bobb AJ, Castellanos FX, Addington AM, Rapoport JL (2004) Molecular genetic studies of ADHD: 1991 to 2004. *Am J Med Genet B Neuropsychiatr Genet* **132**: 109–125.

Cardon LR, Smith SD, Fulker DW, Kimberling WJ, Pennington BF, DeFries JC (1995) Quantitative trait locus for reading disability: correction. *Science* **268**: 1553.

Carli M, Robbins TW, Evenden JL, Everitt BJ (1983) Effects of lesions to ascending noradrenergic neurones on performance of a 5-choice serial reaction task in rats; implications for theories of dorsal noradrenergic bundle function based on selective attention and arousal. *Behav Brain Res* **9**: 361–380.

Carrey N, MacMaster FP, Fogel J, Sparkes S, Waschbusch D, Sullivan S, Schmidt M (2003) Metabolite changes resulting from treatment in children with ADHD: a 1H-MRS study. *Clin Neuropharmacol* **26**: 218–221.

Casey BJ, Trainor R, Giedd J, Vauss Y, Vaituzis CK, Hamburger S, Kozuch P, Rapoport JL (1997) The role of the anterior cingulate in automatic and controlled processes: a developmental neuroanatomical study. *Dev Psychobiol* **30**: 61–69.

Castellanos FX (1997) Toward a pathophysiology of attention-deficit/hyperactivity disorder. *Clin Pediatr* **36**: 381–393.

Castellanos FX (2001) Neural substrates of attention-deficit hyperactivity disorder. *Adv Neurol* **85**: 197–206.

Castellanos FX, Giedd JN, Marsh WL, Hamburger SD, Vaituzis AC, Dickstein DP, Sarfatti SE, Vauss YC, Snell JW, Lange N, Kaysen D, Krain AL, Ritchie GF, Rajapakse JC, Rapoport JL (1996) Quantitative brain magnetic resonance imaging in attention-deficit hyperactivity disorder. *Arch Gen Psychiatry* **53**: 607–616.

Castellanos FX, Giedd JN, Berquin PC, Walter JM, Sharp W, Tran T, Vaituzis AC, Blumenthal JD, Nelson J, Bastain TM, Zijdenbos A, Evans AC, Rapoport JL (2001) Quantitative brain magnetic resonance imaging in girls with attention-deficit/hyperactivity disorder. *Arch Gen Psychiatry* **58**: 289–295.

Castellanos FX, Lee PP, Sharp W, Jeffries NO, Greenstein DK, Clasen LS, Blumenthal JD, James RS, Ebens CL, Walter JM, Zijdenbos A, Evans AC, Giedd JN, Rapoport JL (2002) Developmental trajectories of brain volume abnormalities in children and adolescents with attention-deficit/hyperactivity disorder. *JAMA* **288**: 1740–1748.

Comings DE, Gade-Andavolu R, Gonzalez N, Blake H, Wu S, MacMurray JP (1999) Additive effect of three noradrenergic genes (ADRA2a, ADRA2C, DBH) on attention-deficit hyperactivity disorder and learning disabilities in Tourette syndrome subjects. *Clin Genet* **55**: 160–172.

Cook EH, Stein MA, Ellison T, Unis AS, Leventhal BL (1995) Attention deficit hyperactivity disorder and whole-blood serotonin levels: effects of comorbidity. *Psychiatry Res* **57**: 13–20.

Curran S, Mill J, Tahir E, Kent L, Richards S, Gould A, Huckett L, Sharp J, Batten C, Fernando S, Ozbay F, Yazgan Y, Simonoff E, Thompson M, Taylor E, Asherson P (2001) Association study of a dopamine transporter polymorphism and attention deficit hyperactivity disorder in UK and Turkish samples. *Mol Psychiatry* **6**, 425–428.

Curran S, Purcell S, Craig I, Asherson P, Sham P (2005) The serotonin transporter gene as a QTL for ADHD. *Am J Med Genet B Neuropsychiatr Genet* **134**: 42–47.

Daly G, Hawi Z, Fitzgerald M, Gill M (1999) Mapping susceptibility loci in attention deficit hyperactivity disorder: preferential transmission of parental alleles at DAT1, DBH and DRD5 to affected children. *Mol Psychiatry* **4**: 192–196.

Davids E, Zhang K, Tarazi FI, Baldessarini RJ (2003) Animal models of attention-deficit hyperactivity disorder. *Brain Res Brain Res Rev* **42**: 1–21.

Deutch AY, Roth RH (1990) The determinants of stress-induced activation of the prefrontal cortical dopamine system. *Prog Brain Res* **85**: 367–402.

Dougherty DD, Bonab AA, Spencer TJ, Rauch SL, Madras BK, Fischman AJ (1999) Dopamine transporter density in patients with attention deficit hyperactivity disorder. *Lancet* **354**: 2132–2133.

Dresel S, Krause J, Krause KH, LaFougere C, Brinkbaumer K, Kung HF, Hahn K, Tatsch K (2000) Attention deficit hyperactivity disorder: binding of [99mTc]TRODAT-1 to the dopamine transporter before and after methylphenidate treatment. *Eur J Nucl Med* **27**: 1518–1524.

Durston S, Hulshoff Pol HE, Casey BJ, Giedd JN, Buitelaar JK, van Engeland H (2001) Anatomical MRI of the developing human brain: what have we learned? *J Am Acad Child Adolesc Psychiatry* **40**: 1012–1020.

Ebstein RP, Novick O, Umansky R, Priel B, Osher Y, Blaine D, Bennett ER, Nemanov L, Katz M, Belmaker RH (1996) Dopamine D4 receptor (D4DR) exon III polymorphism associated with the human personality trait of Novelty Seeking. *Nat Genet* **12**: 78–80.

47

Ernst M, Zametkin AJ, Phillips RL, Cohen RM (1998) Age-related changes in brain glucose metabolism in adults with attention-deficit/hyperactivity disorder and control subjects. *J Neuropsychiatry Clin Neurosci* **10**: 168–177.

Ernst M, Zametkin AJ, Matochik JA, Pascualvaca D, Jons PH, Cohen RM (1999) High midbrain [18F]DOPA accumulation in children with attention deficit hyperactivity disorder. *Am J Psychiatry* **156**: 1209–1215.

Faraone SV, Biederman J (1998) Neurobiology of attention-deficit hyperactivity disorder. *Biol Psychiatry* **44**: 951–958.

Faraone SV, Biederman J, Weiffenbach B, Keith T, Chu MP, Weaver A, Spencer TJ, Wilens TE, Frazier J, Cleves M, Sakai J (1999) Dopamine D4 gene 7-repeat allele and attention deficit hyperactivity disorder. *Am J Psychiatry* **156**: 768–770.

Faraone SV, Doyle AE, Mick E, Biederman J (2001) Meta-analysis of the association between the 7-repeat allele of the dopamine D(4) receptor gene and attention deficit hyperactivity disorder. *Am J Psychiatry* **158**: 1052–1057.

Fisher SE, Francks C, McCracken JT, McGough JJ, Marlow AJ, MacPhie IL, Newbury DF, Crawford LR, Palmer CG, Woodward JA, Del'Homme M, Cantwell DP, Nelson SF, Monaco AP, Smalley SL (2002) A genomewide scan for loci involved in attention-deficit/hyperactivity disorder. *Am J Hum Genet* **70**: 1183–1196.

Fox GB, Pan JB, Esbenshade TA, Bennani YL, Black LA, Faghih R, Hancock AA, Decker MW (2002) Effects of histamine H(3) receptor ligands GT-2331 and ciproxifan in a repeated acquisition avoidance response in the spontaneously hypertensive rat pup. *Behav Brain Res* **131**: 151–161.

Frank Y, Pavlakis SG (2001) Brain imaging in neurobehavioral disorders. *Pediatr Neurol* **25**: 278–287.

Fuke S, Suo S, Takahashi N, Koike H, Sasagawa N, Ishiura S (2001) The VNTR polymorphism of the human dopamine transporter (DAT1) gene affects gene expression. *Pharmacogenomics J* **1**: 152–156.

Fung YK, Lau YS (1989) Effects of prenatal nicotine exposure on rat striatal dopaminergic and nicotinic systems. *Pharmacol Biochem Behav* **33**: 1–6.

Gainetdinov RR, Wetsel WC, Jones SR, Levin ED, Jaber M, Caron MG (1999) Role of serotonin in the paradoxical calming effect of psychostimulants on hyperactivity. *Science* **283**: 397–401.

Gerson SC, Baldessarini RJ (1980) Motor effects of serotonin in the central nervous system. *Life Sci* **27**: 1435–1451.

Giros B, el Mestikawy S, Godinot N, Zheng K, Han H, Yang-Feng T, Caron MG (1992) Cloning, pharmacological characterization, and chromosome assignment of the human dopamine transporter. *Mol Pharmacol* **42**: 383–390.

Giros B, Jaber M, Jones SR, Wightman RM, Caron MG (1996) Hyperlocomotion and indifference to cocaine and amphetamine in mice lacking the dopamine transporter. *Nature* **379**: 606–612.

Grigorenko EL, Wood FB, Meyer MS, Hart LA, Speed WC, Shuster A, Pauls DL (1997) Susceptibility loci for distinct components of developmental dyslexia on chromosomes 6 and 15. *Am J Hum Genet* **60**: 27–39.

Hawi Z, Dring M, Kirley A, Foley D, Kent L, Craddock N, Asherson P, Curran S, Gould A, Richards S, Lawson D, Pay H, Turic D, Langley K, Owen M, O'Donovan M, Thapar A, Fitzgerald M, Gill M (2002) Serotonergic system and attention deficit hyperactivity disorder (ADHD): a potential susceptibility locus at the 5-HT(1B) receptor gene in 273 nuclear families from a multi-centre sample. *Mol Psychiatry* **7**: 718–725.

Heinz A, Goldman D, Jones DW, Palmour R, Hommer D, Gorey JG, Lee KS, Linnoila M, Weinberger DR (2000) Genotype influences in vivo dopamine transporter availability in human striatum. *Neuropsychopharmacology* **22**: 133–139.

Hess EJ, Rogan PK, Domoto M, Tinker DE, Ladda RL, Ramer JC (1995) Absence of linkage of apparently single gene mediated ADHD with the human syntenic region of the mouse mutant Coloboma. *Am J Med Genet* **60**: 573–579.

Hesslinger B, Tebartz van Elst L, Mochan F, Ebert D (2003) Attention deficit hyperactivity disorder in adults—early vs. late onset in a retrospective study. *Psychiatry Res* **119**: 217–223.

Hill DE, Yeo RA, Campbell RA, Hart B, Vigil J, Brooks W (2003) Magnetic resonance imaging correlates of attention-deficit/hyperactivity disorder in children. *Neuropsychology* **17**: 496–506.

Holmes J, Payton A, Barrett JH, Hever T, Fitzpatrick H, Trumper AL, Harrington R, McGuffin P, Owen M, Ollier W, Worthington J, Thapar A (2000) A family-based and case–control association study of the dopamine D4 receptor gene and dopamine transporter gene in attention deficit hyperactivity disorder. *Mol Psychiatry* **5**: 523–530.

Hynd GW, Semrud-Clikeman M, Lorys AR, Novey ES, Eliopulos D (1990) Brain morphology in developmental dyslexia and attention deficit disorder/hyperactivity. *Arch Neurol* **47**: 919–926.

Ilgin N, Senol S, Gucuyener K, Gokcora N, Sener S (2001) Is increased D2 receptor availability associated with response to stimulant medication in ADHD? *Dev Med Child Neurol* **43**: 755–760.

Inoue-Murayama M, Adachi S, Mishima N, Mitani H, Takenaka O, Terao K, Hayasaka I, Ito S, Murayama Y (2002) Variation of variable number of tandem repeat sequences in the 3′-untranslated region of primate dopamine transporter genes that affects reporter gene expression. *Neurosci Lett* **334**: 206–210.

Jacobs BL, Heym J, Trulson ME (1981) Behavioral and physiological correlates of brain serotoninergic unit activity. *J Physiol* **77**: 431–436.

Jiang S, Xin R, Wu X, Lin S, Qian Y, Ren D, Tang G, Wang D (2000) Association between attention deficit hyperactivity disorder and the DXS7 locus. *Am J Med Genet* **96**: 289–292.

Jiang S, Xin R, Lin S, Qian Y, Tang G, Wang D, Wu X (2001) Linkage studies between attention-deficit hyperactivity disorder and the monoamine oxidase genes. *Am J Med Genet* **105**: 783–788.

Jin Z, Zang YF, Zeng YW, Zhang L, Wang YF (2001) Striatal neuronal loss or dysfunction and choline rise in children with attention-deficit hyperactivity disorder: a [1]H-magnetic resonance spectroscopy study. *Neurosci Lett* **315**: 45–48.

Kang AM, Palmatier MA, Kidd KK (1999) Global variation of a 40-bp VNTR in the 3′-untranslated region of the dopamine transporter gene (SLC6A3). *Biol Psychiatry* **46**: 151–160.

Kazmi MA, Snyder LA, Cypess AM, Graber SG, Sakmar TP (2000) Selective reconstitution of human D4 dopamine receptor variants with Gi alpha subtypes. *Biochemistry* **39**: 3734–3744.

Kent L, Middle F, Hawi Z, Fitzgerald M, Gill M, Feehan C, Craddock N (2001) Nicotinic acetylcholine receptor alpha4 subunit gene polymorphism and attention deficit hyperactivity disorder. *Psychiatr Genet* **11**: 37–40.

Kim BN, Lee JS, Cho SC, Lee DS (2001) Methylphenidate increased regional cerebral blood flow in subjects with attention deficit/hyperactivity disorder. *Yonsei Med J* **42**: 19–29.

Krause KH, Dresel SH, Krause J, Kung HF, Tatsch K (2000) Increased striatal dopamine transporter in adult patients with attention deficit hyperactivity disorder: effects of methylphenidate as measured by single photon emission computed tomography. *Neurosci Lett* **285**: 107–110.

Levin ED, Simon BB (1998) Nicotinic acetylcholine involvement in cognitive function in animals. *Psychopharmacology* **138**: 217–230.

Levy F, Hay DA, McStephen M, Wood C, Waldman I (1997) Attention-deficit hyperactivity disorder: a category or a continuum? Genetic analysis of a large-scale twin study. *J Am Acad Child Adolesc Psychiatry* **36**: 737–744.

Lou HC (1996) Etiology and pathogenesis of attention-deficit hyperactivity disorder (ADHD): significance of prematurity and perinatal hypoxic–haemodynamic encephalopathy. *Acta Paediatr* **85**: 1266–1271.

Lowe N, Kirley A, Hawi Z, Sham P, Wickham H, Kratochvil CJ, Smith SD, Lee SY, Levy F, Kent L, Middle F, Rohde LA, Roman T, Tahir E, Yazgan Y, Asherson P, Mill J, Thapar A, Payton A, Todd RD, Stephens T, Ebstein RP, Manor I, Barr CL, Wigg KG, Sinke RJ, Buitelaar JK, Smalley SL, Nelson SF, Biederman J, Faraone SV, Gill M (2004) Joint analysis of the DRD5 marker concludes association with attention-deficit/hyperactivity disorder confined to the predominantly inattentive and combined subtypes. *Am J Hum Genet* **74**: 348–356.

Manor I, Eisenberg J, Tyano S, Sever Y, Cohen H, Ebstein RP, Kotler M (2001) Family-based association study of the serotonin transporter promoter region polymorphism (5-HTTLPR) in attention deficit hyperactivity disorder. *Am J Med Genet* **105**: 91–95.

Mascalchi M, Filippi M, Floris R, Fonda C, Gasparotti R, Villari N (2005) Diffusion-weighted MR of the brain: methodology and clinical application. *Radiol Med* **109**: 155–197.

Michelhaugh SK, Fiskerstrand C, Lovejoy E, Bannon MJ, Quinn JP (2001) The dopamine transporter gene (SLC6A3) variable number of tandem repeats domain enhances transcription in dopamine neurons. *J Neurochem* **79**: 1033–1038.

Milberger S, Faraone SV, Biederman J, Testa M, Tsuang MT (1996) New phenotype definition of attention deficit hyperactivity disorder in relatives for genetic analyses. *Am J Med Genet* **67**: 369–377.

Milberger S, Biederman J, Faraone SV, Wilens T, Chu MP (1997) Associations between ADHD and psychoactive substance use disorders. Findings from a longitudinal study of high-risk siblings of ADHD children. *Am J Addict* **6**: 318–329.

Mill J, Asherson P, Browes C, D'Souza U, Craig I (2002a) Expression of the dopamine transporter gene is regulated by the 3′ UTR VNTR: Evidence from brain and lymphocytes using quantitative RT-PCR. *Am J Med Genet* **114**: 975–979.

Mill J, Curran S, Kent L, Gould A, Huckett L, Richards S, Taylor E, Asherson P (2002b) Association study

49

of a SNAP-25 microsatellite and attention deficit hyperactivity disorder. *Am J Med Genet* **114**: 269–271.

Mill J, Richards S, Knight J, Curran S, Taylor E, Asherson P (2004) Haplotype analysis of SNAP-25 suggests a role in the aetiology of ADHD. *Mol Psychiatry* **9**: 801–810.

Mill J, Xu X, Ronald A, Curran S, Price T, Knight J, Craig I, Sham P, Plomin R, Asherson P (2005) Quantitative trait locus analysis of candidate gene alleles associated with attention deficit hyperactivity disorder (ADHD) in five genes: DRD4, DAT1, DRD5, SNAP-25, and 5HT1B. *Am J Med Genet B Neuropsychiatr Genet* **133**: 68–73.

Miller GM, Madras BK (2002) Polymorphisms in the 3′-untranslated region of human and monkey dopamine transporter genes affect reporter gene expression. *Mol Psychiatry* **7**: 44–55.

Mitchell RJ, Howlett S, Earl L, White NG, McComb J, Schanfield MS, Briceno I, Papiha SS, Osipova L, Livshits G, Leonard WR, Crawford MH (2000) Distribution of the 3′ VNTR polymorphism in the human dopamine transporter gene in world populations. *Hum Biol* **72**: 295–304.

Mostofsky SH, Newschaffer CJ, Denckla MB (2003) Overflow movements predict impaired response inhibition in children with ADHD. *Percept Mot Skills* **97**: 1315–1331.

Murphy DG, Critchley HD, Schmitz N, McAlonan G, Van Amelsvoort T, Robertson D, Daly E, Rowe A, Russell A, Simmons A, Murphy KC, Howlin P (2002) Asperger syndrome: a proton magnetic resonance spectroscopy study of brain. *Arch Gen Psychiatry* **59**: 885–891.

Needleman HL (1990) The future challenge of lead toxicity. *Environ Health Perspect* **89**: 85–89.

Ogdie MN, MacPhie IL, Minassian SL, Yang M, Fisher SE, Francks C, Cantor RM, McCracken JT, McGough JJ, Nelson SF, Monaco AP, Smalley SL (2003) A genomewide scan for attention-deficit/hyperactivity disorder in an extended sample: suggestive linkage on 17p11. *Am J Hum Genet* **72**: 1268–1279.

O'Neill MF, Dourish CT, Iversen SD (1991) Evidence for an involvement of D1 and D2 dopamine receptors in mediating nicotine-induced hyperactivity in rats. *Psychopharmacology* **104**: 343–350.

Overmeyer S, Bullmore ET, Suckling J, Simmons A, Williams SC, Santosh PJ, Taylor E (2001) Distributed grey and white matter deficits in hyperkinetic disorder: MRI evidence for anatomical abnormality in an attentional network. *Psychol Med* **31**: 1425–1435.

Palmer CG, Bailey JN, Ramsey C, Cantwell D, Sinsheimer JS, Del'Homme M, McGough J, Woodward JA, Asarnow R, Asarnow J, Nelson S, Smalley SL (1999) No evidence of linkage or linkage disequilibrium between DAT1 and attention deficit hyperactivity disorder in a large sample. *Psychiatr Genet* **9**: 157–160.

Payton A, Holmes J, Barrett JH, Hever T, Fitzpatrick H, Trumper AL, Harrington R, McGuffin P, O'Donovan M, Owen M, Ollier W, Worthington J, Thapar A (2001) Examining for association between candidate gene polymorphisms in the dopamine pathway and attention-deficit hyperactivity disorder: a family-based study. *Am J Med Genet* **105**: 464–470.

Pliszka SR, McCracken JT, Maas JW (1996) Catecholamines in attention-deficit hyperactivity disorder: current perspectives. *J Am Acad Child Adolesc Psychiatry* **35**: 264–272.

Quist JF, Barr CL, Schachar R, Roberts W, Malone M, Tannock R, Basile VS, Beitchman J, Kennedy JL (2000) Evidence for the serotonin HTR2A receptor gene as a susceptibility factor in attention deficit hyperactivity disorder (ADHD). *Mol Psychiatry* **5**: 537–541.

Quist JF, Barr CL, Schachar R, Roberts W, Malone M, Tannock R, Basile VS, Beitchman J, Kennedy JL (2003) The serotonin 5-HT1B receptor gene and attention deficit hyperactivity disorder. *Mol Psychiatry* **8**: 98–102.

Raskin LA, Shaywitz BA, Anderson GM, Cohen DJ, Teicher MH, Linakis J (1983) Differential effects of selective dopamine, norepinephrine or catecholamine depletion on activity and learning in the developing rat. *Pharmacol Biochem Behav* **19**: 743–749.

Roman T, Schmitz M, Polanczyk GV, Eizirik M, Rohde LA, Hutz MH (2002) Further evidence for the association between attention-deficit/hyperactivity disorder and the dopamine-beta-hydroxylase gene. *Am J Med Genet* **114**: 154–158.

Rowe DC, Stever C, Giedinghagen LN, Gard JM, Cleveland HH, Terris ST, Mohr JH, Sherman S, Abramowitz A, Waldman ID (1998) Dopamine DRD4 receptor polymorphism and attention deficit hyperactivity disorder. *Mol Psychiatry* **3**: 419–426.

Rubia K (2002) The dynamic approach to neurodevelopmental psychiatric disorders: use of fMRI combined with neuropsychology to elucidate the dynamics of psychiatric disorders, exemplified in ADHD and schizophrenia. *Behav Brain Res* **130**: 47–56.

Rubia K, Overmeyer S, Taylor E, Brammer M, Williams SC, Simmons A, Bullmore ET (1999) Hypofrontality in attention deficit hyperactivity disorder during higher-order motor control: a study with functional MRI. *Am J Psychiatry* **156**: 891–896.

Rubia K, Overmeyer S, Taylor E, Brammer M, Williams SC, Simmons A, Andrew C, Bullmore ET (2000) Functional frontalisation with age: mapping neurodevelopmental trajectories with fMRI. *Neurosci Biobehav Rev* **24**: 13–19.

Rubia K, Taylor E, Smith AB, Oksanen H, Overmeyer S, Newman S, Oksannen H (2001) Neuropsychological analyses of impulsiveness in childhood hyperactivity. *Br J Psychiatry* **179**: 138–143.

Seeman P, Madras BK (1998) Anti-hyperactivity medication: methylphenidate and amphetamine. *Mol Psychiatry* **3**: 386–396.

Seeman P, Madras B (2002) Methylphenidate elevates resting dopamine which lowers the impulse-triggered release of dopamine: a hypothesis. *Behav Brain Res* **130**: 79–83.

Shaywitz BA, Shaywitz SE, Byrne T, Cohen DJ, Rothman S (1983) Attention deficit disorder: quantitative analysis of CT. *Neurology* **33**: 1500–1503.

Shue KL, Douglas VI (1992) Attention deficit hyperactivity disorder and the frontal lobe syndrome. *Brain Cogn* **20**: 104–124.

Smalley SL (1997) Genetic influences in childhood-onset psychiatric disorders: autism and attention-deficit/hyperactivity disorder. *Am J Hum Genet* **60**: 1276–1282.

Smalley SL, Bailey JN, Palmer CG, Cantwell DP, McGough JJ, Del'Homme MA, Asarnow JR, Woodward JA, Ramsey C, Nelson SF (1998) Evidence that the dopamine D4 receptor is a susceptibility gene in attention deficit hyperactivity disorder. *Mol Psychiatry* **3**: 427–430.

Solanto MV (2002) Dopamine dysfunction in AD/HD: integrating clinical and basic neuroscience research. *Behav Brain Res* **130**: 65–71.

Sun L, Zin Z, Zang YF, Zeng YW, Liu G, Li Y, Seidman LJ, Faraone SV, Wang YF (2005) Differences between attention deficit with and without hyperactivity. *Brain Dev* **27**: 340–344.

Swanson JM (2000) Dopamine-transporter density in patients with ADHD. *Lancet* **355**: 1461–1462.

Swanson JM, Sunohara GA, Kennedy JL, Regino R, Fineberg E, Wigal T, Lerner M, Williams L, LaHoste GJ, Wigal S (1998) Association of the dopamine receptor D4 (DRD4) gene with a refined phenotype of attention deficit hyperactivity disorder (ADHD): a family-based approach. *Mol Psychiatry* **3**: 38–41.

Tahir E, Yazgan Y, Cirakoglu B, Ozbay F, Waldman I, Asherson PJ (2000) Association and linkage of DRD4 and DRD5 with attention deficit hyperactivity disorder (ADHD) in a sample of Turkish children. *Mol Psychiatry* **5**: 396–404.

Tannock R (1998) Attention deficit hyperactivity disorder: advances in cognitive, neurobiological, and genetic research. *J Child Psychol Psychiatry* **39**: 65–99.

Teicher MH, Barber NI, Reichheld JH, Baldessarini RJ, Finklestein SP (1986) Selective depletion of cerebral norepinephrine with 6-hydroxydopamine and GBR-12909 in neonatal rat. *Brain Res* **395**: 124–128.

Teicher MH, Anderson CM, Polcari A, Glod CA, Maas LC, Renshaw PF (2000) Functional deficits in basal ganglia of children with attention-deficit/hyperactivity disorder shown with functional magnetic resonance imaging relaxometry. *Nat Med* **6**: 470–473.

Thomas KM, King SW, Franzen PL, Welsh TF, Berkowitz AL, Noll DC, Birmaher V, Casey BJ (1999) A developmental functional MRI study of spatial working memory. *Neuroimage* **10**: 327–338.

Todd RD, Jong YJ, Lobos EA, Reich W, Heath AC, Neuman RJ (2001) No association of the dopamine transporter gene 3′ VNTR polymorphism with ADHD subtypes in a population sample of twins. *Am J Med Genet* **105**: 745–748.

Vaidya CJ, Austin G, Kirkorian G, Ridlehuber HW, Desmond JE, Glover GH, Gabrieli JD (1998) Selective effects of methylphenidate in attention deficit hyperactivity disorder: a functional magnetic resonance study. *Proc Natl Acad Sci USA* **95**: 14494–14499.

Vandenbergh DJ, Persico AM, Hawkins AL, Griffin CA, Li X, Jabs EW, Uhl GR (1992) Human dopamine transporter gene (DAT1) maps to chromosome 5p15.3 and displays a VNTR. *Genomics* **14**: 1104–1106.

Vandenbergh DJ, Thompson MD, Cook EH, Bendahhou E, Nguyen T, Krasowski MD, Zarrabian D, Comings D, Sellers EM, Tyndale RF, George SR, O'Dowd BF, Uhl GR (2000) Human dopamine transporter gene: coding region conservation among normal, Tourette's disorder, alcohol dependence and attention-deficit hyperactivity disorder populations. *Mol Psychiatry* **5**: 283–292.

van Dyck CH, Quinlan DM, Cretella LM, Staley JK, Malison RT, Baldwin RM, Seibyl JP, Innis RB (2002) Unaltered dopamine transporter availability in adult attention deficit hyperactivity disorder. *Am J Psychiatry* **159**: 309–312.

Van Tol HH, Wu CM, Guan HC, Ohara K, Bunzow JR, Civelli O, Kennedy J, Seeman P, Niznik HB, Jovanovic V (1992) Multiple dopamine D4 receptor variants in the human population. *Nature* **358**: 149–152.

Volkow ND, Wang GJ, Fowler JS, Logan J, Angrist B, Hitzemann R, Lieberman J, Pappas N (1997) Effects of methylphenidate on regional brain glucose metabolism in humans: relationship to dopamine D2 receptors. *Am J Psychiatry* **154**: 50–55.

Volkow ND, Wang GJ, Fowler JS, Gatley SJ, Logan J, Ding YS, Hitzemann R, Pappas N (1998) Dopamine transporter occupancies in the human brain induced by therapeutic doses of oral methylphenidate. *Am J Psychiatry* **155**: 1325–1331.

Walitza S, Renner TJ, Dempfle A, Konrad K, Wewetzer C, Halbach A, Herpertz-Dahlmann B, Remschmidt H, Smidt J, Linder M, Flierl L, Knolker U, Friedel S, Schafer H, Gross C, Hebebrand J, Warnke A, Lesch KP (2005) Transmission disequilibrium of polymorphic variants in the tryptophan hydroxylase-2 gene in attention-deficit/hyperactivity disorder. *Mol Psychiatry* **10**: 1126–1132.

Warren RP, Odell JD, Warren WL, Burger RA, Maciulis A, Torres AR (1995) Is decreased blood plasma concentration of the complement C4B protein associated with attention-deficit hyperactivity disorder? *J Am Acad Child Adolesc Psychiatry* **34**: 1009–1014.

Watts VJ, Vu MN, Wiens BL, Jovanovic V, Van Tol HH, Neve KA (1999) Short- and long-term heterologous sensitization of adenylate cyclase by D4 dopamine receptors. *Psychopharmacology* **141**: 83–92.

Wei J, Xu HM, Ramchand CN, Hemmings GP (1997) Is the polymorphic microsatellite repeat of the dopamine beta-hydroxylase gene associated with biochemical variability of the catecholamine pathway in schizophrenia? *Biol Psychiatry* **41**: 762–767.

Wilens TE, Biederman J, Spencer TJ, Bostic J, Prince J, Monuteaux MC, Soriano J, Fine C, Abrams A, Rater M, Polisner D (1999) A pilot controlled clinical trial of ABT-418, a cholinergic agonist, in the treatment of adults with attention deficit hyperactivity disorder. *Am J Psychiatry* **156**: 1931–1937.

Xu C, Schachar R, Tannock R, Roberts W, Malone M, Kennedy JL, Barr CL (2001) Linkage study of the alpha2A adrenergic receptor in attention-deficit hyperactivity disorder families. *Am J Med Genet* **105**: 159–162.

Xu F, Gainetdinov RR, Wetsel WC, Jones SR, Bohn LM, Miller GW, Wang YM, Caron MG (2000) Mice lacking the norepinephrine transporter are supersensitive to psychostimulants. *Nat Neurosci* **3**: 465–471.

Zabetian CP, Anderson GM, Buxbaum SG, Elston RC, Ichinose H, Nagatsu T, Kim KS, Kim CH, Malison RT, Gelernter J, Cubells JF (2001) A quantitative-trait analysis of human plasma–dopamine beta-hydroxylase activity: evidence for a major functional polymorphism at the DBH locus. *Am J Hum Genet* **68**: 515–522.

3
DIAGNOSIS AND ASSESSMENT

Kapil Sayal

The cardinal features of hyperactivity disorders involve symptoms of inattentiveness, over-activity and impulsiveness. However, these behaviours are also common in many children who do not have a disorder. It is likely that these traits exist to varying extents across the population. Given that these features have a continuous distribution (like blood pressure, for example), where should the cut-off be applied to help decide whether or not a disorder (like hypertension) is present? From a clinical perspective, the key question is: when do these behavioural traits cross over a threshold to constitute a disorder that might merit intervention and treatment? As a rule of thumb, these behaviours are considered to meet criteria for disorder when they are inappropriate for the child's developmental age and are associated with impairment.

The scope of this chapter is to consider the factors influencing recognition of symptoms in the community and in clinical settings; to describe a comprehensive approach to assessment for use in a secondary care clinic; and to consider the practical utility of checklists and questionnaires in aiding the assessment process. Subsequent chapters will consider physical and psychological assessment investigations, and diagnostic formulations that take account of possible coexisting disorders.

Classification systems

For hyperactivity disorders, there are two main classification systems in operation, and they incorporate different concepts of a disorder based on inattentiveness, overactivity and impulsiveness (see Chapter 1). The ICD-10 (WHO 1992) category of 'hyperkinetic disorder' (HKD; see Chapter 10) can be conceptualized as a subtype of the broader attention deficit hyperactivity disorder (ADHD). Clinical practice guidance in the UK (Lord and Paisley 2000) describes it in terms of 'severe ADHD'.

In contrast, the DSM-IV classification (APA 1994) is employed in the USA. Its definition of ADHD has broader criteria than hyperkinetic disorder, as described in Chapter 1. From an epidemiological perspective, these differences between the classification systems are reflected in much higher prevalence rates for ADHD than for HKD.

In clinical practice there are advantages conferred by familiarity with and use of both diagnostic systems. In the first instance, the question is whether a diagnosis of ADHD can be made. If the criteria for ADHD are met, the next question is whether symptoms also reach the threshold for a diagnosis of HKD. Following this, the issue of the presence of possible comorbid disorders needs to be considered as this may influence the choice of treatment. On the other hand, if a diagnosis of ADHD cannot be reached, alternative diagnoses need to be considered. It is possible that the child may not meet criteria for any disorder – in these situations the concept of 'pervasive hyperactivity' may be useful. This implies that the symptoms do occur across at least two settings but are not sufficiently severe or pervasive to meet criteria for a diagnosis. From longitudinal work it is known that pervasive hyperactivity is a risk factor for later development (Taylor et al. 1996). Appropriate behavioural advice to parents and school may be helpful, and a follow-up review should be considered to confirm the (lack of) diagnosis – it is possible that, over time, the severity of problems or associated impairment may become more prominent to the extent that diagnostic criteria are met.

Recognition prior to referral

The recognition rates of hyperactivity disorders are much lower than the epidemiological prevalence. Most children who have ADHD have not received a diagnosis and are not receiving specialist services. This is despite increased awareness of the disorder in recent years amongst clinicians, referrers, teachers and parents. Practice guidance in the UK (NICE 2000) recommends that stimulant medication should be initiated only by specialists, so effective intervention for ADHD requires appropriate referral to such specialist services. This is determined by the recognition of symptoms by adults and the views of the professionals to whom these problems are presented. At the primary level, parents and teachers are the key adults who are likely to recognize symptoms. Even if possible symptoms are noticed, several factors influence whether this results in help-seeking. From the parents' perspective, factors such as severity of symptoms, associated impairment for the child, impact on family life, and problems at school determine their level of concern. Teachers are likely to be concerned about disruptive behaviour. Traditionally, recognition rates have been lower in girls, preschoolers, adolescents, and where symptoms of inattention rather than overactivity predominate. The under-referral of girls with ADHD is an example of referral bias – the type of symptomatology might vary between the genders, with girls being more likely to have problems with inattention and learning, and boys problems with overactivity and impulsiveness. These differences reflect the possibility that referral is more likely to occur if there is an impact of symptoms on adults.

As well as these factors operating at the individual level, recognition can be influenced by cultural and social factors. For example, Leung et al. (1996) found that parents of Chinese boys were more likely than parents of English boys to rate them highly on hyperactivity scales, despite the former having lower activity levels when assessed objectively. This suggests that, in certain cultures, externalizing behaviour is regarded as being relatively unacceptable and problematic. Parental concerns and similar cultural factors are likely to influence relevant professionals. The local availability of specialist services and the attitudes of these providers can also influence the recognition practices of potential referrers such as primary health care professionals. In terms of help-seeking, parents usually discuss their concerns with primary tier professionals such as teachers, GPs or health visitors. Following the presentation of problems to primary care, the decision to refer is often based on the level of concern expressed by the parent and severity of problems including associated comorbidity, especially conduct problems (Sayal et al. 2002). Given that many parents may describe their children as being overactive, it is important for primary tier professionals to be able to clarify the nature of the problems and enquire whether symptoms are pervasive across settings. In deciding about the initial management approach (including the possibility of referral to a specialist service), an account about associated impairment in terms of learning, activities, friendships and family life is also helpful. The use of checklists in aiding this process is discussed later.

Clinical assessment

Following referral, pitfalls may occur in obtaining or interpreting the necessary information to make or refute a diagnosis of ADHD. Compared to previously, it is more likely that the possible presence of ADHD will at least be considered – there is now greater awareness of ADHD amongst specialist clinicians and it is more likely to be highlighted as a referral question. For example, applying an earlier ICD classification system to the same case vignettes, Prendergast et al. (1988) demonstrated that clinicians in the USA tended to make a diagnosis of HKD whereas those in the UK tended to diagnose conduct disorder.

This section describes a comprehensive assessment that can aid the diagnostic process and can be used in a secondary care clinic. It needs to be stressed that there are no diagnostic tests for ADHD - in particular, a response to stimulant medication should not be interpreted as implying that a diagnosis of ADHD is accurate. It is a descriptive diagnosis based on a clinical assessment that includes a detailed history, an examination of the child and, ideally, information from another source. When clear diagnostic criteria are used, the diagnosis is reliable. In order to make a diagnosis of ADHD, the assessor should have a working knowledge of child development to enable them to relate elicited information about symptoms to what would be appropriate for a child of that age and developmental level. Symptoms should be interpreted in the context of the child's functional rather than chronological age. A comprehensive assessment is necessary to distinguish the presence of other disorders that might mimic ADHD or occur alongside (be comorbid with) ADHD: these are discussed in detail in Chapter 6. If available, different disciplines are able to make complementary contributions to the assessment process.

If possible, all family members living at home should be invited. Different family members may have unique perspectives of the index child's difficulties. It provides an opportunity to make observations about family interactions and the level of warmth or criticism expressed. The family are also likely to be actively involved in the process of delivering recommended interventions. Following an initial introduction, a brief enquiry about potentially positive aspects such as the child's interests can be useful in putting everyone at ease and engaging the child. The parents' level of interest and reactions in listening to the child can be a useful pointer to their views about the child and the problems. After this introductory phase, if possible, it is useful for the parents and child to be seen separately. The rest of the section describes three further stages of assessment: (1) history from parents; (2) individual interview with the child; (3) use of checklists or questionnaires.

HISTORY FROM PARENTS
The interview with the parent or main carer is the most important component of the diagnostic

55

process. It is essential to obtain details about the nature, frequency and severity of possible symptoms of ADHD in everyday situations.

One approach to collecting this information systematically is to use the hyperactivity section of the Parental Account of Children's Symptoms (PACS; Taylor et al. 1986 – see Appendix 3.1).

Items from the PACS can easily be incorporated into a clinical interview. The PACS is a standardized, semi-structured interview that is a reliable and valid measure of child behaviour at home. The parent is asked for detailed descriptions of what the child has recently done in specific situations. For hyperactivity, this involves two main components. First, descriptions are obtained about attention span, restlessness and fidgeting in age-appropriate situations such as watching television, reading, and both playing alone and with others. 'Attention span' measures the time spent on a single activity; 'restlessness' measures moving about during the same activities; and 'fidgeting' measures movements of parts of the body during these activities. It is important that the parent has observed the child during the situation under scrutiny. Otherwise, for example, there may be a risk of overestimating the duration of activities when the child has been swapping from one activity or game to another. In particular, the duration of playing computer games is a poor indicator of concentration span as it involves frequent changes in demands. Second, descriptions are obtained of activity levels in structured situations such as mealtimes, shopping and outings.

The clinician needs to make a judgement as to whether the symptoms are inappropriate compared to what would be expected for that child. As described earlier, symptoms should be interpreted within the context of the child's developmental age. The presence of associated impairment in terms of the impact of symptoms on peer relationships, activities, home life and school should be established. It is also important to establish the age at onset of symptoms and the presence of symptoms of other disorders. One should also consider whether symptoms of other disorders are mimicking ADHD – misdiagnoses can reflect a range of other disorders including: oppositional defiant or conduct disorder; emotional disorders (anxiety and depression); pervasive developmental disorders; tic disorders; and general and specific (e.g. reading, spelling, arithmetic) problems with learning and motor skills (see Chapters 6 and 11). Although some of these problems may be reported spontaneously, careful enquiry should be made about others such as associated internalizing symptoms.

Further history includes details about the family such as similar symptoms in other family members, other family medical and psychiatric history, parental education and learning problems, and family structure, relationships and support. A detailed developmental history includes information about the pregnancy (including any risk behaviours such as smoking and use of substances), birth, infancy period, attainment of milestones as well as a complete medical history with particular enquiry about fits, faints, illnesses, injuries, vision and hearing (including episodes of otitis media). Further details about current family life, stresses and housing conditions are useful in interpreting the context of the difficulties. If information has not already been gathered about symptoms in earlier nursery or school settings, an educational history should be obtained at this stage. Finally, an account of the child's temperament, personality, interpersonal relationships, and interests and strengths should be obtained.

INTERVIEW WITH THE CHILD

In the novel environment of the clinic, the child may not be particularly inattentive or overactive. This might also reflect them receiving attention from an adult at an individual level. If the symptoms of ADHD are not observed, this should not refute a diagnosis. Conversely, if the described behaviours are witnessed, such observation can be a rich source of information. It may provide an indication of the associated antecedents and consequences and help guide advice for management strategies.

Ideally, the child should also be seen individually. The length and structure of this interview will depend on the child's developmental level. For younger children, this will be done most usefully within a play context. It is important that the child is engaged in this process. Commencing with a general chat about their day-to-day life and interests can help put both parties at ease. It can be informative to obtain an impression about their awareness as to why they have come to the clinic. Although their views about the impact of their symptoms on home life, activities, school work, and relationships with family members, teachers and peers can be illuminating, too much weight should not be placed on the child's account of their symptoms. Research evidence suggests that adults are more accurate informants of such symptoms. It is helpful to obtain an account of any other concerns they might have such as associated distress or other functional difficulties. As appropriate, enquiry should also be made about the child's mood and possible variability of this, and possible symptoms of anxiety or paranoia. Physical examination should incorporate an assessment of general health; growth; neurological status, including assessment of fine and gross motor coordination; and hearing and vision. Any further investigations should be guided by the history and examination (see Chapter 5).

INFORMATION FROM TEACHERS AND USE OF CHECKLISTS

Although the parent may give an accurate indication about the pervasiveness of symptoms, it is essential to obtain an independent account from school to confirm this. This should focus on the presence of symptoms at school as well as their impact with particular regard to friendships and learning. In making a diagnosis of ADHD, information from teachers makes a valuable contribution to the decision-making process. It can be extremely useful to get information across the child's school career as the tolerance and perceptions of different teachers may vary considerably. Information about any specialist educational input should also be obtained. Furthermore, if doubt remains about the diagnosis after the assessment, observation at schools across at least two different types of activities can be informative. Although potentially time-consuming, this can be invaluable in clarifying the diagnosis.

The initial information from schools can be gathered by means of questionnaires, forms with open-ended questions to obtain behavioural descriptions, or a brief telephone interview. It is useful to obtain this information before the assessment takes place. The role of questionnaire rating scales is considered briefly. In referred samples, these can also be used for screening to identify which children might benefit from a detailed diagnostic assessment. However, with such an approach, the risk of false negatives (children who have ADHD but are missed by the questionnaire) needs to be kept in mind. As part of the assessment process, it must be stressed that rating scales should not be used in isolation. These can be useful adjuncts to the clinical assessment but are not diagnostic. Detailed descriptions of behaviours are essential. Although numerous parent and teacher rating scales for ADHD are available, this chapter will focus on the use of two scales commonly used in clinical practice in the UK. Both these scales have similar versions for parents and teachers. For a more detailed review of a range of scales, the reader is referred to Collett et al. (2003).

Scales can be considered in terms of broad-band scales that assess a range of symptoms including ADHD and narrow-band scales that are specific measures to assess ADHD. Broad-band scales can be useful in highlighting the presence of possible comorbidity or differential diagnoses that might require further investigation. The Strengths and Difficulties Questionnaire (SDQ; http://www.sdqinfo.com) is an example of a broad-band scale. It consists of five items to assess symptoms of ADHD. It also provides ratings reflecting conduct and emotional disorders, as well as an impairment score that reflects any symptoms. At a community level, it is useful in identifying which children may benefit from further diagnostic assessment (Sayal et al. 2002). The Conners' Rating Scales – Revised (CRS-R; Conners 1997) is an example of a narrow-band scale. In clinical practice, the short (28 item) version is useful. It provides three subscales that inform about inattention, hyperactivity and oppositional behaviours. In addition, a summary ADHD index scale score is provided.

Overall, rating scales are useful at a community level for screening to help identify which children may benefit from further assessment. They could be used by potential referrers to help decide whether referral for assessment to establish the possible presence of ADHD is appropriate. Within clinics, they may aid the decision-making process as to whether a detailed assessment for ADHD is warranted. Furthermore, they may be useful to assess the response to treatment once a diagnosis is made. However, within the context of assessment for ADHD, they are not diagnostic in their own right and should not be used in isolation to establish a diagnosis.

REFERENCES

APA (1994) *Diagnostic and Statistical Manual of Mental Disorders, 4th edn (DSM-IV)*. Washington, DC: American Psychiatric Association.

Collett BR, Ohan JL, Myers K (2003) Ten-year review of rating scales. V: Scales assessing attention deficit hyperactivity disorder. *J Am Acad Child Adolesc Psychiatry* **42**: 1015–1037.

Conners CK (1997) *Conners' Rating Scales: Revised Technical Manual*. New York: Multi-Health Systems.

Leung PW, Luk SL, Ho TP, Taylor E, Mak FL, Bacon-Shone J (1996) The diagnosis and prevalence of hyperactivity in Chinese schoolboys. *Br J Psychiatry* **168**: 486–496.

Lord J, Paisley S (2000) The clinical effectiveness and cost-effectiveness of methylphenidate for hyperactivity in childhood. Version 2 – for consultation. London: National Institute for Clinical Excellence (online at http://www.nice.org.uk/download.aspx?o=11655).

NICE (2000) Attention deficit hyperactivity disorder (ADHD) – methylphenidate. Technology appraisal guidance no. 13. London: National Institute for Clinical Excellence [Now obsolete, replaced by NICE (2006) Methylphenidate, atomoxetine and dexamfetamine for attention deficit hyperactivity disorder (ADHD) in children and adolescents (review). Technology appraisal guidance no. 98. (online at: http://www.nice.org.uk/page.aspx?o=TA098guidance).]

Prendergast M, Taylor E, Rapoport JL, Bartko J, Donnelly M, Zametkin A, Ahearn MB, Dunn G, Wieselberg HM (1988) The diagnosis of childhood hyperactivity. A U.S.–U.K. cross-national study of DSM-III and ICD-9. *J Child Psychol Psychiatry* **29**: 289–300.

Sayal K, Taylor E, Beecham J, Byrne P (2002) Pathways to care in children at risk of attention deficit hyperactivity disorder. *Br J Psychiatry* **181**: 43–48.

Taylor EA, Schachar R, Thorley G, Wieselberg M (1986) Conduct disorder and hyperactivity: I. Separation of hyperactivity and antisocial conduct in British child psychiatric patients. *Br J Psychiatry* **149**: 760–767.

WHO (1992) *International Statistical Classification of Diseases and Related Health Problems, 10th edn (ICD-10).* Geneva: World Health Organization.

APPENDIX 3.1
INTERVIEWING FOR HYPERACTIVE SYMPTOMS

The *Parental Account of Children's Symptoms* (PACS) is a standardized, investigator-based interview measure, first developed as an instrument for measuring children's behaviour problems as seen at home (Taylor et al. 1986). It is administered by a trained interviewer, and the reliability is in the interviewer's training. Part of the schedule is reproduced below as an example for detailed behavioural interviewing.

Parents are asked, not for their ratings of problems, but for detailed descriptions of what their child has done in specified situations over the previous week. Such situations are defined either by external events – e.g. watching TV, reading a book or comic, playing alone, playing with friends, going to bed, travelling – or by behaviours shown – e.g. crying, worried talk, tempers, fighting with siblings. The interviewers then make their own ratings, on the basis of formal training and written definitions of the behaviours to be rated. Inter-rater reliability for trained interviewers is high, with product–moment correlations for pairs of interviewers ranging from 0.79 to 0.96; and it predicts well to diagnostic judgements of ADHD and to external measures of activity and attention (Chen and Taylor 2006).

Situations that have not occurred are not scored, so the scale score is the mean for the items that can be validly completed out of sections 1 through 8. The scores should not be considered as having been normed; but as a rough guide, scores above 1.2 are considered to indicate hyperactive behaviour in the home situation for children at the peak presenting ages of 7–9 years [the mean for children with hyperactivity in one study was 1.4 vs a mean for ordinary population controls of 0.5 (SD 0.4) – Taylor et al. 1991). If such a score is combined with a score above cut-off on a teacher rating scale of hyperactivity then a diagnosis of ADHD is likely. Scores fall during adolescence. (There is also a computer algorithm for research diagnosis.)

The full interview includes several subscales – one for hyperactivity and inattention, which is reproduced below, and others for defiance/oppositional behaviours (temper tantrums, lying, stealing, defiance, disobedience, truanting, destructiveness), emotional disorder (misery, worrying, fears, hypochondriasis, somatic symptoms), and commonly associated problems such as tics and symptoms of attachment disorder and autistic spectrum disorders.

REFERENCES

Chen W, Taylor E (2006) Parental Account of Children's Symptoms (PACS), ADHD phenotypes and its application to molecular genetic studies. *Prog ADHD Res* (in press).

Taylor E, Sandberg S, Thorley G, Giles S (1991) *The Epidemiology of Childhood Hyperactivity. Maudsley Monograph No. 33.* Oxford: Oxford University Press.

Taylor E, Schachar R, Thorley G, Wieselberg M (1986) Conduct disorder and hyperactivity: I. Separation of hyperactivity and antisocial conduct in British child psychiatric patients. *Br J Psychiatry* **149**: 760–767.

PACS SCALE FOR ACTIVITY LEVEL AND INATTENTIVE BEHAVIOUR

1. WATCHING TV

Can you think about a time in the past week or recently when X was watching TV or a video? How long did he/she watch for?
If the answer is vague: **Would it be for more or less than half an hour? Is X able to watch a programme right the way through? Would that be a typical length of time for X to watch something he/she is interested in?**
USUAL ATTENTION SPAN while watching TV:

More than 30 minutes	0
Between 15 and 30 minutes	1
Between 6 and 15 minutes	2
5 minutes or less	3

When you last saw X watching TV, did he/she stay in one place or get up and move around the room? **How often did X get up from the watching position?**
If the answer is vague: **Was it every 15 minutes or less often than that? Is that amount of moving around typical of X when watching TV?**
USUAL RESTLESSNESS while watching TV:

No restlessness	0
Once every 15 minutes	1
More than once every 15 minutes but less than once every 5 minutes	2
Once every 5 minutes or stays in place for less than 5 minutes	3

The last time you saw X watching TV did he/she fidget, e.g. swing legs, tap fingers, fiddle with an object or clothing?
If the answer is vague: **Did he/she fidget throughout the watching time, more than half the time or less than half the time? Is that the usual amount of fidgeting X does when watching TV?**
USUAL FIDGETING while watching TV:

No fidgeting	0
Less than half the time	1
More than half the time but not throughout	2
Continuous fidgeting	3

Did X talk while watching TV?
If the answer is vague: **Did X talk all the time he/she was watching? More than half the time or less than half the time? Is that how talkative X usually is when watching something he/she is interested in?**
USUAL TALKATIVENESS while watching TV:

No talking or the occasional comment	0
Talked for less than half the time	1
More than half the time but not throughout	2
Talked continuously	3

Did X make any other sort of noise while watching? What kind of noise? Is this usual for X?
USUAL NOISINESS while watching TV:

No noise	0
Noisy less than half the time	1
More than half the time but not throughout	2
Continual noise throughout	3

2. READING

Can you think about a time in the past week or recently when X was reading a book, magazine or comic? How long did he/she read for on that occasion? Is that the usual amount of time he/she would sit and read for?
USUAL ATTENTION SPAN while reading:

More than 30 minutes	0
Between 15 and 30 minutes	1
Between 6 and 15 minutes	2
5 minutes or less	3

Note: *Only rate independent reading. Do not rate reading a school book aloud to a parent.*

When you last saw X reading did he/she stay in one place or move around the room? How often did X do this?
If the answer is vague: **Did X sit in one place for more than five minutes while reading? Is that amount of moving around typical of X when he/she reads?**
USUAL RESTLESSNESS while reading:

No restlessness	0
Moves from position once every 15 minutes	1
More than once every 15 minutes but less than once every 5 minutes	2
Once every 5 minutes or stays in place for less than 5 minutes	3

The last time you saw X reading did he/she fidget?

If the answer is vague: **Did he/she fidget all the time while reading? More than half the time or less than half the time? Is that typical of the amount of fidgeting X usually does while reading?**

USUAL FIDGETING while reading:

No fidgeting	0
Less than half the time	1
More than half the time but not throughout	2
Continuous fidgeting	3

Did X talk while reading?

If the answer is vague: **Did X talk all the time he/she was reading? More than half the time or less than half the time? Is that how talkative X usually is when reading?**

USUAL TALKATIVENESS while reading:

No talking or the occasional comment	0
Talked for less than half the time	1
More than half the time but not throughout	2
Talked continuously	3

Did X make any other sort of noise while reading? What kind of noise? Is this usual for X?

USUAL NOISINESS while reading:

No noise	0
Noisy less than half the time	1
More than half the time but not throughout	2
Continual noise throughout	3

3. SOLITARY PLAY

Can you think about a time in the past week or recently when X was playing alone, e.g. drawing, painting, building models, needlework? How long did he/she spend doing this? Is that typical of the amount of time he/she would do something on his/her own for?

If the answer is vague: **Can X keep him/herself occupied for half-an-hour or would it be for less than that?**

USUAL ATTENTION SPAN during solitary play:

More than 30 minutes	0
Between 15 and 30 minutes	1
Between 6 and 15 minutes	2
5 minutes or less	3

Note: *If the duration span differs for different activities, rate the longest duration. Do not include activities shared with another person.*

During this task, did X stay in one place or get up and move around? How often did he/she do that? Is that amount of moving around typical of X when doing something on his/her own like this?

RESTLESSNESS during solitary play:

No restlessness	0
Once every 15 minutes	1
More than once every 15 minutes but less than once every 5 minutes	2
Once every 4 minutes or stays in place for less than 5 minutes	3

Did X fidget while doing this task?

If the answer is vague: **Did X fidget throughout, more than half the time or less than half the time? Is that the usual amount of fidgeting X does when doing things on their own?**

USUAL FIDGETING during solitary play:

No fidgeting	0
Less than half the time	1
More than half the time but not throughout	2
Continuous fidgeting	3

Did X talk while doing this?
If the answer is vague: **Did he/she talk all the time? More than half the time or less than half the time? Is that how talkative X usually is when doing something on his/her own?**
USUAL TALKATIVENESS during solitary play:

No talking or the occasional comment	0
Talked for less than half the time	1
More than half the time but not throughout	2
Talked continuously	3

Did X make any other sort of noise while doing this? What kind of noise? Is this usual for X during this sort of activity?
USUAL NOISINESS during solitary play:

No noise	0
Noisy less than half the time	1
More than half the time but not throughout	2
Continual noise throughout	3

4. JOINT PLAY WITH OTHER CHILDREN

Can you think of a time recently or in the past week when X was doing things with other children, perhaps friends or brothers or sisters? What were they doing? On that occasion, how long did they play for? Is that typical of the amount of time X would spend doing things with other children?
USUAL ATTENTION SPAN during joint play:

More than 30 minutes	0
Between 15 and 30 minutes	1
Between 6 and 15 minutes	2
5 minutes or less	3

On that occasion was X running around unnecessarily, eg. in and out of rooms, or clambering over furniture? If so, how often? Is that what usually happens when he/she is playing with other children?
USUAL RESTLESSNESS during joint play:

No restlessness	0
Once every 15 minutes	1
More than once every 15 minutes but less than once every 5 minutes	2
Once every 5 minutes or more	3

Did X talk much while playing with the others?
If the answer is vague: **Did he/she talk all the time he was playing? More than half the time or less than half the time? Is that how talkative X usually is when playing with other children?**
USUAL TALKATIVENESS during joint play:

Appropriate level of conversation	0
Talked for less than half the time	1
More than half the time but not throughout	2
Talked continuously	3

Did X make any other sort of noise while playing? What kind of noise? Is this usual for X?
USUAL NOISINESS during joint play:

Appropriate level of noise	0
Noisy less than half the time	1
More than half the time but not throughout	2
Continual noise throughout	3

5. MEALTIMES

Can you think of a time in the past week or recently when X was sitting eating a meal? Did he/she get up and down from the seat at all?
Note: If the parent didn't allow the child to get up, rate 0. Do not rate getting up for useful purposes, e.g. to get a glass of water or salt, etc.
If the answer is vague: **Would X usually get up once or twice or more during a meal?**

USUAL RESTLESSNESS at mealtimes:

No restlessness	0
Once only	1
2 to 5 times	2
More than 5 times	3

Did X fidget while having the meal?
If the answer is vague: **Did X fidget throughout, more than half the time or less than half the time? Is that the usual amount of fidgeting at the dinner table?**
USUAL FIDGETING during solitary play:

No fidgeting	0
Less than half the time	1
More than half the time but not throughout	2
Continuous fidgeting	3

Did X talk much during the meal?
If the answer is vague: **Did he/she talk all the time? More than half the time or less than half the time? Is that how talkative X usually is when sitting having a meal?**
USUAL TALKATIVENESS at mealtimes:

Appropriate level of conversation	0
Talked for less than half the time	1
More than half the time but not throughout	2
Talked continuously	3

Did X make any other sort of noise during the meal? What kind of noise? Is this usual for X?
USUAL NOISINESS at mealtimes:

Appropriate level of noise	0
Noisy less than half the time	1
More than half the time but not throughout	2
Continual noise throughout	3

6. SHOPPING TRIPS

Can you think of an occasion recently when X has gone shopping with you? Did he/she stay with you or run away from you?
If he/she did run away from you, how many times did he/she do that? Is that what usually happens when you take him/her shopping?
USUAL RESTLESSNESS while shopping:

No restlessness	0
Every 5 minutes or less	1
Every 2 to 5 minutes	2
More often than every 2 minutes	3

Notes: • *Include disturbing other shoppers by pushing trolley around in an uncontrolled way*
• *Do not rate if child goes away from parent to fetch an item and bring it back*
• *If the parent has stopped taking the child shopping because of disruptive behaviour, rate 3*

Did X talk much during the shopping trip?
If the answer is vague: **Did he/she talk all the time? More than half the time or less than half the time? Is that how talkative X usually is when at the shops with you?**
USUAL TALKATIVENESS while shopping:

Appropriate level of conversation	0
Talked for less than half the time	1
More than half the time but not throughout	2
Talked continuously	3

Did X make any other sort of noise when you were out shopping? What kind of noise? Is this usual for X?
USUAL NOISINESS while shopping:

Appropriate level of noise	0
Noisy less than half the time	1

| More than half the time but not throughout | 2 |
| Continual noise throughout, complaints from others | 3 |

7. FAMILY OUTINGS

Has X recently been with you on a family outing or to visit relatives? On this occasion did he/she run around excessively or climb on things? If the answer is YES: How many times during the visit did X do this? Did this behaviour disturb other people? Is this behaviour you have described what usually happens when you take him/her on an outing?
USUAL RESTLESSNESS on outings:

No restlessness	0
Every 10 minutes or less	1
Every 5 to 10 minutes	2
More often than every 5 minutes	3

Notes: • *If no outings in last 6 months, rate 8*
   • *If the parent has stopped taking the child on outings because of disruptive behaviour, rate 3*

Did X make any other sort of noise on this occasion? What kind of noise? Is this usual for X?
USUAL NOISINESS on outings:

Appropriate level of noise	0
Noisy less than half the time	1
More than half the time but not throughout	2
Continual noise throughout	3

8. IMPULSIVITY

Have there been times recently when X has needed to wait his/her turn in a queue? What happens then?
If the answer is vague: **Is X happy to wait his/her turn or does he/she get impatient?**

Little or no difficulty waiting	0
Becomes impatient very quickly but can wait	1
Often butts in or goes before his/her turn	2

Have there been times recently when X has needed to wait his/her turn to be served food? What happens then?
If the answer is vague: **Is he/she happy to wait their turn or does he/she get impatient?**

Little or no difficulty waiting	0
Becomes impatient very quickly but can wait	1
Often butts in or goes before his/her turn	2

Have there been times recently when X has needed to wait in a game where players take turns? What happens then?
If the answer is vague: **Is X happy to wait his turn or does he/she get impatient?**

Little or no difficulty waiting	0
Becomes impatient very quickly but can wait	1
Often butts in or goes before his turn	2

Can you think of a time recently when you have asked X a question, eg about his/her day at school or in a quiz? Does X wait until you have finished asking before answering? Is this typical of what happens when you ask a question?

Waits until the question is completed	0
Is somewhat hasty but listens to the question first	1
Blurts out the answer before the question is completed	2

If there was a time when you were talking to someone else and X was in the room, what happened? Did X interrupt the conversation or make unnecessary comments?

No interruptions	0
Some interrupting	1
Constant interrupting so as to make conversation impossible	2

PARENTAL PERCEPTIONS OF HYPERACTIVITY/IMPULSIVITY

You have told me that X is *(restate reported problem[s] and confirm with parent).* **Do you see this as a problem? Does it give you cause for concern?**
• *If the answer is No:*   Rate 0
• *If the answer is Yes:*   **Would you say that it is a serious or a minor problem?**
Note: *If there were several problems ask, "Do any of these worry you?" and code the worst.*

PERCEIVED SEVERITY
No problem perceived, no parental concern	0
Minor problem perceived, slight/intermittent concern	1
Serious problem perceived, much/constant concern	2

ONSET
How old was X when you first noticed this happening?
Write age in years.   —

CONTROL
Do you think X can control this difficulty?
• *If Yes:*   **Why do you think this? Can you give me an example of this happening recently?**
• *If No:*   **Does he/she ever try to stop it happening? Can you describe what happens then?**
Can almost always control behaviour / can modify on most occasions	0
Sometimes has control over behaviour / can often modify or stop	1
No control over behaviour / cannot modify or stop	2

IMPACT
Is this causing X distress, or getting him/her into trouble at school, or affecting relationships with friends or family members?
No impairment	1
Impaired at times or minor impairment	2
Serious impairment	3

ABNORMALITY
Interviewer's abnormality rating here – is this inappropriate to the child's age and developmental level? (One rating to encompass severity and frequency.)
Normal	0
Mildly abnormal	1
Markedly abnormal	2
Severely abnormal	3

8. INATTENTIVE BEHAVIOUR

A. Can you think of a time recently when X was given a structured task to do at home? This could be something like laying the table or tidying or washing up. What exactly was he/she expected to do? Was this the usual way that he/she would go about things?
Note: *Adjust the examples in accordance with the child's age. Code the usual pattern.*

Was X reluctant to begin this task?
Eager, or at least cooperative at first	0
Somewhat reluctant at first but no further complaints when started	1
Strong initial resistance or continued to complain throughout the task	2
Strong continued resistance or complete avoidance of the task	3

Did X pay attention to detail during the task? (e.g. places laid correctly, task finished)
Yes	0
Effort to get things right, but occasional lapses	1
Showed little attention to detail	2
No attention to detail at all, task unfinished or sloppily done	3

Did X make mistakes during the task?
No mistakes	0

Understood the task but made 1 or 2 unnecessary mistakes	1
Failed to pay close attention resulting in repeated careless mistakes	2
Was so careless that the task could not be completed or had to be done again	3

Did X listen to your instructions and understand what you told him/her to do?

Listened and understood the instructions	0
Did not seem to listen but showed by actions that he/she had heard the instructions and understood	1
Did not seem to listen and showed by actions that he/she had only partly understood the instructions	2
Showed a marked lack of attention to and clearly misunderstood instructions	3

If rated 0 or 1, ask the following two questions. If rated 2 or 3 do not ask the following two questions but rate 8.

i. How well did X follow the instructions?

Followed all instructions completely	0
Followed the most important instructions but failed to follow others	1
Failed to follow most instructions including the most important ones	2
Not applicable	8

ii. Did X complete the task?

Completed the task	0
Completed most of task but left unfinished	1
Gave up very quickly or had to be forced to complete task	2
Not applicable	8

Was X easily distracted from the task, e.g. by noises from the street, background conversations or other people coming into the room?

Not at all distracted	0
Temporarily distracted but returned to task of their own accord	1
Had to be told to return to task or abandoned task	2
Not applicable	8

B. Can you think of a time recently when X brought home a task from school to do as homework? What exactly was he/she expected to do?

Was X reluctant to begin this task?

Eager, or at least cooperative at first	0
Somewhat reluctant at first but no further complaints when started	1
Strong initial resistance or continued to complain throughout the task	2
Strong continued resistance or complete avoidance of the task	3

Did X pay attention to detail during the task?

Yes	0
Effort to get things right, but occasional lapses	1
Showed little attention to detail	2
No attention to detail at all, task unfinished or sloppily done	3

Did X make mistakes during the task?

No mistakes	0
Understood the task but made 1 or 2 unnecessary mistakes	1
Failed to pay close attention resulting in repeated careless mistakes	2
Was so careless that the task could not be completed or had to be done again	3

Had X listened to instructions at school and understood what to do; or listened to you if you told him/her what to do?

Listened and understood the instructions	0
Did not seem to listen but showed by actions that he/she had heard the instructions and understood	1
Did not seem to listen and showed by actions that he/she had only partly understood the instructions	2
Showed a marked lack of attention to and clearly misunderstood instructions	3

If rated 0 or 1, ask the following two questions. If rated 2 or 3 do not ask the following two questions but rate 8.

i. How well did X follow the instructions?

Followed all instructions completely	0

Followed the most important instructions but failed to follow others	1
Failed to follow most instructions including the most important ones	2
Not applicable	8

ii. Did X complete the task?

Completed the task	0
Completed most of task but left unfinished	1
Gave up very quickly or had to be forced to complete task	2
Not applicable	8

Was X easily distracted from the task eg by noises from the street, background conversations or by other people coming into the room?

Not at all distracted	0
Temporarily distracted but returned to task of their own accord	1
Had to be told to return to task or abandoned task	2
Not applicable	8

C. Now can you think of a time recently when X had to do something that needed organization? Something like having to get paper and pencils together for homework or drawing or getting cleaning materials together for a household task? On occasions like this how well does X organize?

Collects everything needed before starting a task	0
Frequently has to get things after a task has been started	1
Never thinks beforehand about what is needed for the task	2

On this occasion, did X arrange the things that were needed to work on the task, e.g. clothes, toys, pencils or books? Is X usually able to find things?

Never loses things	0
Loses things occasionally but does not make a habit of it	1
Loses things frequently, materials scattered or carelessly handled	2

Has there been an occasion recently when X has forgotten things, e.g. people's names or his/her lunch, or football, swimming or gym kit? Does this happen often?

Never or rarely forgetful	0
Forgetful occasionally but does not make a habit of it	1
Forgets things frequently	2

PARENTAL PERCEPTIONS OF INATTENTIVENESS

You have told me that X is *(restate reported problem[s] and confirm with parent).* **Do you see this as a problem? Does it give you cause for concern?**
• *If the answer is No:*   Rate 0
• *If the answer is Yes:*   **Would you say that it is a serious or a minor problem?**
Note: *If there were several problems ask, "Do any of these worry you?" and code the worst.*

PERCEIVED SEVERITY

No problem perceived, no parental concern	0
Minor problem perceived, slight/intermittent concern	1
Serious problem perceived, much/constant concern	2

ONSET

How old was X when you first noticed this happening?
Write age in years.   —

CONTROL

Do you think X can control this difficulty?
• *If Yes:*   **Why do you think this? Can you give me an example of this happening recently?**
• *If No:*   **Does he/she ever try to stop it happening? Can you describe what happens then?**

Can almost always control behaviour/ can modify on most occasions	0
Sometimes has control over behaviour/ can often modify or stop	1
No control over behaviour/ cannot modify or stop	2

IMPACT
Is this causing X distress, or getting him/her into trouble at school, or affecting relationships with friends or family members?

No impairment	1
Impaired at times or minor impairment	2
Serious impairment	3

ABNORMALITY
Interviewer's abnormality rating here – is this inappropriate to the child's age and developmental level? (One rating to encompass severity and frequency.)

Normal	0
Mildly abnormal	1
Markedly abnormal	2
Severely abnormal	3

COPING AND CONSISTENCY FOR HYPERACTIVITY, IMPULSIVENESS AND INATTENTIVENESS

MOTHER'S COPING with activity level/inattentiveness
What did you do when X behaved like that? What do you usually do? Does that work? Have you tried anything else? What was the result?
If there is more than one response made, ask what is it that makes the parent react one way or the other?

Highly efficient; problems always or nearly always anticipated and avoided	0
Efficient; proven plans in place even though they may not work every time	1
Problems are not avoided but ineffective strategies have been replaced with more effective ones	2
Ineffective strategies only, but do not aggravate the problem	3
Lack of response to a problem (e.g. uninvolved); but not making it worse	4
Parental actions are making the problem worse or adding new problem	5
Parental actions lead to the problem getting out of hand	6
Parental actions are abusive	7

FATHER'S COPING with activity level/inattentiveness
What did you do when X behaved like that? What do you usually do? Does that work? Have you tried anything else? What was the result?
If there is more than one response made, ask what is it that makes the parent react one way or the other?

Highly efficient; problems always or nearly always anticipated and avoided	0
Efficient; proven plans in place even though they may not work every time	1
Problems are not avoided but ineffective strategies have been replaced with more effective ones	2
Ineffective strategies only, but do not aggravate the problem	3
Lack of response to a problem (e.g. uninvolved); but not making it worse	4
Parental actions are making the problem worse or adding new problem	5
Parental actions lead to the problem getting out of hand	6
Parental actions are abusive	7

Note: *In the father's absence the rating should be based on the mother's report. If the mother's report (of the father's coping) is considered unreliable, rate 9 (unknown).*

PARENTAL CONSISTENCY
Do you and your partner agree or disagree over how to handle X when he/she behaves like this? Do you handle the behaviour in different ways or overrule each other's orders? Do you and your partner ever argue about how to handle X. Do you argue when he/she is present?
Note: *Don't ask these questions if the parent has already volunteered the information when discussing coping skills.*

No disagreements	0
Differences of opinion but not of style	1
Differences in behaviour towards child	2
Parents overrule, countermand, or argue openly	3

Note: *For one-parent families, rate the absent partner's coping and the parental consistency 8.*

SCHOOL BEHAVIOURS (ADHD)
Over the past year how has X been getting on at school? With other children? With teachers?
Academic: How has the work been going? Concentration, finishing projects? Daydreaming?
Have you heard complaints about hyperactive behaviour (e.g. silly, nuisance, noisy in class, restless, fidgeting)?
Has there been any special educational provision? Suspension? Exclusion?
Source of information?
Child –
Teacher –
Other (please specify) –
Interviewer's abnormality rating here – is this inappropriate to the child's age and developmental level? (One rating to encompass severity and frequency.)

Normal	0
Mildly abnormal	1
Markedly abnormal	2
Severely abnormal	3

4
PSYCHOLOGICAL ASSESSMENT

Jody Warner-Rogers

Hyperactivity refers to a constellation of inattentive, overactive and impulsive behaviours generally seen in children. Individuals whose behaviour gets labelled as 'hyperactive' tend to experience marked difficulties in day-to-day functioning, as they seem unable to control their behaviour in relation to expectations. As toddlers in a playgroup, such children change activities frequently, rushing from toy to toy. When their playmates are sat at a table for a drink, they wriggle, get out of their chair and run about. In reception class, they struggle to remain still during sedentary activities. In early primary years, they call out frequently in class, exasperate the teacher and irritate other pupils with their intrusive and disruptive behaviour on the playground. When misdeeds are brought to their attention, they seem genuinely sorry. They promise not to do it again, but in a similar situation, they tend to they behave in exactly the same way. In secondary school they appear more settled and less boisterous, but their concentration in the classroom is vulnerable. They feel restless and struggle to complete assignments, and in less structured and supervised settings, such as being out with their friends, they act impulsively without consideration of the consequences of their behaviours.

Professionals from many different disciplines can be involved in the assessment of hyperactivity. Assessment of any kind involves gathering data about something in order to better understand it. Increased understanding leads to better-informed interventions.

A multimodal (i.e. more than one method) and multi-informant (i.e. more than one person) approach to the assessment of hyperactivity is essential. Goodman and Scott (1997) propose that five key areas should be addressed in any comprehensive assessment: (1) symptoms ("What are the problems?"); (2) impact ("How much impairment does it cause?"); (3) risks ("What factors may have initiated or maintained the problems?"); (4) strengths ("Where are the strengths and resources which can be drawn upon?"); and (5) explanatory models ("What expectations and beliefs do the family and individual bring with them?"). Psychological assessment involves the use of four key methods to collect information across these areas. These methods are norm-referenced tests, interviews, observations and informal evaluation. Clinical skills are then relied upon to analyse and integrate this information (Sattler 2001). This chapter reviews how psychological assessment methods are used to facilitate the understanding and management of the problems associated with hyperactivity. It focuses on norm-referenced tests, as observations, interviews and rating scales are reviewed in Chapter 3. Data from norm-referenced testing, when integrated with other clinical information, can provide a more thorough understanding of an individual's cognitive and emotional strengths and vulnerabilities than a diagnostic interview (Roth and Saykin 2004).

When does hyperactivity become a 'problem'?

No one behaves impeccably in all situations. Almost everyone exhibits overactive, inattentive or impulsive behaviour on occasion. Hyperactivity is a trait inherent in most people's behavioural repertoire and appears to be normally distributed in the general population (Taylor et al. 1991). There is a continuum of hyperactivity expression, with some individuals showing quite a low level of hyperactivity and others evidencing a higher level. In the general population, approximately 17% of school-aged children show 'high levels' of hyperactivity (Taylor et al. 1991).

Expectations for behavioural control differ across developmental levels, situations and cultures, with hyperactivity even being an asset in certain environments. Ascertaining *what is expected* in a given setting, *controlling one's behaviour accordingly*, and *modifying behaviour as needed* are essential skills, which are acquired gradually by most individuals. The frequency with which hyperactivity presents itself tends to decrease as children mature. Preschoolers are inherently more hyperactive than youngsters in middle school, and children in primary school cannot concentrate as long as teenagers in secondary school. Young adults put more thought into their actions and are better able to inhibit their impulses than adolescents.

Hyperactivity becomes a problem when an individual's behaviour is at odds with the demands of the situation and the expectations of others. This occurs when the individual is seen to be chronologically old enough to regulate their behaviour in response to a situation, but consistently fails to do so. When this happens repeatedly over time (i.e. chronically), in more than one situation (i.e. pervasively) and impairs the functioning of the individual *or those around them*, then the hyperactive behaviours tend to get labelled as 'problematic'. Children with pervasive and significant hyperactivity face a serious developmental challenge. If left unaddressed, hyperactivity has the potential to compromise long-term educational, social and behavioural functioning (Barkley et al. 1990).

What kinds of difficulties are associated with hyperactivity?

The consequences of hyperactivity, both in the short and long term, vary widely and are influenced by a multitude of factors. Direct, causal links between hyperactivity and outcome can be difficult to make because the condition often occurs in conjunction with other problems. Between 50% and 80% of children with clinically significant hyperactivity will also exhibit another disorder, such as conduct disorder or reading problems (Jensen et al. 1997, Tannock 1998). Such children may also show poor fine motor skills (Pitcher et al. 2003). Gender may also play a role. Girls with hyperactivity, for example, may have more psychological difficulties than boys, such as depression, anxiety and stress (Rucklidge and Tannock 2001). Features of the immediate environment, including the level of organization and structure in the home and classroom, the behaviour management strategies used by parents and teachers, and the resources of the school, workplace or community may provide much needed support or cause additional strain.

Adolescents who were hyperactive in childhood are likely to experience worse psychosocial outcomes (e.g. emotional difficulties, social problems) than their nonaffected peers (Wilson and Marcotte 1996). Persistence of the symptoms of hyperactivity into adulthood is associated with adjustment and behavioural difficulties, substance misuse, increased involvement with mental health services and erratic employment (Murphy and Barkley 1996). Relationship problems, including marital discord, and driving violations are also more common amongst adults with hyperactivity compared to the general population (Murphy and Barkley 1996). Individuals that display the most impulsivity may be at particular risk for later maladjustment (Murphy et al. 2002).

Over the last several decades, research evidence has consistently concluded that hyperactivity can reliably be identified by school age. Fortunately, the core symptoms of inattention, overactivity and impulsiveness can be reduced through medical and psychological interventions (MTA Cooperative Group 1999). This reduction may, in turn, lead to improvements in developmental outcome. The tools of psychological assessment are being used in combination with other medical procedures, such as magnetic resonance imaging (MRI) of the brain and genetic testing to shed light on the relationship between behaviour and brain function. This research is vital to the understanding of the underlying causes of behavioural problems.

How can psychological assessment enhance the understanding of hyperactivity?

Hyperactivity is an observable phenomenon. One can see whether a child is out of their seat, looking out of the window when they are supposed to be focusing on the teacher, or interrupting the flow of conversation. But what *causes* a child to behave this way? Identifying the core deficits that underpin hyperactivity is an area of intense research. Psychological assessment is a vital tool in this endeavour and allows competing theories of causation to be examined. Several of the psychological tests that have been useful in research for enhancing our understanding of the problems do not yet have adequate normative data or information on other psychometric properties (e.g. reliability) to be used diagnostically (for a review, see Nichols and Waschbusch 2004).

Shedding light on the causes of hyperactive behaviour

Weaknesses, deficits or delays in certain cognitive processes may underpin hyperactive behaviour. 'Cognitive processes' denote the means by which children acquire knowledge, solve problems, make plans and control their behaviour (Sattler 2001). They reflect the way the brain works and as such are covert, i.e. hidden from simple observation. Psychological tests have been designed to tap into these cognitive processes and provide standardized means for turning a covert process (e.g. attention) into something observable (i.e. a test score).

Psychological tests are available for assessing a variety of cognitive functions, including memory, attention, perception, planning, reasoning, receptive and expressive language skills, and overall intellectual ability. The most clinically useful of these tests are those that are norm-referenced. An individual's score can be compared to data from the 'normative group', which provides information on the performance of a large group of matched individuals (Sattler 2002). Norm-referenced tests are the hallmark of psychological assessment and have been used extensively to search for deficits in cognitive processes that may lead to hyperactivity.

Much of the early research on hyperactivity was directed at pinpointing the actual deficits in attention. Attention is a multidimensional construct that can be applied to a host of cognitive processes and behaviours. 'Inattentive behaviour' may include a lack of persistence in activities, orientation to stimuli irrelevant to the task at hand, or frequent changes of activity (Taylor 1994). 'Cognitive attention' encompasses level of arousal, attending to one aspect of the environment in the presence of distractors (selective attention), or focusing attention over time (concentration). No one aspect of attention has been identified as consistently deficient in hyperactive children. They may perform poorly on tests of attention, but so do children without hyperactivity. Thus, attentional 'deficits', or any cognitive impairments, although displayed by many affected by hyperactivity, are not sufficiently specific to this problem and their presence cannot function as a diagnostic marker (Matier-Sharma et al. 1995, Doyle et al. 2000).

Currently, a major theoretical view posits that deficits in 'executive functioning' underpin hyperactive behaviour. Executive functions are the group of cognitive processes thought to be responsible for purposeful, goal-directed and problem-solving behaviour. Executive functions can be divided into two subdomains. The first involves the ability to regulate or manage behaviour. This includes initiating behaviour, inhibiting competing actions, selecting relevant task goals, and planning and organizing thoughts to solve complex problems. Shifting strategies and being flexible when necessary are also involved. The second subdomain is working memory. This is where information is temporarily held 'on line' in one's mind in order to use it to complete a particular task (Dawson and Guare 2004).

Barkley (1997) suggests that deficits in three core areas of executive functioning, which specifically underpin behavioural inhibition, may give rise to hyperactive behaviour. These areas include: difficulty inhibiting a prepotent response, stopping an on-going response, and controlling 'interference' (Barkley 1997). This interference arises in situations where individuals actually have stopped a prepotent or ongoing response, but cannot use this window of opportunity effectively because it is easily disrupted by alternative events or competing responses.

Youngsters with elevated levels of hyperactivity seem to show a specific difficulty on psychological tests of inhibitory control – that is, the ability to hold back a response. In preschool years, hyperactivity has been associated with specific deficits in inhibitory control as opposed to other aspects of executive skills (Sonuga-Barke et al. 2002, Roth and Saykin 2004). Executive deficits and slowness in speed of information processing have also been demonstrated in 'real-life' activities of youngsters with ADHD (Lawrence et al. 2004). Deficits in executive functioning do seem particularly characteristic of young people with hyperactivity, as individuals with other externalizing and disruptive behaviour problems do not show such deficits (Clark et al. 2000). A review of studies focusing on hyperactivity in adults concluded that those with hyperactivity show problems in several cognitive domains, including attention, inhibition and memory (Hervey et al. 2004).

Although problems in inhibitory control are now well recognized as characterizing most children with hyperactivity, some researchers (e.g. Sonuga-Barke 1996, 2002) propose that not all individuals with hyperactivity show deficits in behavioural inhibition. Rather, these individuals evidence an atypical motivational style, which can masquerade as behavioural disinhibition on certain tests. For these individuals, an altered sensitivity to rewards, especially in situations that involve a delay of reward, may be operating.

Ongoing and future studies will no doubt further our understanding of the causes of hyperactivity, and this will in turn improve our ability to manage the behaviour and its consequences. But in order to access the benefits from evidence-based treatments, affected individuals first must be identified and the manner in which their functioning is specifically compromised must be clarified. At an individual level, appreciating how a young person is uniquely affected by hyperactivity serves as the first and most effective step towards addressing their difficulties and supporting their development.

Unfortunately, researchers and test developers have not yet produced a psychological assessment device on which poor performance is sufficiently specific to hyperactivity or ADHD that it can be used as a diagnostic instrument in clinical practice (Grodzinsky and Barkley 1999, McGee et al. 2000). Nonetheless, psychological assessment still plays a very valuable role in diagnostic decisions.

Contributing to diagnostic decisions

If hyperactivity is sufficiently pervasive and severe, then one must consider whether diagnosis of a psychiatric condition, such as attention deficit hyperactivity disorder (ADHD; APA 1994) or hyperkinetic disorder (HKD, WHO 1988), is indicated. The diagnostic criteria for both ADHD and HKD require that the constellation of inattentive, overactive and impulsive behaviours occur "often", "impair functioning", and be out of keeping with an individual's developmental level. In order to make decisions about whether these criteria are met, detailed information regarding the frequency of hyperactive behaviours, the range and extent of functional impairment and the individual's developmental level is required. In addition, diagnosing ADHD or HKD involves actively considering and ruling out differential diagnoses, such as conduct disorder, pervasive developmental disorder, global learning difficulties or sensory impairment.

Psychological assessment provides a reliable and valid means for examining and quantifying behaviour, impairment and developmental functioning across a range of ability areas. It also provides a way to determine an individual's unique pattern of cognitive strengths and weaknesses, as well as their learning style. A comprehensive assessment of cognitive abilities will determine an individual's developmental level. Evaluation of academic attainment can detect specific learning disabilities. Tests of cognitive attention, response inhibition, memory and visuospatial abilities highlight areas of potential neuropsychological deficit. The data yielded by psychological assessment help to establish whether the presenting problems reach a level of diagnostic significance and if other issues or disorders offer a better explanation for the behaviours.

Delineating cognitive and adaptive profiles and learning styles

Hyperactivity and ADHD are usually associated with some level of educational impairment. Compared to children without behavioural difficulties, children with hyperactivity may score slightly lower on tests of general intellectual ability (e.g. Tripp et al. 2002). Children with ADHD have been shown to have deficits in adaptive functioning that are not predicted by their overall level of intellectual ability (Stein et al. 1995). Young adults with a childhood diagnosis of ADHD are more likely to have had special educational input in secondary school (Murphy et al. 2002), and lower overall academic attainment than individuals without

ADHD (Wilson and Marcotte 1996) and adolescents with ADHD are more likely to drop out of high school (Hansen et al. 1999). Although many adults with ADHD might function well enough academically to attend university, their grades tend to be lower than those of their unaffected peers and they encounter more learning difficulties (Heiligenstein et al. 1999). They are also less likely to graduate from college (Murphy et al. 2002).

Psychological tests allow one to determine whether an individual's performance in a particular area assessed is better, worse or about the same as that expected in others their age. At the end of an assessment, one can draw up a profile, or 'balance sheet' (Levine 2002), of assets and areas of vulnerability. Knowledge about a child's profile serves both to highlight co-occurring problems and to ensure that one appreciates any strengths that an individual may have that may help them compensate for problems in other areas. If the core symptoms of ADHD are reduced, but other difficulties are left unaddressed, then obstacles to a child's development will still remain.

How do results from psychological assessment compare to 'real-life'?

Validity refers to the extent to which an assessment measures what it is supposed to measure. No one profile of psychological assessment results is specifically indicative of hyperactivity or ADHD. Scores within the normal limits on a test of attention would not preclude the presence of hyperactivity, nor would it imply that the child was being lazy, naughty or unmotivated. Rather, they might suggest that whilst the child may have no discernible cognitive impairment, they do show a functional impairment – they are unable to access their skills in real life, when and where they need them.

Psychological assessment is not just about test scores. Administering tests provides an excellent context for observing behaviour under standardized conditions. As the tests are given in the same way to all individuals, psychologists can compare the behaviour of the individual in front of them to that of others they have evaluated. In particular, the individual's general attitude, response to success and frustration, whether they approach tasks quickly and haphazardly or thoughtfully and in an organized fashion, their activity level, eye contact, general compliance and motivation are important to note. Psychologists also consider these observations in light of other extended samples of behaviour taken from more naturalistic environments (e.g. reports from teachers and parents).

It is important to emphasize, however, that novel, well-structured and supervised situations – such as being in a clinic and working one-on-one with a psychologist – will often function to suppress hyperactivity symptoms. The lack of symptoms during assessment or the failure of cognitive tests to identify any deficit in underlying psychological processes does not infer lack of problem in real life. It is also crucial to note whether a child with hyperactivity is receiving treatment at the time of assessment. If an individual is on stimulant medication, for example, this may improve their performance on certain psychological tests (e.g. Kempton et al. 1999).

The evaluation of children and families in their natural environment probably provides the most valid indication of their functioning in these settings. Direct observation is one of the major tools of psychological assessment, as it provides the opportunity to identify associations between aspects of the immediate environment and the occurrence of behavioural difficulties. Factors and situations that elicit or maintain problematic patterns of behaviour may be noted.

Direct observation can be particularly helpful if information from different sources seems contradictory (e.g. good performance on attainment tests but poor performance in the classroom, or high scores on parent-completed rating scales but low scores on teacher-completed versions). However, it is not always possible to directly observe behaviour. Some formal coding schemes exist for quantifying observations of hyperactive symptoms (see Barkley 1988), but they can be time-consuming.

Clinical interviews also generate useful information. Children and young people can discuss their emotional and social abilities, but they tend to underreport difficulties in the areas of inattention, overactivity and impulsivity (Danckaerts et al. 1999). Indeed children with ADHD seem to overestimate their competencies in those areas that are actually most problematic (Hoza et al. 2004).

The consideration of 'real life' should include the impact of hyperactivity on those living, learning and working with affected individuals. Their well-being also needs to be addressed in any assessment. Parenting any child can be stressful at times. Parenting a child with hyper-activity can be stressful most of the time. The amount of support parents receive can be an important factor in how well they will be able to address their child's needs. Poor parental coping is one factor that influences whether children with hyperactivity actually get referred for assessment (e.g. Woodward et al. 1997), and the presence of a support network as well as the level and frequency of support can influence a family's use of mental health services (Bussing et al. 2003).

How can psychological assessment enhance the management of hyperactivity?
The overarching goals of treatment are to reduce the symptoms of hyperactivity and to encourage a child's general development. Although the main behavioural difficulties of a child with hyperactivity may be in attention, impulsivity and hyperactivity, it is likely that the impact of these behaviours is observed in many areas, particularly in the classroom and in social situations. It is therefore not surprising that in the longer term, educational attainment, family and peer relationships, and self-esteem can be adversely affected. Because the difficulties associated with ADHD are so varied, treatment plans must be tailored accordingly. Treatment plans should be individualised and comprehensive. A plan is more likely to address the needs of the child across all areas of development and touch on the family's ability to cope with and manage the child, if it is based on assessment results gathered in a systematic and detailed manner (Warner-Rogers 1998).

Identifying treatment targets
When a psychological assessment produces a profile of an individual's emotional, behavioural and cognitive strengths and weaknesses, potential targets for intervention become clear. An holistic treatment plan can be devised whereby *all* of an individual's needs are considered.

Monitoring treatment effects
Once treatment targets are identified and intervention is underway, it is essential to monitor

behavioural change in order that the efficacy of treatment can be determined. Ongoing assessment of intervention effectiveness necessitates clearly defined treatment targets and outcome goals, as well as a timetable and methods for measurement. When these features are in place, it is easy to quantify behavioural change. Psychological assessment can play a valuable role in monitoring treatment effects and tracking overall developmental progress.

What should be the targets of psychological assessment and what tools are available for clinicians?

The actual targets and tools of any given assessment will depend on many factors, including specific reasons for the assessment, time available to spend on the psychological component of the evaluation, and the resources of the assessment centre (e.g. staff, equipment). A comprehensive psychological assessment should be undertaken by a psychologist. Such an assessment may take up to three hours to complete. Decisions about the real need for a detailed (and thus time-consuming and expensive) psychological assessment may need to be made on an individual basis if resources are limited (Warner-Rogers 2002). At the very least one should expect that children whose ADHD is associated with problems at school should have an assessment of intellectual potential; an 'attention problem' has to be judged in the light of mental age as well as chronological age.

At present, there is no one single evidence-based psychological assessment protocol for hyperactivity. Our experience indicates that psychological assessment should include an evaluation of overall cognitive functioning, examination of academic attainment and an appraisal of specific cognitive processes of attention and response inhibition. Several commercially available assessment batteries contain subtests that index these cognitive processes. A core set of five to six assessment devices would suffice to tap into the relevant aspects of cognitive functioning. Different psychologists may have preferences for one device over another. The author's recommendations follow.

GENERAL INTELLECTUAL ABILITY

Target

Tests of general intellectual ability, or 'intelligence tests', provide information regarding a child's global level of overall cognitive functioning and yield data about cognitive strengths and vulnerabilities. When developmental functioning is quantified in this manner, it may help determine whether symptoms of hyperactivity are significantly 'out of keeping' with other mental abilities.

Tools

For school-aged children, the Wechsler Intelligence Scale for Children – 4th edition (WISC-IV; Wechsler 2003) is the most widely used battery of tests of general intellectual ability. The full assessment consists of 12 subtests of verbal and nonverbal abilities. These tests have been standardized on a nationally representative sample of British children. Individual subtests contribute to either a Verbal IQ score or a nonverbal (Performance) IQ score. A Full Scale IQ is a composite of the Verbal and Performance scores. The WISC-IV is different in content and structure to the previous edition (WISC-III; Wechsler 1992). Estimates suggest that Full Scale IQ scores are likely to be about 3 points lower on the WISC-IV than on the WISC-III (Sattler and Dumont 2004). The Wechsler series also contains versions for younger children (3 years to 7 years 3 months: Wechsler Preschool and Primary Scale of Intelligence – 3rd edition [WPPSI-III]; Wechsler 2002) and adults (Wechsler Adult Intelligence Test – 3rd edition [WAIT-III]; Wechsler 1997).

Subtests from the WISC-III can be used to generate index scores such as 'Freedom from Distractibility', which, though at face value sound indicative of ADHD-type problems, do not have sufficient discriminative validity to be useful diagnostically (e.g. Anastopolous et al. 1994). No one particular profile of WISC-III scores has been reliably associated with ADHD (for more detailed comment regarding WISC-III ADHD profiles, see Kaufman 1994).

The British Abilities Scales: 2nd edition (BAS II; Elliott et al. 1996) and the Differential Ability Scales (DAS; Elliott 1990) are used, in the UK and USA respectively, as alternatives to the WISC-IV to assess overall cognitive ability.

ACADEMIC FUNCTIONING

Target

It is hoped that those children who are struggling with the acquisition of literacy and numeracy skills will already be known to their teachers and their school's special educational needs services. School systems have their own policies and procedures for evaluating, supporting and monitoring children's special education needs. Depending on the level of need, the local education authority and educational/school psychologist may be involved.

However, it is not uncommon, particularly when learning difficulties are less obvious or obscured by maladaptive or disruptive behaviour, for a child's learning needs to have gone unrecognized. Cognitive profiling can provide information about learning styles and can determine whether there is any *discrepancy* between a child's *actual level* of academic attainment in literacy and numeracy and the *level predicted* from their overall intellectual ability. This is the first step in establishing whether a specific learning problem (e.g. developmental reading disorder, 'dyslexia') may exist.

Depending on an individual's age, formal assessment of literacy skills might tap letter identification, word attack skills, sight recognition, reading fluency, or reading comprehension. Evaluation of numeracy skills should focus on actual calculation abilities as well as familiarity with more general mathematical concepts, such as size, measurement, graphs, and money. Informal evaluation of academic attainment should include some assessment of an individual's level of work production and consistency and handwriting.

Tools

The Wechsler Individual Achievement Test – 2nd edition (WIAT-II; Wechsler 2001) provides the means to comprehensively assess children's achievement across several domains. When used in conjunction with the WISC-IV, one can determine whether discrepancies between potential and achievement exist and warrant further investigation. In addition, information should also be sought from schools. End of term reports can also be extremely helpful in gauging a teacher's perception of an individual's abilities. Any formal data collected by the school (e.g. standard assessment test results) can also shed light on a child's ability to keep pace academically with their peers.

ATTENTION AND EXECUTIVE FUNCTION

Targets

As noted earlier, cognitive attention can be parcelled into several different processes, including overall arousal level, sustained (i.e. maintaining attention over time), selective/focused (i.e. maintaining attention to a particular aspect of the environment despite distractions), and divided attention (i.e. paying attention to two or more aspects of the environment simultaneously), as well as attention control/switching (i.e. shifting attention to different aspects of the environment as needed). Some clinicians find it useful to think of attention in three forms: control over mental energy, control over input (of information) and control over output (work and behaviour) (Levine 2002). The nature of the overt behavioural impairments can inform the choice of which aspects of cognitive attention should be considered for an assessment. For example, if concentration is problematic, then one might pursue assessment of sustained attention abilities.

Tools

Several tests of attention are commercially available. Continuous performance tests (CPTs) are perhaps the most widely known. No one standard CPT exists, but most involve presentation of stimuli to the child at different rates or intervals over the course of a set time (e.g. 9 or 20 minutes). The child is expected to respond to particular target stimuli only. Scores are usually calculated for several indices, including how many target stimuli the child responded to and missed ('attention'), and how many non-target stimuli they responded to (i.e. 'impulsive responding'). Some require attention to visual stimuli, others are auditory in nature. Although associations have been demonstrated between teacher ratings of hyperactivity and poor performance on CPTs (McGee et al. 2000), such tests are still not sufficiently specific to be used diagnostically for hyperactivity. The information provided nonetheless can contribute to understanding cognitive vulnerabilities.

The Test of Everyday Attention for Children (TEA-Ch; Manly et al. 1998) has normative data for British children and contains nine subtests that tap different aspects of attention and response inhibition. No global score is calculated, so the selected subtests can be administered in isolation depending on the focus of the assessment. This device also has parallel forms, making it an ideal task when repeated assessment is indicated.

The NEPSY is a collection of neuropsychological subtests specifically developed to tap processes, such as attention, that contribute to a child's ability to learn (Korkman et al. 1998). Six subtests of this measure specifically index attentional processes. The NEPSY can be used with children between the ages of 3 and 12 years.

Many tests are available to assess the attentional capacities of adults (for an excellent review of options, see Spreen and Strauss 1998). The Thames Valley Test Company publishes the Test of Everyday Attention (TEA; Robertson et al. 1994, 1996), which is an adult version of the TEA-Ch and contains parallel forms.

One should not overlook the importance of behavioural observation of a child's performance on any assessment task that requires concentrated and sustained effort. This gives a qualitative indication of their ability to attend over shorter periods of time and may be more consistent with the demands of day-to-day activities. For example, the WISC-III contains two subtests (Coding and Symbol Search) that require the child to work independently for two minutes. An inability to remain on task for the duration of these subtests in the highly supervised testing situation would certainly be a warning sign for vulnerabilities in attentional control. The TEA-Ch contains two subtests that tap selective attention, but are designed so the child is required to work until they believe they have found all the targets (which usually takes about two minutes). Informally, it may be an indication of behavioural inhibition or delay aversion if the child signals that they have completed the task before they have identified all target stimuli.

IMPULSIVENESS AND BEHAVIOURAL INHIBITION
Targets
It is useful to include some measure of behavioural inhibition in a psychological assessment, as research suggests that cognitive deficits are strongly associated with behavioural impairment (Sonuga-Barke et al. 2002). At a behavioural level, the ability to inhibit action, withhold responding, and act thoughtfully and carefully appears to be lacking in children and adults with hyperactivity. At the level of testing, one must be sure that the competing (or parallel) theories of deficient behavioural control and delay aversion are considered when interpreting assessment results. Elevated scores on a test of inhibition might actually reflect delay aversion as the child responded haphazardly and prematurely because they realized the task ended more rapidly if they did. Comparing and contrasting examiner-controlled conditions (e.g. child must work for allotted time) to examinee-controlled conditions (e.g. child works until task is finished) may shed some light on this area.

Tools
Both the TEA-Ch and the NEPSY contain tasks that specifically tap into behavioural inhibition. Wright et al. (2003) have designed an assessment of inhibition that can be used with children as young as 3 years of age. Assessment of impulsiveness in adults generally is included in batteries designed to measure executive functioning (for an overview, see Spreen and Strauss 1998).

OTHER NEUROPSYCHOLOGICAL PROCESSES
Depending on the nature of a child's presenting difficulties, additional assessment of their learning and memory skills may be useful. Several tests are available, including the widely used Children's Memory Scale (CMS; Cohen 1997). Examination of memory for information presented verbally can be contrasted with the retention of materials presented visually. It is also important to consider whether differences exist in an individual's ability to recognize information compared to their free recall ability. This can have important ramifications for educational assessment of classroom learning.

Speech and language problems are not uncommon in children with hyperactivity (Taylor et al. 1991). Receptive skills reflect the ability to understand words through hearing or reading. Expressive ability denotes communicating effectively through speaking or writing. The NEPSY contains seven subtests designed to assess different aspects of language functioning, including: repeating nonsense words, understanding instructions; speeded naming; ability to produce rhythmic oral sequences (Korkman et al. 1998). If significant concerns are evidenced on these devices, referral to a speech and language therapist for more specialized assessment is indicated.

Specific motor deficits may be found in children with hyperactivity, but, like other measures of neuropsychological functioning, such difficulties are not specific predictors of the presence of ADHD (Steger et al. 2001) or developmental coordination disorder (DCD; Henderson and Henderson 2003). If significant difficulties are noted in coordination, referral to an occupational therapist may be warranted, although Dunford et al. (2004) argue that it would be prudent not to presuppose a diagnosis of DCD, as psychologists in particular are apparently fairly inaccurate in identifying the disorder.

When both attention and coordination deficits co-occur in conjunction with perceptual problems, the label 'deficits in attention, motor control and perception' (DAMP) is sometimes applied (Kadesjo and Gillberg 1988). Visuospatial skills may include visualization, judgement of line and angle orientation, discrimination of left and right, appreciation of location and directionality, and ability to rotate objects mentally and to use maps and routes (Korkman et al. 1998). The NEPSY contains several subtests that can screen for sensorimotor impairment. These include the ability to process basic tactile information, to imitate hand positions, to reproduce repetitive and sequential hand movements, and to use a pencil rapidly and accurately (Korkman et al. 1998). The concept of DAMP is fairly controversial and the label is more widely used in Scandinavian countries than in the UK or USA.

PSYCHOLOGICAL SCREENING
Targets
Not all clinics will have 'in-house' psychological services. In this situation, a mechanism for basic screening should be in place so individuals who may require more comprehensive assessment can be referred elsewhere. A screening protocol should be quick to administer and score (i.e. less than 30 minutes). Some screening tests do not even require a psychologist to administer them. The target of screening should be to rule out major developmental delay and reading disorders.

Tools
Several tools are available to screen for overall intellectual functioning. The Wechsler Abbreviated Scale of Intelligence (WASI; Wechsler 1999) contains four subtests and can be used for people from 6 to 89 years of age. The Kaufman Brief Intelligence Test (K-BIT; Kaufman and Kaufman 1990) contains two subtests and provides a measure of verbal and nonverbal abilities for individuals between the ages of 4 and 90 years. The Raven's Progressive Matrices (Raven et al. 1986) taps nonverbal reasoning ability, though it should be used in conjunction with a test of verbal capacity (e.g. British Picture Vocabulary Scale) when screening intellectual ability (Sattler 2001). Review of school-based attainment results should also be mandatory.

Conclusions

Psychological assessment has much to contribute to how professionals, families and young people understand, identify and manage hyperactivity. Research using the tools of psychological assessment continues to illuminate potential underlying cognitive and neuroanatomical mechanisms of the behavioural component of the condition. Clinically, although there is no specific, evidence-based assessment protocol, standard psychological measures can be employed to document overall cognitive abilities, academic attainment and profiles of neuropsychological assets and weaknesses.

REFERENCES

Anastopolous AD, Spisto MA, Maher MC (1994) The WISC-III Freedom from Distractibility factor: Its utility in identifying children with attention deficit hyperactivity disorder: *Psychol Assess* **6**: 368–371.

APA (1994) *Diagnostic and Statistical Manual of Mental Disorders, 4th edn (DSM-IV)*. Washington, DC: American Psychiatric Association.

Barkley RA (1988) Attention deficit disorders with hyperactivity. In: Mash EJ, Terdal LG (eds) *Behavioral Assessment of Childhood Disorders, 2nd edn*. New York: Guilford Press, pp. 69–104.

Barkley RA (1997) Behavioral inhibition, sustained attention, and executive functions: Constructing a unifying theory of ADHD. *Psychol Bull* **121**: 65–94.

Barkley RA, Fischer M, Edelbrock CS, Smallish L (1990) The adolescent outcome of hyperactive children diagnosed by research criteria. I. An 8-year prospective follow-up study. *J Am Acad Child Adolesc Psychiatry* **29**: 546–557.

Bussing R, Zima BT, Gary FA, Mason DM, Leon CE, Sinha K, Garvan CW (2003) Social networks, caregiver strain, and utilization of mental health services among elementary school students at high risk for ADHD. *J Am Acad Child Adolesc Psychiatry* **42**: 842–850.

Clark C, Prior M, Kinsella GJ (2000) Do executive function deficits differentiate between adolescents with ADHD and oppositional defiant/conduct disorder? A neuropsychological study using the Six Elements Test and Hayling Sentence Completion Test. *J Abnorm Child Psychol* **28**: 403–414.

Cohen M (1997) *Children's Memory Scale (CMS)*. San Antonio: Psychological Corporation.

Danckaerts M, Heptinstall E, Chadwick O, Taylor E (1999) Self-report of attention deficit hyperactivity disorder in adolescents. *Psychopathology* **32**: 81–92.

Dawson P, Guare R (2004) *Executive Skills in Children and Adolescents: A Practical Guide to Assessment and Intervention*. London: Guilford Press.

Doyle AR, Biederman J, Seidman LJ, Weber W, Faraone SV (2000) Diagnostic efficiency of neuropsychological test scores for discriminating boys with and without attention deficit hyperactivity disorder. *J Consult Clin Psychol* **68**: 477–488.

Dunford C, Street E, O'Connell H, Kelly J, Sibert JR (2004) Are referrals to occupational therapy for developmental coordination disorder appropriate? *Arch Dis Child* **89**: 143–147.

Elliott CD (1990) *Differential Ability Scales (DAS)*. San Antonio: Psychological Corporation.

Elliott CD, Smith P, McCullouch K (1996) *British Abilities Scales, 2nd edn (BAS II)*. Windsor: nfer-Nelson.

Goodman R, Scott S (1997) *Child Psychiatry*. Oxford: Blackwell Scientific.

Grodzinsky GM, Barkley RA (1999) Predictive power of frontal lobe tests in the diagnosis of attention deficit hyperactivity disorder. *Clin Neuropsychol* **13**: 12–21.

Hansen C, Weiss D, Last CG (1999) ADHD boys in young adulthood: Psychosocial adjustment. *J Am Acad Child Adolesc Psychiatry* **38**: 165–171.

Heiligenstein E, Guenther G, Levy A, Savino F, Fulwiler J (1999) Psychological and academic functioning in college students with attention deficit hyperactivity disorder. *J Am Coll Health* **47**: 181–185.

Henderson SE, Henderson L (2003) Toward an understanding of developmental coordination disorder: Terminological and diagnostic issues. *Neural Plast* **10**: 1–13.

Hervey AS, Epstein JN, Curry JF (2004) Neuropsychology of adults with attention deficit hyperactivity disorder: A meta-analytic review. *Neuropsychology* **18**: 485–503.

Hoza B, Gerdes AC, Hinshaw SP, Arnold LE, Pelham WE, Molina BS, Abikoff HB, Epstein JN, Greenhill LL, Hechtman L, Odbert C, Swanson J, Wigal T (2004) Self-perceptions of competence in children with

ADHD and comparison children. *J Consult Clin Psychol* **72**: 382–391.

Jensen PS, Martin BA, Cantwell DP (1997) Comorbidity in ADHD: Implications for research, practice and DSM-IV. *J Am Acad Child Adolesc Psychiatry* **36**: 1065–1079.

Kadesjo B, Gillberg C (1998) Attention deficits and clumsiness in Swedish 7-year-old children. *Dev Med Child Neurol* **40**: 796–804.

Kaufman AS (1994) *Intelligent Testing with the WISC-III.* New York: John Wiley.

Kaufman AS, Kaufman NL (1990) *Kaufman Brief Intelligence Test.* Circle Pines, MN: American Guidance Service.

Kempton S, Vance A, Marfuff P, Luk E, Costin J, Pantelis C (1999) Executive function and attention deficit hyperactivity disorder: Stimulant medication and better executive function performance in children. *Psychol Med* **29**: 527–538.

Korkman M, Kirk U, Kemp S (1998) *NEPSY: A Developmental Neuropsychological Assessment: Manual.* New York: Psychological Corporation.

Lawrence V, Houghton S, Douglass G, Durkin K, Whiting K, Tannock R (2004) Executive function and ADHD: a comparison of children's performance during neuropsychological testing and real-world activities. *J Atten Disord* **7**: 137–149.

Levine M (2002) *A Mind at a Time.* New York: Simon & Schuster.

Manly T, Robertson IH, Anderson V, Nimmo-Smith I (1998) *Test of Everyday Attention for Children (TEA-Ch).* Bury St Edmunds: Thames Valley Test Company.

Matier-Sharma K, Perachia N, Newcorn JD, Sharma V, Halperin JM (1995) Differential diagnosis of ADHD: Are objective measures of attention, impulsivity and activity level helpful? *Child Neuropsychol* **2**: 118–127.

McGee RA, Clark SE, Symons DK (2000) Does the Conners' Continuous Performance Test aid in ADHD diagnosis? *J Abnorm Child Psychol* **28**: 415–424.

MTA Cooperative Group (1999) A 14-month randomized clinical trial of treatment strategies for attention-deficit/hyperactivity disorder. *Arch Gen Psychiatry* **56**: 1073–1086.

Murphy K, Barkley RA (1996) Attention deficit hyperactivity disorder adults: comorbidities and adaptive impairments. *Compr Psychiatry* **37**: 393–401.

Murphy K, Barkley RA, Bush T (2002) Young adults with attention deficit hyperactivity disorder: subtype differences in comorbidity, educational, and clinical history. *J Nerv Ment Dis* **190**: 147–157.

Nichols SL, Waschbusch DA (2004) A review of the validity of laboratory cognitive tasks used to assess symptoms of ADHD. *Child Psych Hum Dev* **34**: 297–315.

Pitcher TM, Pick JP, Hay DA (2003) Fine and gross motor abilities in males with ADHD. *Dev Med Child Neurol* **45**: 525–535.

Raven JC, Court JH, Raven J (1986) *Manual for Raven's Progressive Matrices and Vocabulary Scales (Section 2) – Coloured Progressive Matrices.* London: HK Lewis.

Robertson IH, Ward T, Ridgeway V, Nimmo-Smith I (1994) *Test of Everyday Attention.* Bury St Edmunds: Thames Valley Test Company.

Robertson IH, Ward T, Ridgeway V, Nimmo-Smith I (1996) The structure of normal human attention: The Test of Everyday Attention. *J Int Neuropsychol Soc* **2**: 525–534.

Roth RM, Saykin AJ (2004) Executive dysfunction in attention-deficit/hyperactivity disorder: Cognitive and neuroimaging findings. *Psychiatr Clin N Am* **27**: 83–96.

Rucklidge JJ, Tannock R (2001) Psychiatric, psychosocial, and cognitive functioning of female adolescents with ADHD. *J Am Acad Child Adolesc Psychiatry* **40**: 530–540.

Sattler JM (2001) *Assessment of Children: Cognitive Applications, 4th edn.* Le Mesa, CA: Jerome M Sattler.

Sattler JM (2002) *Assessment of Children: Behavioral and Clinical Applications, 4th edn.* Le Mesa, CA: Jerome M Sattler.

Sattler JM, Dumont R (2004) *Assessment of Children: WISC-IV and WPPSI-III Supplement.* San Diego, CA: Jerome M Sattler.

Sonuga-Barke EJ (1996) When "impulsiveness" is delay aversion; a reply to Schweitzer and Sulzer-Azaroff (1995). *J Child Psychol Psychiatry* **37**: 1023–1025.

Sonuga-Barke EJ (2002) Psychological heterogeneity in AD/HD—a dual pathway model of behaviour and cognition. *Behav Brain Res* **130**: 29–36.

Sonuga-Barke EJ, Dalen L, Daley D, Remington B (2002) Are planning, working memory, and inhibition associated with individual differences in preschool ADHD symptoms? *Dev Neuropsychol* **21**: 255–272.

Spreen O, Strauss E (1998) *A Compendium of Neuropsychological Tests: Administration, Norms and Commentary.* Oxford: Oxford University Press.

Steger J, Imhof K, Coutts E, Gundelfinger R, Steinhausen HC, Brandeis D (2001) Attentional and neuromotor deficits in ADHD. *Dev Med Child Neurol* **43**: 172–179.

Stein MA, Szumowski E, Blondis TA, Roizen NJ (1995) Adaptive skills dysfunction in ADD and ADHD children. *J Child Psychol Psychiatry* **36**: 663–670.

Tannock R (1998) ADHD: Advances in research. *J Child Psychol Psychiatry* **39**: 65–100.

Taylor E (1994) Syndromes of attention deficit and overactivity. In: Rutter M, Taylor E, Hersov L (eds) *Child and Adolescent Psychiatry: Modern Approaches, 3rd edn.* Oxford: Blackwell Scientific.

Taylor EA, Sandberg S, Thorley G, Giles S (1991) *The Epidemiology of Childhood Hyperactivity. Maudsley Monographs No. 33.* Oxford: Oxford University Press.

Tripp G, Ryan J, Peace K (2002) Neuropsychological functioning in children with DSM-IV combined type Attention Deficit Hyperactivity Disorder. *Aust NZ J Psychiatry* **36**: 771–779.

Warner-Rogers J (1998) Attention deficit hyperactivity disorder. In: Howlin P (ed) *Behavioural Approaches to Problems in Childhood. Clinics in Developmental Medicine No. 146.* London: Mac Keith Press, pp 28–53.

Warner-Rogers J (2002) Attention deficit hyperactivity disorder. In: Howlin P, Udwin O (eds) *Outcomes in Neurodevelopmental and Genetic Disorders.* Cambridge: Cambridge University Press, pp 1–25.

Wechsler D (1992) *Wechsler Intelligence Scale for Children, 3rd edn UK.* Sidcup, Kent: Psychological Corporation.

Wechsler D (1997) *Wechsler Adult Intelligence Scale – 3rd edn.* San Antonio: Psychological Corporation.

Wechsler D (1999) *Wechsler Abbreviated Scale of Intelligence.* San Antonio: Psychological Corporation.

Wechsler D (2001) *Wechsler Individual Achievement Test – 2nd edn.* San Antonio: Psychological Corporation.

Wechsler D (2002) *Wechsler Preschool and Primary Scale of Intelligence – 3rd edn.* San Antonio: Psychological Corporation.

Wechsler D (2003) *Wechsler Intelligence Scale for Children – 4th edn.* San Antonio: Psychological Corporation.

WHO (1988) *The ICD-10 Classification of Mental and Behavioural Disorders.* Geneva: World Health Organization.

Wilson JM, Marcotte AC (1996) Psychosocial adjustment and educational outcome in adolescents with a childhood diagnosis of attention deficit disorder. *J Am Acad Child Adolesc Psychiatry* **35**: 579–587.

Woodward L, Downey L, Taylor E (1997) Child and family factors influencing the clinical referral of children with hyperactivity: A research note. *J Child Psychol Psychiatry* **38**: 479–485.

Wright I, Waterman M, Prescott H, Murdoch-Eaton D (2003) A new Stroop-like measure of inhibitory function development: Typical developmental trends. *J Child Psychol Psychiatry* **44**: 561–575.

5
MEDICAL INVESTIGATIONS AND TESTS

Angie Stevens and Gillian Baird

The purpose of medical investigation is to identify underlying and/or associated medical conditions, not to diagnose ADHD (the latter being based on history and structured behavioural observations across contexts). Whilst this may be obvious to professionals, it is not necessarily so for parents, who may think that the term 'investigation of ADHD' encompasses diagnosis of ADHD and comorbidities. It may be important to clarify this in talking to families about planned investigations. In other developmental disorders, parents usually ask "why?" and want investigations of causation as a high priority. This is less so in ADHD where parental concern is for diagnosis and treatment, including that of the associated developmental/learning and behavioural problems.

What parents want from professionals in response to concerns about their child's ADHD is clear from consultation with families (ADDISS 2003):
• Belief of parent report and response to their concerns
• Professional competence, knowledge and belief in the condition
• Clear pathway of referral for diagnosis
• Systematic assessment of strengths and weaknesses including learning difficulties and other coexisting conditions
• Information, explanation and intervention
• Integrated professional working including education
• Family support including for siblings
• Disability-specific knowledge and skills in any key worker
• Other treatments to be available – behaviour advice/strategies, anger management.

What reasons are there for medical investigation of a child with ADHD? The rationale for proceeding with medical investigations in any developmental or behavioural disorder is to detect any *treatable condition* or a disorder with *genetic implications*. The treatment threshold is a clinical decision, preferably one that is evidence based.

If a medical condition is found on investigation, it could be for one of three reasons. First, there may be a causal relationship (i.e. the medical condition is directly responsible for the ADHD symptomatology). Second, it may be that a single aetiology results in both ADHD and the identified condition. Finally it may be that the medical condition is an incidental comorbid finding, arising from a separate cause.

There are two approaches to thinking about investigations – the evidence-based approach and consensus practice which may be evidence based to a greater or lesser extent. In evaluating the evidence base for deciding on the medical investigations in any condition, it is be helpful to turn to studies that have asked "how often do investigations in condition A

86

uncover medical conditions previously unknown that have treatment or genetic implications?" But when searching the literature it is found that studies usually ask, "how often are medical conditions associated with A, or how often is A found in a particular medical condition?" and "what is the yield of a particular test?" 'Test' needs to be defined, it could be a physical examination or a laboratory test. The sensitivity and specificity of the particular test also need to be known.

In evaluating any relevant studies it is necessary to look at the population studied, the *extent* of investigations and the ascertainment of comorbidity. A study that estimates the prevalence of a range of medical conditions in a clinical sample may not be relevant to the particular child under consideration. A child presenting with ADHD in a primary care setting may be different in a number of respects from one presenting in a tertiary setting.

It is common in developmental and behavioural disorders to find a very limited evidence base, and many clinicians turn to a consensus view of tests to be done. Their selection will depend on their experience and seniority – the more senior, the more embarrassing it is to miss a medical diagnosis!

Comorbid developmental and neuropsychiatric conditions are very commonly associated with ADHD (70% in the NIMH Multimodal Treatment Study of Children with ADHD [MTA] – MTA Cooperative Group 1999). Learning disability, either general (mental retardation in USA parlance) or specific, or both, is a particularly common accompanying impairment in ADHD (see Chapter 13). The degree of mental retardation is a more powerful 'signpost' for underlying medical disorders than the ADHD.

In deciding which tests are worthwhile, the clinician makes a clinically sensible estimate of the patient's pre-test probability of any particular test being positive, i.e. of their having the condition being tested for (equivalent to the baseline prevalence in the population): to this end, adequate knowledge of the sensitivity and specificity of the test is needed (Sackett et al. 2000). The pre-test probability can be substantially influenced by history and examination, and by factors such as IQ. This is most obviously shown in considering a blood test for fragile X. For example, Hartley et al. (2002) discuss the efficacy of a six-item screening checklist for fragile X in decisions about tests for developmental delay (mild to moderate mental retardation). The checklist is highly sensitive, allowing individuals scoring <5 to be effectively ruled out of having the diagnosis. This allows substantial numbers of children to be spared molecular testing. A score ≥5 still produces only a small likelihood ratio, and hence a small increase in the probability of having the disorder. A child with IQ <70, autism and one other feature (elongated face, large or prominent ears, ADHD, or maternal history of X-linked mental retardation) would be likely to score 5 or above, and fall into the population meriting molecular testing. This also highlights another consideration in deciding what tests to do, which is *the clinical risk of missing a single positive result*, and hence an important calculation is the number of unaffected children that can reasonably be screened to effect a small but important yield, e.g. missing fragile X would be extremely important for a family. Because the definitive molecular test for fragile X has high sensitivity (i.e. it does not produce false negatives) and because a positive result has important implications for genetic counselling and takes the clinician above the 'treatment/action' threshold, it is justified to test a larger number of non-affected children to capture the few with the disorder.

Studies informing practice

Dooley et al. (2003) found in 500 consecutive referrals to a tertiary paediatric neurology clinic that examination and investigations did not influence the management of children with a number of disorders including ADHD.

Early studies had suggested an increased prevalence of thyroid abnormalities in ADHD, although none required medication; however, more recent studies (Valentine et al. 1997, Stein and Weiss 2003) found no clinically significant thyroid abnormalities in ADHD, leading to the conclusion that routine thyroid tests are not warranted, although specific examination findings may change that decision.

Height and weight measurement are essential prerequisites to any medical management. Spencer et al. (1996) in a cross-sectional study looked at Z scores of height and weight of children and adolescents with and without ADHD. Small but significant differences in height were evident in early but not late adolescence. (Parental heights were not significantly different.) Maturational lag was one hypothesis.

There are theoretical reasons for considering iron deficiency (using serum ferritin as a measure of iron stores) as relevant in ADHD as iron has some influence on dopamine function. Konofal et al. (2004) found a correlation between serum ferritin and Connors scale scores (but also greater cognitive deficits) and reported an individual case where iron treatment improved ADHD symptoms.

Routine neuroimaging and electroencephalography have not shown consistent differences between cases and controls, certainly nothing diagnostic or that leads to treatment, although differences in morphology and functioning have been proposed, e.g. that fronto-striatal–thalamic pathways and areas involved in working memory are differently modulated (Jucaite et al. 2005).

Recommended procedure in ADHD

Physical examination is regarded as routine good practice when any child is referred with a problem affecting behaviour or development. Information from the physical examination thus informs decision making with regard to further medical tests. It is also assumed that assessment will have proceeded through a careful pre-, peri- and postnatal history, as well as a family history, and that information will be available about the level of learning disability (mental retardation). Figure 5.1 gives a suggested algorithm. Assessment should proceed through the following stages:

• Presenting symptoms and behavioural diagnosis
• Assess any other comorbidities, developmental and neuropsychiatric, including IQ
• Systematic enquiry about sleep disturbance (see Chapter 10)
• Physically examine child
• Decide on any additional tests.

A Clinical Practice Guideline has been published by the American Academy of Pediatrics (2000).

PHYSICAL EXAMINATION

The main purpose of physical examination in children is to look for evidence of specific

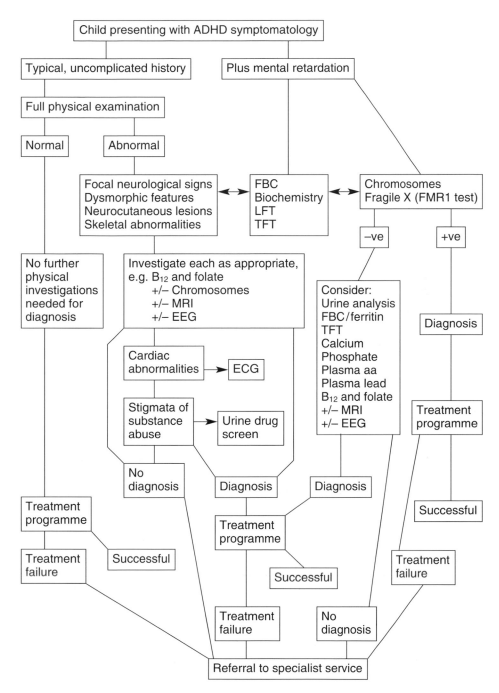

Fig. 5.1. Algorithm for physical investigations of ADHD.
Abbreviations: FBC = full blood count; LFT = liver function tests; TFT = thyroid function tests; ECG = echocardiogram; aa = amino acids; MRI = magnetic resonance imaging; EEG = electroencephalogram.

medical syndromes, illnesses and signs of abuse or neglect. The presence of comorbid conditions, especially low IQ, will enhance the likelihood of diagnostic findings.

Height and weight should be entered onto standard charts suitable for the population, as these will provide a baseline for monitoring subsequent treatment regimes. Crossing centiles, i.e. trajectory of measures, is usually the important consideration in the ADHD clinic. Head circumference should be entered onto standard charts. Although nonspecific, micro- and macrocephaly are associated with specific disorders, e.g. microcephaly and fetal alcohol syndrome. Most children with large heads have parents with large heads. The skin should be examined for stigmata suggestive of neurocutaneous syndromes, e.g. ash leaf macules (tuberous sclerosis), axillary freckling, café au lait patches and fibroangiomas (neurofibromatosis), or bruises that require explanation. Woods light in a darkened room highlights the ash-leaf depigmented areas of tuberous sclerosis. The hands should be examined for skin crease patterns and any digit abnormalities. Any areas of deliberate self-injury should be noted. In those adolescents where there is a suspicion of substance abuse, the presence of stigmata of drug use should be sought.

Systemic examination should include the cardiovascular system (blood pressure and pulse for baseline monitoring), and the respiratory system. There is no evidence that routine cardiac investigations in the absence of symptoms are likely to yield diagnostic information. It is helpful to know if the child is taking medication, e.g. for asthma, as exacerbations of behaviour may occur with illness and medications.

Neurological assessments include: gait, coordination (gross and fine motor skills), balance, muscle bulk, tone and strength (but see comments above about yield). 'Soft signs', e.g. walking on the outside of the feet, mirror movements or dysdiodochokinesis, are nonspecific.

Vision and hearing assessments may have been carried out as part of the health services' surveillance programme but if there is any doubt about hearing, refer for full audiometry. The physical appearance of the ears should be noted. Inspection of the eyes provides clues for a range of neurological conditions.

The presence of any motor and/or vocal tics should be noted.

Physical demeanour and facial expression also provide important clues as to mood, etc.

MEDICAL TESTS
The child/young person with ADHD with no abnormal findings on examination and a normal IQ
In a child who presents with typical ADHD, in whom the age of onset is also typical and in whom there is no evidence of developmental delay (either physical or cognitive), if the physical examination is entirely normal then there is no justification for further medical investigations. In this case the minimal investigation is a comprehensive physical examination (including height, weight, head circumference and blood pressure), to provide baseline measurements prior to commencing treatment (Stephen and Kindley 2006).

The child/young person with ADHD and developmental delay and/or mental retardation with no dysmorphic features and no findings on physical examination
In the preschool years particularly, children may present with a mixed developmental

problem in which several impairments appear to co-occur and where it may be difficult to establish the exact IQ. In this situation there have been several attempts at trying to decide, either on the basis of evidence or by consensus, what the appropriate medical tests/investigations should be for developmental delay (Gringras 1998) It used to be the case that a full mental retardation screen was considered necessary. However, in recent years there has been a move away from this intensive investigation, due largely to the observation that many of the tests in the screening protocol have very low detection rates (Curry et al. 1997).

There are consensus views of what investigations should be undertaken in mild mental retardation without physical findings on examination, but there will inevitably be variation across professionals depending on their experience, e.g. whether they are paediatric neurologists or psychiatrists who may see only severe cases and consequently may have a biased view both of yield and about their professional views of what they should do. That consensus view will also depend upon the context of work and whether the child is likely to have had perinatal screening for phenylketonuria and thyroid abnormality, which would be the situation in the UK but is not universal across the world. In the absence of any physical abnormality but in the presence of global delay in a preschool child, most would carry out a creatinine kinase assay to exclude a muscle disorder, and karyotype and DNA analysis for fragile X. Ferritin levels may be considered in the child with a very limited or abnormal diet.

In the school-aged child presenting with ADHD, mild mental retardation and no physical findings, only karyotype and DNA analysis for fragile X would be justified on treatment outcomes.

The child with ADHD, learning disorder (mental retardation) and dysmorphic features or abnormal findings on physical examination
Abnormal physical features may suggest particular syndromes. Abnormal head circumference is a feature of, for example, fetal alcohol syndrome (microcephaly) and Sotos syndrome (macrocephaly). Further specific indications for particular tests may be elicited, which will again affect the likelihood of a positive test, and combined with the outcome of a positive test will lead the clinician to perform it. Dysmorphic features are often seen in velocardiofacial syndrome, Prader–Willi syndrome, Williams syndrome and fragile X syndrome. Other findings suggesting specific tests include: a history of pica/marked change of behaviour – blood lead; loss of skills – mucopolysaccharides, thyroid function tests; metabolic illness – metabolic screen of amino/organic acids; markedly abnormal diet – full blood count/serum ferritin.

ADHD and other developmental/psychiatric comorbidities
Other psychiatric conditions that occur alongside ADHD include the pervasive developmental disorders, conduct disorder, abnormal affective states (e.g. bipolar affective disorder), Tourette syndrome and post-head-trauma states. The differential diagnosis of such conditions is considered in Chapter 6 but with respect to physical examination, the principles remain the same. The choice of investigations is based on the presenting history and the physical examination, and where the diagnosis remains unclear, referral to a specialist centre is the preferred option.

Epilepsy

The diagnosis of epilepsy is established by history, paying particular attention to details of the episodes, day or night. An EEG may be requested as part of epilepsy investigation, but it should be borne in mind that a normal EEG does not exclude a diagnosis of epilepsy and the EEG is no substitute for sound clinical assessment. Often the person in a position to give the best account of absence seizures is the classroom teacher. Other seizures that may have relevance in the investigation of ADHD are complex partial seizures, and again an EEG can be very helpful in delineating these phenomena. The accurate diagnosis of epilepsy is important, and there has been recent publicity about inaccuracies of diagnosis. Guidelines for the investigation and management of epilepsy in young people have been published by NICE (2004). Decisions about epilepsy when complicated by ADHD and other learning difficulties require expert opinion, but epilepsy is not a contraindication to treating ADHD. ADHD plus epilepsy requires particularly careful physical examination using Wood's light looking for tuberous sclerosis.

ADHD and loss of skills

Should any loss of previously existing skills be noted in a child with ADHD, further assessment of history, life events and experiences, physical examination and possibly medical investigations should be undertaken. True regression of skills is an indication for further referral to tertiary neurology/neuropsychiatry services. If indicated clinically, one might also consider a drug and alcohol screen.

NEUROIMAGING

Routine neuroimaging is not recommended in ADHD. In some children with focal epilepsy, focal neurological signs, neurocutaneous stigmata, or a changing neurological or neuropsychiatric picture, neuroimaging may be indicated but the general clinician should not hesitate to refer such a child for tertiary assessment.

Summary

All children referred for developmental difficulties should have a physical examination as well as a full medical, developmental and social history sufficient to formulate an explanation of their difficulties. Such a physical examination assesses normal growth and development and is a baseline for treatment monitoring. No medical tests are indicated in uncomplicated ADHD with absence of comorbidity and no physical findings. The presence of comorbidities with and without features found on physical examination does change the indication for further tests that have treatment and/or genetic implications. Of these, in the UK the most important are karyotype and DNA analysis for fragile X.

REFERENCES

ADDISS (2003) *Parents, Provision and Policy. A Consultation with Parents.* London: ADDISS (online at: http://www.addiss.co.uk/factsheets.htm).
American Academy of Pediatrics (2000) Clinical practice guideline: diagnosis and evaluation of the child with attention-deficit/hyperactivity disorder. *Pediatrics* **105**: 1158–1170.

Curry CJ, Stevenson RE, Aughton D, Byrne J, Carey JC, Cassidy S, Cunniff C, Graham JM, Jones MC, Kaback MM, Moeschler J, Schaefer GB, Schwartz S, Tarleton J, Opitz J (1997) Evaluation of mental retardation: recommendations of a consensus conference. *Am J Med Genet* **72**: 468–477.

Dooley JM, Gordon KE, Wood EP, Camfield CS, Camfield PR (2003) The utility of the physical examination and investigations in the pediatric neurology consultation. *Pediatr Neurol* **28**: 96–99.

Gringras P (1998) Choice of medical investigations for developmental delay: a questionnaire survey. *Child Care Health Dev* **24**: 267–276.

Hartley L, Salt A, Dorling J, Gringras P (2002) Invesigation of children with "developmental delay". *West J Med* **176**: 29–33.

Jucaite A, Fernell E, Halldin C, Forssberg H, Farde L (2005) Reduced midbrain dopamine transporter binding in male adolescents with attention deficit hyperactivity disorder: association between striatal dopamine markers and motor hyperactivity. *Biol Psychiatry* **57**: 229–238.

Konofal E, Lecendreux M, Arnulf I, Mouren MC (2004) Iron deficiency in children with attention deficit hyperactivity disorder. *Pediatr Adolesc Med* **158**: 1113–1115.

MTA Cooperative Group (1999) A 14-month randomized clinical trial of treatment strategies for attention-deficit/hyperactivity disorder. *Arch Gen Psychiatry* **56**: 1073–1086.

NICE (2004) *The Epilepsies: Diagnosis and Management of the Epilepsies in Adults and Children in Primary and Secondary Care.* London: National Institute for Clinical Excellence (online at: http://www.nice.org.uk/guidance/CG20).

Ross DM, Ross SD (1982) *Hyperactivity: Current Issues, Research and Theory.* New York: Wiley.

Sackett DL, Straus SE, Richardson WS, Rosenberg W, Hayners RB (2000) *Evidence-Based Medicine: How to Practice and Teach EBM.* Edinburgh: Churchill Livingstone.

Spencer TJ, Beiderman J, Harding M, O'Donnell D (1996) Growth deficits in ADHD children revisited: evidence for disorder-associated growth delays. *J Am Acad Child Adolesc Psychiatry* **35**: 1460–1469.

Stein MA, Weiss RE (2003) Thyroid function tests and neurocognitive functioning in children referred for attention deficit/hyperactivity disorder. *Psychoneuroendocrinology* **28**: 304–316.

Stephen E, Kindley AD (2006) Should children with ADHD and normal intelligence be routinely screened for underlying cytogenetic abnormalities? *Arch Dis Child* **91**: 860–861.

Valentine J, Rossi E, O'Leary P, Parry TS, Kurinczuk JJ, Sly P (1997) Thyroid function in a population of children with attention deficit hyperactivity disorder. *J Pediatr Child Health* **33**: 117–120.

6
MAKING A CASE FORMULATION: DIFFERENTIAL DIAGNOSIS AND RECOGNIZING COMORBIDITY

Wai Chen

Clinical formulation is the summing up of a case. It weighs up evidence and provides an analysis that identifies the most likely diagnosis from a set of possible 'contenders' (differential diagnoses).

A good formulation summarizes the salient features of the case, drawing relevant information from the mental state examinations and histories (mainly from informants in child psychiatry, but including self-reported histories in older children and adolescents). The purpose is to arrive at a working diagnosis: that is, pinpointing the most likely diagnosis given the evidence hitherto available. A working diagnosis implies that it is provisional, and may be revised when additional information comes to light from further tests, observations or assessments. Naturally, at initial assessments, other possible disorders giving rise to a similar clinical picture have to be considered. The discussion on differential diagnosis hence embodies comparing and contrasting the 'possible' in order to identify the most 'probable'.

However, a set of comorbidities is distinct from a set of differential diagnoses. Differential diagnoses are a list of possible disorders exhibiting similar clinical features, with only one condition being the most probable diagnosis. In this list of 'differentials', all conditions exhibit certain common features. But each condition may have its own telltale signs, which allow differentiation and distinction from one another. That is, out the choice of several conditions, only one is 'genuine', while the others are 'fakes'. The goal of a clinical formulation is to identify the 'best fit' condition, and dismiss the 'fakes' or 'impostors', while offering an argument together with evidence to support that choice. In contrast, comorbidities are other coexisting conditions, which overlap, superimpose or mask the primary disorder. That is, several 'genuine' conditions are superimposed upon one another. The task of the clinician here is to detect as many as there are, no more and no less.

For an analogy, differential diagnoses are like an identity parade. The witness has to pick out the real criminal from a line-up of suspects and actors. 'Comorbidities' are more like catching as many criminals as possible involved in a gang robbery. The former is selecting the 'best fit', and the latter is 'counting heads'. The latter is more characteristic of the DSM-IV system (APA 1994) than of the World Health Organization's ICD-10 (WHO 1992). In the ICD-10 system, there is a preference for making a single diagnosis that captures the full clinical picture. For instance, a case with both hyperkinetic and conduct disorders is preferentially diagnosed as 'hyperkinetic conduct disorder', rather than listed as two separate disorders.

Attention deficit hyperactivity disorder (ADHD) is a neurodevelopmental disorder characterized by age-inappropriate levels of inattentiveness, hyperactivity and impulsivity, with an onset in early to middle childhood. Symptoms should be persistent over time, and impairment should be pervasive across settings. There are a number of conditions that also give rise to symptoms of inattention, excess of motor movements or agitation that resemble hyperactivity – such as anxiety disorder, tic disorder, stereotypies, mania, depression, conduct disorder, learning difficulties and other specific learning difficulties giving rise to secondary inattentiveness. They can therefore resemble ADHD, and create a need for differential diagnosis. These and other conditions can also be associated with ADHD (coexist with it). They may be aetiologically linked with ADHD, or represent the complications of ADHD, or the reasons for their association with ADHD are still unknown. These conditions include specific developmental disorders, such as dyspraxia, specific language disorders, oppositional defiant disorder, conduct disorder, substance abuse and later antisocial personality disorder. These are called comorbidities or comorbid conditions. The word 'comorbidity' is misleading; in medicine it is usually used to refer to the simultaneous presence of two distinct disorders, but in this context it is not always clear that they are indeed distinct disorders.

Conditions and ADHD: as differential diagnoses or comorbid diagnoses
SECONDARY INATTENTIVENESS DUE TO GLOBAL LEARNING DIFFICULTIES AND SPECIFIC LEARNING DISORDERS
As a differential diagnosis
One common misdiagnosis of ADHD is 'secondary inattentiveness', which is inattention secondary to an unrecognized learning difficulty: either a *global* learning difficulty or a *specific* learning difficulty. The distinguishing hallmark here is situational, rather than pervasive, inattention: that is, the inattentiveness is situational to a setting that overburdens the cognitive ability of these children, while for tasks appropriate to their cognitive levels, they do not exhibit inattentive symptoms.

Amongst global learning difficulties, children with borderline low IQ (around 55–70) are often not detected. They can appear 'normal' to both teachers and parents, especially those with an extrovert temperament. Their global learning difficulties can be masked by friendliness, charm and talkativeness. The reasons for their inattention are twofold: (1) they are functioning at a lower mental age than their actual chronological age, i.e. their attention span is shorter, in keeping with a younger mental age; and (2) the class work (appropriate for children of their chronological age) is too challenging for their cognitive abilities – analogous to giving an adult's jigsaw puzzle to a normal toddler, who will soon lose interest and become distractible.

Amongst specific learning difficulties, several conditions can give rise to inattentiveness: for instance, specific reading difficulties (commonly referred to as 'dyslexia'), specific mathematics difficulties and specific language disorders. Yet the inattentiveness is again situational to settings where the children have to perform tasks taxing that particular skill. Typically, these children can concentrate on most tasks, but become inattentive, progressing to restlessness when confronted with tasks that challenge their specific deficits, and they can become agitated and even disruptive in order to avoid these tasks. Typically they are calm, sit still and concentrate well when they are engaging in activities of their own choice and appropriate to their cognitive level. In other words, their inattentiveness is not pervasive (or across settings), but situational. Such specific learning disabilities are distinguished from global learning difficulties, because the cognitive deficit is circumscribed to an isolated cognitive ability, out of keeping with the general IQ.

Many children with specific learning difficulties have not been detected by the educational system. They are often mislabelled as 'bright but lazy', 'hyperactive' or 'disruptive'. Some are referred to clinics with a label of 'ADHD'. Specific learning difficulties are strongly associated with conduct disorder, educational failure, later maladjustments and delinquency. It is therefore desirable for specialist clinics to screen for learning difficulties, before confirming the diagnosis of 'ADHD'.

There is an important caveat to bear in mind. Sometimes, children with very high IQ can show symptoms of secondary restlessness and inattentiveness at school. This is because the assigned class work is too simple, and therefore uninteresting and unchallenging for them. These cases are especially difficult to recognize, when the secondary inattentiveness has become a chronic problem. In such cases, these bright children will perform poorly academically, and may become disengaged from schoolwork, or depressed, or demoralized. There may therefore be few external signs to indicate their superior intelligence. Shy and introverted children, who have much self-doubt, are particularly at risk. These children often appear unhappy, bored and suffer from low self-esteem. Formal IQ testing can make an accurate estimate of their true cognitive abilities.

As a comorbidity
ADHD is associated with both global learning difficulties and specific learning disorders. Borderline IQ may coexist with ADHD, in particular the inattentive subtype. Specific language disorder, specific reading disorder, specific spelling disorder and dyspraxia (or specific motor developmental disorder) are also associated with ADHD, especially for boys. For these children, their learning difficulties require additional interventions, such as educational statementing or a classroom assistant, after their ADHD symptoms have been controlled by medication or other forms of treatment. The importance of cognitive screening cannot be overemphasized.

OPPOSITIONAL DEFIANT DISORDER AND CONDUCT DISORDER
As a differential diagnosis
Oppositional and defiant behaviours are common and normal for young children aged between 2 and 3 years, often referred to as 'the terrible twos'. Children at that age assert their independence: they typically reject adults' intervention and reply "no" to adults' requests. These are developmentally normal behaviours, which will subside with maturity.

Some children, however, display a persistent (at least six months) pattern of negativistic, hostile and defiant behaviours, which are both quantitatively and qualitatively above and beyond that of normative range. Their behaviours are characterized by frequent displays of any four or more of the following symptoms: (1) losing temper, (2) being argumentative, (3) defying adults' requests, (4) deliberately annoying others, (5) blaming others, (6) being 'touchy' and easily annoyed, (7) being spiteful or vindictive, and (8) being angry or resentful. They reach the threshold for an *oppositional defiant disorder* (ODD) if there are sufficient number and severity of symptoms, which cause impairments to their daily functioning. Whether it should be seen as an illness is debatable, but it is useful to have such a category for classification.

Conduct disorder (CD) is characterized by behaviour problems such as: (1) aggression to people and/or animals, involving threats, actual harm and victimization of others; (2) deliberate destruction of others' property, and fire-setting with intention to cause serious damage; (3) deceitfulness, 'break-ins' or theft; and (4) serious violation of rules, including truancy from school (before age 13), running away from home or staying out at night despite parental prohibitions. In other words, the transgression violates the rights of others, with intent and awareness. The DSM-IV specifies a list of 15 behavioural criteria within the above four domains. The presence of three (or more) items in any of the domains within the past 12 months, with at least one in the past 6 months, will meet the diagnostic threshold.

Children with CD can be disruptive both at home and at school, or confined to one setting only. Typically, problems start at home, and then generalize to settings outside the home, such as school. They can be classified as childhood-onset subtype (before age 10) or adolescent-onset subtype (from age 10 or later). Epidemiological studies indicate that the early-onset form runs a more severe and persistent life-course with greater risk for crimes and maladjustments in later life.

ADHD children can be unruly and out of control. They are also impulsive, with poor self-control and low tolerance for frustration: they are therefore prone to display some overlapping symptoms, such as throwing temper tantrums, being disruptive or breaking rules. These challenging behaviours arise out of their poor self-control. CD children, in contrast, typically break rules out of defiance, spite and violation of others' rights, typically with anger, aggression and malicious intent with or without premeditation. They may have little empathy or regards for their victims' feelings and well-being. They may lack remorse, blame others and be unable to take responsibility for their own actions.

ADHD children, on the other hand, are more likely to commit these acts out of impulsiveness. When confronted with the consequences of their actions or the impact on others, they are capable of experiencing remorse, regret and distress. ADHD children may exaggerate or tell lies, but in an impulsive way. Often they derive no personal gain from their wild stories. CD children, in contrast, tell lies with intent to deceive and make personal gain, often with premeditation. ADHD children may 'steal' property, but more out of impulsivity, forgetfulness, and a lack of reflection and self-monitoring. The items they have stolen may have no use or value to them. CD children, on the other hand, steal to gain, with the knowledge and awareness of the antisocial nature of their actions.

As a comorbidity
Both ODD and CD are associated with ADHD. That is, two or all three of these conditions may occur together in the same individual.

The reason for such an association with CD is interesting, but not fully understood. Different theories have been proposed: for instance, the comorbid form represents a more severe variant of ADHD (i.e. with greater loading of genetic risks); a dose–response relationship (i.e. the more severe and persistent the ADHD, the more likely the child also has CD); an aetiologically distinct entity (i.e. mediated by different genetic and environmental factors); or a result of critical parenting (that is, amongst dysfunctional parents, ADHD symptoms provoke negative parental expressed emotions, which in turn produce CD symptoms).

A child with ADHD is diagnosed with an additional CD or ODD when his or her disruptive and rule-breaking behaviour has gone beyond the confines of ADHD. That is, the types of transgression and the manners in which these were carried out are beyond that typical of ADHD-alone children.

Epidemiological studies show that these children with comorbidity are at particular risk of later educational failure, substance abuse, maladjustment and involvement with crime. Some studies suggest that the development of CD amongst ADHD children is related to dysfunctional parenting. The latter includes critical parental remarks, hostile and rejecting attitudes and inconsistencies in expected behavioural standards, as well as inconsistencies in rewards and discipline. For some cases, the ADHD symptoms in the child drive the critical and negative parental attitudes; and the effective use of medication, which reduces ADHD symptoms in the child, improves parenting. It is thus worthwhile reviewing the cases for persistence of ODD and CD symptoms after ADHD symptoms are fully controlled.

The recent Multimodal Treatment Study of Children with ADHD (MTA Cooperative Group 1999) indicates that children with comorbid ODD or CD diagnosis should not be treated with behavioural or psychological treatment alone. Medication is usually needed for the effective control of symptoms.

ANXIETY DISORDER

As a differential diagnosis

Anxiety disorders can be broadly divided into two groups: (1) those with generalized 'free-floating' anxiety, and (2) those whose symptoms of anxiety are elicited by specific triggers. *Specific anxiety disorders* can be subclassified by the triggers involved, such as animal phobia, social phobia, claustrophobia, agoraphobia, school phobia, toilet phobia and so on. They are referred to as 'fears' in lay language. In the absence of the trigger, the child is anxiety-free. The anxiety problem is thus *situational*, *episodic* and *immediate (responding to a cue)*. *Generalized anxiety disorder*, on the other hand, means that the child's anxiety is not triggered by environmental cues, but by an over-anxious internal state. Thus the anxiety state is likely to be *persistent*, *generalized* and *anticipatory*. In this condition, the external focus as the perceived source of anxiety can be shifting. This is referred to as 'worries' in lay language. For instance, a child is worried about the exams, then about abandonment if parents come home late, then about the possibility that an accident might happen, and then about a catastrophe that might occur. It is sometimes graphically labelled as 'free-floating' anxiety, as though the anxiety is floating in the air and latching onto whatever concrete objects come along. The anxiety is also characteristically anticipatory, i.e. something that might happen: like a threat, though the focus at a given time can be concrete or abstract. *Separation anxiety disorder* occupies the overlap area of these two, partly situational and partly anticipatory. Other anxiety disorders include panic disorder and obsessive–compulsive disorder (OCD). Some abused and neglected children display anxiety symptoms together with symptoms of *post-traumatic stress disorder*, characterized by the triad of hypervigilance, avoidance and experiencing flashbacks.

An anxious child is restless, fidgety and unsettled. Their mind is preoccupied with the perceived threat – concrete, real or imagined. S/he is thus inattentive, distractible and forgetful. The distinction from ADHD is based on the salient features in the history and mental state.

As a comorbidity

The recent MTA study has shown that about 33% of their subjects with ADHD also met DSM-III-R criteria for an anxiety disorder (excluding simple phobias) (MTA Cooperative Group 1999). These children may respond both to behavioural treatment and to stimulant medication. Improvements were most evident in outcome measures on (1) parent-reported hyperactivity and inattention, (2) parent–child relationships, and (3) teacher-rated social skills. Perhaps children with anxiety symptoms are biologically more sensitive and hence responsive to conditioning. The moderating effect of anxiety would then favour the inclusion of psychosocial treatment for them. Indeed, the MTA study found that the presence of anxiety with ADHD (regardless of conduct disorder) increased the likelihood of response to behavioural treatment. As a simple 'rule of thumb' for predicting treatment response, ADHD subjects with coexistent anxiety are likely to respond to any of the three treatments: behavioural alone, medication alone, or a combination of medication and behavioural intervention. However, for the doubly comorbid group who show anxiety and CD, as well as ADHD, combination interventions appear to offer substantial advantages over other treatment.

AUTISM, ASPERGER SYNDROME AND AUTISM SPECTRUM DISORDER
As a differential diagnosis

Autism is a neurodevelopmental disorder characterized by the triad of social impairments, communication impairments, and rigidity and circumscribed repetitive interests, with an onset prior to age 3 years. Asperger syndrome is defined by the same triad, but with an additional criterion that stipulates normal early developmental language acquisition – that is, no developmental history of language delay. In these children, the acquisition of language may be normal; yet the social use of the acquired language is not. Children meeting only two symptom domains of the triad are diagnosed as having atypical autism. Those with borderline symptoms of varying patterns of combination are designated as having 'pervasive developmental disorder, not otherwise specified' (PDD-NOS). The precise diagnosis of complex cases of autism requires the specialized skills of subspecialty experts and is not discussed here in detail. For simplicity, unless specified, 'autism spectrum disorders' (ASDs) as a collective term will be used in this section to include all variants of the disorder.

Children with an ASD may be mistaken as having ADHD for several reasons: temper tantrums, repetitive behaviours, stereotyped mannerisms, avoidance of eye contact and inattention to activities outside of their circumscribed preoccupations. First, they are liable to temper tantrums when their rigid routines are disrupted. These temper tantrums, however, are driven by their intolerance of change, and severe anxiety when their routines are disrupted, rather than by oppositionality or defiance. Second, ASD children may engage in repetitive behaviours, such as opening and closing drawers again and again; or they may have stereotyped mannerisms such as hand flapping or rubbing their hands on their ears. These may be misinterpreted as restlessness or hyperactivity. Third, children with ASD often avoid eye contact and are oblivious of their carers even when their names are called. Carers find it difficult to elicit joint attention, or direct their attention. These behaviours can be misinterpreted as distractibility and inattention. Fourth, children with ASD engage in activities strictly on their own terms; as a result, activities outside of their circumscribed interests are often ignored or abandoned after a brief trial. They can therefore be mistaken as having attention deficits. Finally, both ADHD children and ASD children have social impairments and are often rejected by peers. ADHD children are rejected because of their impulsive, erratic, domineering and intrusive interaction styles. ASD children can simply be disinterested in other children. Some will act in a remote, aloof and eccentric manner. If they are interested in their peers, their gauche social overtures and ill-judged responses often lead to rebukes, ridicule and rejection. Key differentiating features are discussed in the next section. Typically, the deficits of ADHD children are improved by stimulants, while ASD symptoms can be worsened. Children with ASD may be hypersensitive to stimulants, so these need very careful dose titration.

As a comorbidity
ASD can coexist with ADHD. These cases can be notoriously difficult to diagnose. Often the ADHD symptoms mask the ASD symptoms until ADHD symptoms are controlled by medications. This is especially so when ADHD is severe: these children are so hyperactive and inattentive that they will not engage with any activities for an extended period of time, so there is little evidence of circumscribed interests or preoccupations. Once they are given stimulants, their ASD symptoms start to emerge: they then start to display symptoms of over-focused concentration, circumscribed preoccupations and repetitive behaviours. This emergence of underlying ASD symptoms can be misconstrued as a side-effect of stimulants.

In milder ADHD cases, the autistic preoccupations can give a false impression of good concentration span. These children can show very good concentration, but only in the areas of their circumscribed interests. Outside these, the child has very poor concentration. In these cases, a seemingly contradictory clinical picture may arise, such that clinicians may be given conflicting accounts of the child's concentration span by different informants. The distinguishing feature is that the intense concentration is highly situational to areas of preoccupied interests. It is as though the ASD can override the ADHD in specific areas of their preoccupations: "Most of the time, he will only concentrate for about 5–10 minutes, but he can watch certain specific video tapes, like Thomas the Tank Engine, for several hours repetitively." The hallmark is that his over-focused attention is restricted to certain objects. Furthermore, the manner in which he watches that video is qualitatively abnormal, i.e. he would rewind and watch a short segment again and again.

Early indicators of overlapped ASD and ADHD cases include: the children may have remote aloofness, a lack of concern for others' feelings, failure to show concern and comfort to others when it would be appropriate, having an exceptional memory for details, displaying stereotypic utterances, and insistence on having things done on their own terms. They may become distressed when the usual teacher has been substituted by a replacement, furniture has been rearranged at home or at school, or they are travelling home via a different route. These children are often hypersensitive to stimulants. At a relatively low dose, they can become overfocused, and develop marked symptoms of autism. Their medication regime therefore requires careful fine-dose titration: that is, starting at a very low dose, then slowly increasing by small increments. One needs to monitor the response with caution. In suspected comorbid cases, it is essential to prepare their parents for such an additional diagnosis, explain the possibility, give the reasons for fine-dose titration, and warn of possible adverse effects in advance. For some case, stimulants cannot be used. Then, second- and third-line medications are required, such as clonidine, atomoxetine, atypical neuroleptics, imipramine, SSRIs or meclobamide.

SUBSTANCE ABUSE

Substance abuse disorder is associated with ADHD, more as a late developmental outcome than a childhood or adolescent comorbidity. However, illicit drug experimentation and substance misuse are more common in ADHD in late childhood and in adolescence.

Substance abuse disorder is characterized by a maladaptive pattern of substance use, leading to clinically significant impairment or distress, as manifested by three of the following in the last 12 months: tolerance, withdrawal, using large dosage (including chronic use), or binge usage. Consequences include spending a great deal of time in procuring the substance, with detrimental effects on social, educational and occupational functioning; the person often continues to misuse substances despite knowledge of possible harm and a wish to stop. When substance abuse is present, the adolescent needs to be managed by a specialist. Sometimes, young persons use alcohol and illicit psychotropics to self-medicate symptoms of depression, social phobia or OCD. These comorbid conditions should be assessed and managed.

MOOD DISORDER

As a differential diagnosis

Depression can cause cognitive impairment: inattention, distractibility and forgetfulness (due to poor registration of information rather than true memory loss). The adult form of depression is rare in childhood, but increases towards adult levels of prevalence after puberty, especially amongst girls. Conduct disorder can be associated with low mood and depression.

The adult form of depression is defined by having five of the following symptoms during the same two-week period: low mood (irritability); diminished interests/pleasure; weight loss or failure to gain weight; insomnia or hypersomnia; psychomotor agitation or retardation; fatigue; feelings of worthlessness; recurrent thoughts of death; and cognitive impairment in thinking, concentrating and decision making.

Depression with agitation and irritability may resemble symptoms of inattention and over-activity. However, the onset of depression is likely to be discrete, and can be differentiated from ADHD by the chronic nature of ADHD with onset predating age 7 years.

As a comorbidity

Mood disorder may present in adolescents with ADHD. Comorbid depression need to be recognized, assessed, diagnosed and treated promptly, and should be not be dismissed as 'adolescent turmoil'. Untreated depression can exacerbate inattention problems as well as social and occupational impairments. As depression is associated with deliberate self-harm, untreated depression is a potentially life-threatening illness, and its ensuing risks must be taken very seriously.

Bipolar disorder and mania

In recent years, a childhood variant form of 'bipolar disorder' has been recognized, and its symptoms are quite similar to some of those of ADHD. ADHD is often associated with irritability, over-reaction and an explosive temperament. Adults with ADHD often report marked and rapid escalation of anger when frustrated. They are also prone to have marked dejection when encountering a disappointment and to become over-joyous when a minor positive event occurs. This tendency of exaggerated emotional reactions to minor or trivial changes in external environment is known as 'emotional over-reactivity'. Increasingly, it has been recognized that children can also display these emotional features: their moods can appear labile and volatile; and they can show explosive anger and marked emotional reactivity. These symptoms are not listed in the DSM or ICD criteria as core features of ADHD true bipolar symptomology.

There is accordingly an unresolved controversy about whether these symptoms should be seen as part of ADHD, or as a form of bipolar disorder, or as a separate condition. In the UK, the National Institute of Clinical Excellence (NICE) has reviewed the published literature (Lord and Paisley 2000). It has arrived at a conservative conclusion: that there is not yet sound evidence to establish a new category of paediatric bipolar disorder. Only bipolar I disorder, the review recommends, should be recognized in childhood.

A "bipolar I disorder" requires episodes of mania. This is a distinct period of abnormally and persistently elevated, expansive or irritable mood, lasting at least 1 week. During this period, the individual experiences an inflated self-esteem, a sense of grandiosity. There are also other features, including a decreased need for sleep, pressured speech, excessive talk, flights of ideas, racing thoughts, distractibility, psychomotor agitation, and, in adults, e.g. excessive pleasurable indulgence: foolish business investments, sexual indiscretions, buying sprees, or grandiose actions involving poor judgement.

Mania has common features with ADHD in excessive activity, poor judgement, impulsive behaviour and distractibility. However, ADHD can be distinguished by having an early onset, chronic course and no expansive mood. Childhood bipolar disorder should not be diagnosed outside a subspecialty centre specializing in mood disorders, due to the treatment implications of using a mood-stabilizer.

REACTIVE ATTACHMENT DISORDER

Reactive attachment disorder is by definition a condition caused by pathogenic care, and characterized by abnormal social attachment behaviours and an inability to establish selective attachment. Pathogenic care is defined as abnormal early nurturing with disregard of a child's basic needs, including (1) physical needs, (2) emotional need for comfort, stimulation and affection, and (3) need for selective attachment through repeated changes of primary caregiver, preventing the formation of stable attachment.

Clinically, there are two subtypes of reactive attachment disorder: inhibited and disinhibited. The inhibited subtype is characterized by withdrawal and persistent failure to respond to social interactions. The disinhibited subtype is characterized by over-familiarity, indiscriminate sociability, and attempts to form a social attachment after a very brief acquaintance. Children with attachment problems have difficulties sustaining engagement with a given activity for a prolonged period, thereby appearing to be inattentive. However, their apparent 'hyper-activity' is driven by their urge to initiate and establish social relatedness with new people. Thus they fret from person to person. They are rather changeable in their interests and brief in their activities. Yet their 'hyperactivity' is seldom severe.

TOURETTE SYNDROME AND TIC DISORDERS
As a differential diagnosis
Tourette syndrome is characterized by the *combined* presence of vocal and motor tics, which are persistent over a year, without remission for more than three consecutive months within that year. A tic is a sudden, rapid, recurrent, nonrhythmic, stereotyped motor move-ment (motor tic) or vocalization (vocal tic). If either persistent motor tics or persistent vocal tics occur in isolation, then the diagnosis is either *chronic motor* or *vocal tic disorder*. If the tics last less than a year, then *transient tic disorder* is diagnosed. Tics involving an isolated group of muscle are called 'simple tics', e.g. a simple jerk of the neck. Those involving the combination of several muscle groups are called 'complex tics', e.g. thumping sideways, which movement involves the shoulder muscles, extension of the elbow and forearm, and the small muscles of the hand to make a fist.

A child with tics can be mistaken as having ADHD, because of their excessive motor movements or vocalizations. A wrong diagnosis can be harmful, because the stimulant medication treatment used for ADHD can worsen tics. The reverse is also true, as sometimes ADHD children are mistaken as having a tic disorder, because of their hyperactivity, restlessness and fidgetiness. The key differentiating feature is that tics are stereotyped and repetitive: that is, the same movement (involving the same muscle group in 'simple tics', or the same combination of muscle groups in 'complex tics') repeated again and again with little variation. In contrast, the hyperactivities of ADHD are highly variable in forms and frequency: that is, involving different muscle groups, variable combinations of muscle groups, and exerting with variable magnitudes, intensities and strengths. There is also a rapid alteration involving successive groups of muscles in ADHD. Furthermore, the involvement of neck, facial and ocular muscles, such as neck jerking, twitching of mouth, repetitive retracting eyelids, or forced gaze sideways, are typical of tics. In doubt, the differential diagnosis between tics and ADHD should be made by specialist clinics, with experience and expertise in diagnosing tic disorders.

As a comorbidity
Tourette syndrome is a relatively rare condition, occurring at about 5 in 10,000 individuals.

It is more common in boys, with onset peaking at around age 7–9 years, though it can start as early as 2 years. Tourette syndrome is associated with ADHD: that is, many children with Tourette syndrome also have ADHD.

When the clinical syndrome of ADHD is superimposed upon the Tourette syndrome, a dual diagnosis has to be made. This is best achieved in a specialist clinic, as complex treatments are involved. Stimulants conventionally used for ADHD may or may not exacerbate tics. Clonidine can be used to treat both conditions simultaneously, but is less effective in correcting the cognitive symptoms of ADHD. Sometimes, a polypharmacy approach has to be adopted. In addition, Tourette syndrome will run a fluctuating course, and it is important to cut back on its medication when symptoms subside otherwise an escalating dosage of anti-tic medication will be prescribed with accumulating risk of side-effects. Tourette syndrome is also associated with CD, OCD and substance abuse. All these conditions require separate assessments and treatments, but must be carried within an overview of a coherent management strategy. The expertise involved is nontrivial.

HYPERKINESIS WITH STEREOTYPIES

This condition may be encountered in children with significant learning difficulties but without autism or related disorder. More typically, the degree of learning difficulties is in the moderate to severe range (i.e. IQ <50). The presentation is dominated by repetitive and stereo-typed motor behaviours. These activities can be semi-purposeful, while the overactivity is highly repetitive and stereotypical rather than fretting from one task to another. Stimulants are ineffective in these children; an SSRI or an atypical neuroleptic agent can be tried.

REFERENCES

APA (1994) *Diagnostic and Statistical Manual of Mental Disorders, 4th edn (DSM-IV)*. Washington, DC: American Psychiatric Association.

Lord J, Paisley S (2000) The clinical effectiveness and cost-effectiveness of methylphenidate for hyperactivity in childhood. Version 2 – for consultation. London: National Institute for Clinical Excellence (online at www.nice.org.uk/download.aspx?o=11655).

MTA Cooperative Group (1999) A 14-month randomized clinical trial of treatment strategies for attention-deficit/hyperactivity disorder. *Arch Gen Psychiatry* **56**: 1073–1086.

WHO (1992) *International Statistical Classification of Diseases and Related Health Problems. 10th edn (ICD-10)*. Geneva: World Health Organization.

7
EDUCATION AND ADVICE

Maxine Sinclair

Longitudinal studies report that ADHD persists into adolescence in more than half of affected children (Klein and Mannuzza 1991, Weiss and Hechtman 1993, Mannuzza et al. 1998). The majority of these young people will be educated in mainstream schools, rather than requiring the alternative educational provisions associated with special schools, but they often need certain accommodations to support them in their educational environment.

Impaired attention and impulse control, along with overactivity limit the ADHD child's opportunity to benefit from educational instruction. These behaviours detrimentally affect listening skills, organization, planning, mental effort, etc. – the on-task behaviours essential for accruing and using new learning. Studies reporting the academic achievements of children with ADHD indicate that they are more likely than normally developing peers to receive lower grades in academic subjects and to score lower on standard measures of reading and mathematics (Barkley et al. 1990, Wener 1990). Anderson et al. (1987) reported that more than 80% of 11-year-olds with ADHD were at least 2 years behind in reading, spelling, math or written language. These learning difficulties are thought to contribute to follow-up evidence that over half of the children with ADHD who are taught in regular schools will experience school failure or fail at least one grade in adolescence (Minde et al. 1971, Brown and Borden 1986, Barkley et al. 1990) and over half will fail to finish secondary school (Weiss and Hechtman 1993). Their risk of failure is two to three times greater than for other children of similar intellectual ability (Rubenstein and Brown 1981). Failure at school may lead to disaffection with the school process, poor self-esteem and social isolation, which in turn may eventually result in school drop-out, increased exposure to delinquent groups and antisocial activity. There is a great challenge to devise effective school-based strategies to minimize the potentially negative effects on learning.

There is some controversy whether a whole school approach is necessary. Cooper and O'Regan (2001) think not, but in my opinion it is advisable. The classroom is not a vacuum and the child is one member of the whole school community. It is valuable to ensure that the child's developmental conditions, and their potential effects on academic and non-academic activities, are understood by all staff likely to come into contact with the child. Only then will they be able to work together effectively to support the child in the classroom and in the less structured environment of the playground. Educational psychologists, clinical psychologists, paediatricians and psychiatrists can play important roles in collaborating with general educators with the joint aim of optimizing functioning of children with ADHD.

The specific characteristics of ADHD that manifest themselves in the school environment vary greatly, both within and between individuals and over time. Despite this, the behaviours

can generally be grouped in the following categories:
- Attention and concentration
- Reasoning and information processing
- Memory
- Executive functioning (problem solving, planning, organizing).

School-based approaches to address the needs of children with ADHD should be comprehensive to ensure appropriateness, i.e. to effectively limit difficulties experienced in all the above areas. The integration of school, family and biological factors into an explanatory and intervention model will encourage effective action plans. This ecological approach should ensure that consideration is given to:
- Environmental management
- Instructional accommodation
- Self-regulation
- Medical management
- Effective home–school communication.

Environmental management

This refers to "all the teacher directed activities that support efficient operations of the classroom and lead to the establishment of optimal conditions for learning" (Smith et al. 1995).

Teacher-directed activities should consider:
- Psychosocial factors – child, teacher, peers, parents
- Instruction factors – timetable, transitions, homework
- Procedural factors – classroom rules and procedures
- Physical factors – seating arrangements, assistive technology
- Behavioural modification strategies – building and increasing adaptive behaviours, decreasing undesirable ones
- Personnel – SENCO, class teacher, teaching support assistant, extended school staff, educational psychologist, etc.

PSYCHOSOCIAL FACTORS

Psychosocial factors include the attitudes held by teaching staff about the children and/or their diagnoses. Shores et al. (1993) and Chazan (1994) found that, given the increasing demands and limited resources in mainstream schools, regular educators were less willing to tolerate pupils with challenging and provocative behaviour than special educators were. Similarly, teachers' attitudes and management skills concerning behavioural problems are important factors in the success or failure of mainstreaming children with learning disabilities or behavioural difficulties (Meijer and Foster 1988).

Knowledge about ADHD is helpful, and Appendix A provides a handout for teachers. A school-based intervention also seeks to provide teachers with the necessary skills to manage behaviours associated with ADHD. Teachers who believe that they can effectively manage behavioural problems tend to report fewer problems. Teachers' attitudes about the children may therefore be a powerful determinant of the success of school-based interventions. Parent-related factors include parental attitude to learning, socio-economic status, and willingness to participate in and support the school-based programme. The most effective interventions are able to foster continuity of expectation and contingency reinforcement across settings. Child-related factors may include motivation, previous school history and problems with learning, amongst a whole host of other influences. These will necessarily be primary targets of any intervention. The number of children in the class and whether other children require special accommodation (and the funding arrangements to support these) will inevitably influence the adequacy of any strategy.

Teaching staff will need to be able to appraise, analyse and develop responses to the behavioural, emotional and academic needs of the child. Understanding of behavioural management principles and experience with developing behavioural management programmes are obviously desirable, but should not be seen as requirements for all, providing they have recourse to people who do have this knowledge (e.g. educational psychologist, behavioural support team, clinical psychologist). The emphasis should be on contingent behavioural reinforcement using frequent and immediate rewards for desirable behaviours with the judicious use of sanctions for undesirable ones.

INSTRUCTIONAL ACCOMMODATION

This refers to the demands placed on the child. There needs to be a balance between the ability of the child and the requirements of the curriculum. The child with ADHD may be more productive if the demands placed upon him or her are perceived to be achievable. These may include some flexibility in the time spent on a task. Children with ADHD selectively attend to novelty, finding activities or situations that require sustained attention difficult. Zentall (1985) found that the longer the duration of the task without breaks, the more problems children with ADHD had compared to their non-ADHD peers. The quality of work can be increased by: breaking long assignments into smaller manageable parts with staggered due dates for plan, notes, rough draft, introduction, final copy; and reducing the amount of homework by focusing on the time spent on homework rather than the work achieved. The length of academic tasks should therefore correspond to the child's attention span. Barkley et al. (2000) suggest that, as a rule of thumb, one should assign the amount of work that would be appropriate for a child 30% younger.

Zentall and his colleagues (Zentall and Zentall 1976; Zentall 1985a,b, 1986) found that when tasks involved repeated exposure to stimuli of decreasing novelty (and most classroom activity would fit this category), children with ADHD showed increased activity and impulsive responding. Increasing novelty and interest level of the task through increased stimulation (practicals, sensory modalities, computers, etc.) reduce disruptive behaviour and facilitate on-task behaviour and motivation. Similarly, setting up a personal cueing signal has been found to improve on-task behaviours effectively. The cue should ideally be unobtrusive and within the classroom repertoire, for example placing a hand on the child's desk. Alternating between low-interest or table-top tasks, and high-interest or practical assignments, may optimize attention and concentration – especially when these can be predicted by the child, for example by displaying the day's or week's schedule in a conspicuous place. Problems with sustained attention may mean more errors during later performance, including later on in the school day. Consequently, it may be advisable to schedule difficult subjects at the start of the day, as one would predict less attention control and behavioural inhibition as the day progresses.

PROCEDURAL FACTORS

Basic rules and consequences are fundamental to classroom management and/or behavioural management plans. Children, including children with ADHD, need to know what is expected of them and what the consequences will be if they do not adhere to these rules.

Smith et al. (1995) suggest that in general:

- Rules should be stated simply – they should be clearly and explicitly stated so that the children know exactly what is expected from them. The rationale for keeping rules (or any information/instruction) brief and simple comes in part from research indicating that performance deficits are observed in children with ADHD when they are forced to distinguish relevant and important information embedded in information that is superfluous to the task or instruction
- Rules should be stated in the positive – so that there can be no ambiguity over what is expected from the child, e.g. "Raise your hand and wait until you are asked to speak" or "Stay in your seat unless given permission to stand or walk about during lessons"
- The number of rules should be kept to a manageable amount – a few rules, usually less than six – that are rehearsed and frequently referred to, so as to improve automatic recall and limit demands made on limited capacity memory
- Rules should be posted conspicuously – as a cued recall strategy
- Rules should be enforced and consistently applied – consequences for rule adherence as well as contravention should be reinforced.

PHYSICAL FACTORS

As noted, children with ADHD attend preferentially to novelty and may become distracted by irrelevant features in their environment. Simple physical management can help to reduce this type of off-task behaviour. The child should be placed in the least distracting place, away from wall displays, cupboards, doors, main thoroughfares and windows but within easy sight of the teacher. Close physical proximity to the teacher makes it easier to implement cueing strategies to help the child refocus on a task, and it also increases the ability to monitor both on-task and off-task behaviours so that these can be reinforced immediately. Traditionally, children are seated in vertical rows or small groups, and whilst this arrangement is usually dictated by the dimensions of the classroom, it provides ample opportunity for pupils to physically interact with one another. A large group circle provides an alternative arrangement with the added benefits of limiting opportunities for physical interaction and allowing the teacher to see all students easily. Seating the ADHD child between good role models may also allow the teacher to take advantage of peer support and/or peer-pressure especially when combined with whole-class incentives, a useful strategy for engendering group responsibility.

BEHAVIOURAL MANAGEMENT

Research has focused primarily on the efficacy of behaviour management as a classroom strategy for increasing on-task behaviour, task completion, compliance, impulse control and social skills, while reducing hyperactivity, off-task behaviour, disruptive behaviour and aggression. The evidence indicates that positive reinforcement can be effective in reducing activity levels, increasing time on-task and improving academic performance of students with ADHD (O'Leary et al. 1975, 1979; Rosenbaum et al. 1975). Other investigators have questioned the relative effectiveness of behavioural therapy compared to stimulant medication (Gittelman-Klein et al. 1976). These investigators found that methylphenidate was more effective in improving conduct, attention, hyperactivity and disruption than a positive reinforcement programme, and that combining behaviour therapy with methylphenidate was no different to methylphenidate alone. This suggested that behavioural therapy had nothing to add to medication; but medication is not always acceptable to some parents and/or their children, and we need alternative strategies in our repertoire.

A number of studies have examined the effect of prudent negative consequences or reprimands on the performance of children with ADHD. The results indicate efficacy in decreasing off-task behaviour and to a lesser extent in increasing academic productivity. Worland (1976) compared positive feedback, negative feedback and no feedback, and found that children with ADHD were on-task significantly more under negative feedback than under the other two conditions. Abramowitz et al. (1988) demonstrated that short reprimands resulted in significantly lower rates of off-task behaviours than long reprimands. A similar trend, though not significant, was found for improvement in academic functioning. They surmise that long reprimands may serve as positive reinforcers because they involve more adult attention. Abramowitz and O'Leary (1990) found that immediate sanctions were associated with lower rates of interactive (involving another pupil) off-task behaviours than were delayed sanctions. Moreover, the sudden introduction and maintenance of strong sanctions may result in more overall suppression of undesirable behaviours and reduced the overall level of negative consequences needed than a gradually strengthening series of sanctions. This provides empirical support for Barkley's (2000) supposition that children with ADHD need more powerful contingencies than their non-ADHD peers.

A combination of positive and negative reinforcement, 'response–cost', can be effective in improving attention, on-task behaviour and completion of academic assignments. Sullivan and O'Leary (1990) found that both positive reinforcement and response–cost were effective in producing immediate improvements in children's on-task behaviours, but only students in the response–cost arm of their study maintained these benefits when the programmes were faded out.

The most important facet of any behavioural management intervention is the ability to catch children being good. As a general rule the second time a teacher gives a child a verbal warning or sanction this should act as a cue to catch that child being good and positively reinforce this behaviour.

Examples of reinforcers include:
- Positive reinforcement
- Free time
- Tangibles (real or concrete rewards, e.g. toys or food, provided by parents
- Certificate/stickers

- Time in the gym
- Intermediate reinforcers – e.g. tokens, marbles – that can be exchanged for an activity or tangible of the child's choice.

The child should be involved in the selecting of rewards. Any reward needs to be more powerful and valued than the advantage to the child of continued engagement in undesirable behaviours.

NEGATIVE REINFORCEMENTS

Time out

One normally recommends that a 'time out' period should be for a few minutes only and depend on the child's age (one minute per year of age). The initial time out period used in a large North American study (MTA Cooperative Group 1999) was 20 minutes, much longer than is usually recommended. However, children were able to earn a 50% reduction for complying with this sanction without protest. The rationale was that this might increase compliance and prevent the escalation of negative behaviours (Wells et al. 2000a,b).

Loss of privilege

Loss of break time appears to be a favoured sanction in some schools. However, when children with ADHD are deprived of an opportunity to let off steam during break, their concentration and classroom behaviour often deteriorate as a consequence. It also deprives them of crucial social skill building opportunities, and the aim of any intervention should be not only to decrease undesirable behaviours but also to increase desirable ones.

PERSONNEL

This refers to the people involved in applying and supporting the programme. It is essential that roles are clearly designated and that sufficient reviews take place to evaluate progress and make the necessary modifications to ensure positive progress for the young person.

Effective home–school communication

A substantial body of evidence demonstrates the benefits associated with home–school partnership practice in mainstream education. Lee (1994) reported higher student attendance, better grades and more homework effort. Hoover-Dempsey and Sandler (1995, 1997) suggest that parents were most active in supporting school initiatives if they experienced a sense of personal self-efficacy for helping their child succeed in school. Those who believe they are capable of influencing achievement-related outcomes are those most likely to support school-based programmes. Concomitant parent training might be one route into facilitating this process. Other programmes include a component of parental involvement, usually with the parent providing rewards for positive behaviour.

Self-regulation

This refers to interventions that, having been taught by the teacher, are intended to be implemented independently by the child. The underlying principle is informed by cognitive behavioural principles employing the use of self-directed internalized speech. The empirical evidence for the use of cognitive behavioural therapy in ADHD populations is equivocal. A review by Hinshaw et al. (1998) indicated little evidence to support its efficacy; but when used in conjunction with traditional behavioural techniques it may have a part to play.

Zentall (1993) identifies a number of difficulties associated with ADHD that might be ameliorated by a more cognitive format. These include:
- Academic errors arising from the child's failure to consider alternative information in problem solving
- Failure to wait, leading to poor test performance, poor skill in planning, limited organizational skills, and failure to read instructions
- Reduced likelihood of asking for help, especially when this leads to delay, extending their time on a task.

A number of educational interventions have been developed to promote self-regulation, e.g. Stop–Think–Do, STAR (Stop–Act–Review), COPS (Capitalization–Organization–Punctuation–Spelling), PLAN (Preview the assignment; List main topics to write about; Assign an order to these topics; Note ideas in complete sentences). These focus on:
- Increasing selective attention
- Modifying impulsive responding
- Using verbal mediation to assist in academic and social problem solving
- Teaching self-instructional statements to facilitate analysis and synthesis of problems
- Providing strategies that may lead to improved peer relationships and the development of prosocial (socially desirable) behaviour.

The methods can be used to make children more consciously aware of – and ultimately take more responsibility for changing – unwanted behaviours. They are essentially self-management/organizational techniques. The strategies teach self-assessment, self-monitoring, self-instruction and self-reinforcement skills through role play and monitoring. The steps are rehearsed and accompanied, first by externalized speech, then sub-vocalization and ultimately progressing to internalized speech.

Self-instructions include focusing on the task and defining the problem. The child must then plan a strategy that will assist in solving the problem, including generating possible solutions and selecting one of these. Finally the performance is evaluated and the child reinforces him/herself if successful.

Medical management
Whilst school staff are not the professionals who coordinate or prescribe medication they are an important resource for the medical management team. Monitoring behaviour pre- and post-assessment and pre- and post-intervention is an integral part of medical or multimodal management.

Attributional training
The failure experience of the typical underachieving ADHD child is often related to lower self-esteem and negative self-attributions, with the causes of success and failure often perceived as external and uncontrollable (Lin and Hodge 1982, Rosenbaum and Baker 1984). Children who perceive past successes and failures as being caused by events outside

their control are less likely to use effort in new situations than are children who see events as within their control. Teaching children to attribute their failures to the controllable cause of insufficient effort results (when combined with success experiences) in greater motivation and improved performance (Dweck 1975, Licht et al. 1985). Teachers can therefore be provided with information on self-regulation, specific strategy training and attributional training to support the parallel sessions received by the children in cognitive therapy, so they can support the students to implement their knowledge in the classroom.

Recent studies have linked interpersonal relationships between teachers and students to motivational outcomes (Pianta 1992, Birch and Ladd 1996). Several authors have suggested that feelings of belonging and of being cared for can foster the adoption and internalization of goals and values of caregivers (Connell and Wellborn 1991, Noddings 1992, Baumeister and Leary 1995). According to Noddings (1992), the academic objectives cannot be met unless teachers provide students with a caring and supportive environment.

Educating parents and child

Education should not just be confined to the academic process. One essential part of ADHD management provides information about the condition to the child and parents at a level that they are able to accept and understand. This might include direct psychoeducation and/or reading materials and reference information. There are several excellent books describing ADHD from the child's perspective that will interest even the most reluctant reader.

Feeding back to the family after the child's assessment should be considered as part of the psychoeducation process. It is an opportunity to discus the diagnosis, prognosis and treatment options. It is often a relief to parents to be given a diagnosis but this is often the first step of the journey. For some parents the diagnosis will be official confirmation of their suspicions and they are usually very well informed. Others parents may need more educating. Given the media coverage that surrounds this disorder it is essential to their understanding of the condition to correct any misinformation they have been given. Whilst it is important that the child and his/her family have correct information about ADHD, it is just as important to stress the positive aspects of the child's development to provide a balanced view of the child that will ultimately help foster his/her self-esteem.

REFERENCES

Abramowitz AJ, O'Leary SG (1990) Effectiveness of delayed punishment in an applied setting. *Behav Ther* **21**: 231–239.
Abramowitz AJ, O'Leary SG, Futtersak MW (1988) The relative impact of long and short reprimands on children's off-task behaviour in the classroom. *Behav Ther* **19**: 243–247.
Anderson JC, Williams S, McGee R, Silva PA (1987) DSM-III disorders in preadolescent children. Prevalence in a large sample from the general population. *Arch Gen Psychiatry* 44: 69–76.
Barkley RA, Fisher M, Edelbrook CS, Smallish L (1990) The adolescent outcome of hyperactive children diagnosed by research criteria: I. An 8-year prospective follow-up study. *J Am Acad Child Adolesc Psychiatry* **29**: 546–557.
Barkley RA, Shelton TL, Crosswait C, Moorehouse M, Fletcher K, Barrett S, Jenkins L, Metevia L (2000) Multi-method psycho-educational intervention for preschool children with disruptive behavior: Preliminary results at post-treatment. *J Child Psychol Psychiatry* **41**: 319–332.

Baumeister RF, Leary MR (1995) The need to belong: Desire for interpersonal attachments as a fundamental human motivation. *Psychol Bull* **117**: 497–529.

Birch SH, Ladd GW (1996) Interpersonal relationships in the school environment and children's early school adjustment: The role of teachers and peers. In: Juvonen J, Wentzel K, eds. *Social Motivation: Understanding Children's Adjustment.* New York: Cambridge University Press, pp. 199–225.

Brown RT, Borden KA (1986) Hyperactivity at adolescence: some misconceptions and new directions. *J Clin Child Psychol* **15**: 194–209.

Chazan M (1994) The attitudes of mainstream teachers towards pupils with emotional and behavioural difficulties. *Eur J Special Needs Educ* **9**: 261–274.

Connell JP, Wellborn JG (1991) Competence, autonomy, and relatedness: A motivational analysis of self-system processes. In: Gunnar MR, Sroufe LA, eds. *Minnesota Symposium on Child Psychology, vol. 23.* Hillsdale, NJ: Erlbaum, pp. 43–77.

Cooper P, O'Regan FJ (2001) *Educating Children with AD/HD: A Teacher's Manual.* London: Routledge Falmer.

Dweck CS (1986) Motivational processes affecting learning. *Am Psychol* **41**: 1040–1048.

Gittelman-Klein R, Klein DF, Abikoff H, Katz S, Gloisten AC, Kates W (1976) Relative efficacy of methylphenidate and behavior modification in hyperkinetic children: an interim report. *J Abnorm Child Psychol* **4**: 361–379.

Hinshaw S, Klein R, Abikoff H (1998) Childhood attention-deficit/hyperactivity disorder: nonpharmacologic and combination treatments. In: Nathan PE, Gorman JM, eds. *A Guide to Treatments That Work.* Oxford: Oxford University Press, pp. 26–41.

Hoover-Dempsey, Sandler HM (1995) Parental involvement in children's education. Why does it make a difference? *Teachers Coll Rec* **95**: 310–335.

Hoover-Dempsey, Sandler HM (1997) Why do parents become involved in their children's education? *Rev Educ Res* **67**: 3–42.

Klein RG, Mannuzza S (1991) Long term outcome of hyperactive children: a review. *J Am Acad Child Adolesc Psychiatry* **30**: 383–387.

Lee S (1994) Family–school connections and students' education: Continuity and change of family involvement from the middle grades to high school. DPhil dissertation, Johns Hopkins University, Baltimore.

Licht BG, Kistner JA, Ozkaragoz T, Shapiro S, Clausen L (1985) Causal attributions of learning disabled children: Individual differences and their implications for persistence. *J Educ Psychol* **77**: 208–216.

Lin RT, Hodge GK (1982) Locus of control in childhood hyperactivity disorder. *J Consult Clin Psychol* **50**: 592–593.

Mannuzza S, Klein RG, Bessler A, Malloy P, Hynes ME (1997) Educational and occupational outcome of hyperactive boys grown up. *J Am Acad Child Adolesc Psychiatry* **36**: 1222–1227.

Mannuzza S, Klein RG, Bessler P, Malloy M (1998) Adult psychiatric status of hyperactive boys grown up. *Am J Psychiatry* **155**: 493–498.

Meijer C, Foster S (1988) The effect of teacher self-efficacy on referral chance. *J Special Educ* **22**: 378–385.

Minde K, Lewin D, Weiss G, Lavigueur H, Douglas V, Sykes E (1971) The hyperactive child in elementary school. A five year controlled follow-up. *Except Child* **38**: 215–221.

MTA Cooperative Group (1999) A 14-month randomized clinical trial of treatment strategies for attention-deficit/hyperactivity disorder (ADHD). *Arch Gen Psychiatry* **56**: 1073–1086.

Noddings N (1992) *The Challenge to Care in Schools.* New York: Teachers College Press.

O'Leary KD (1975) Behavioral assessment: an observational slant. In: Weinberg RA, Wood FH, eds. *Observation of Pupils and Teachers in Mainstream and Special Education Settings: Alternative Strategies.* Minneapolis: University of Minnesota Press, pp. 181–191.

O'Leary KD (1979) Behavioral assessment. *Behav Assess* **1**: 31–36.

Pianta RC (1992) Conceptual and methodological issues in research on relationships between children and non-parental adults. *New Dir Child Dev* **57**: 121–129.

Rosenbaum A, O'Leary KD, Jacob RJ (1975) Behavioural intervention with hyperactive children: Group consequences as a supplement to individual contingencies. *Behav Ther* **6**: 315–323.

Rosenbaum M, Baker E (1984) Self-control behavior in hyperactive and nonhyperactive children. *J Abnorm Child Psychol* **12**: 303–317.

Rubinstein R, Brown R (1981) An evaluation of the validity of the diagnostic category of ADD. *Am J Ortho-psychiatry* **54**: 398–414.

Shores R, Jack S, Gunter D, Ellis D, DeBriere T, Wehby J (1993) Classroom interactions of children with behaviour disorders. *J Emot Behav Disorder* **1**: 27–39.

Smith TEC, Polloway EA, Patton JR, Dowdy CA (1995) *Teaching Students with Special Needs in Inclusive Settings.* Boston: Allyn & Bacon

Sullivan MA, O'Leary SG (1990) Maintenance following reward and token programs. *Behav Ther* **21**: 139–149.

Weiss G, Hechtman LT (1993) *Hyperactive Children Grown Up, 2nd edn.* New York: Guilford Press.

Wells KC, Epstein JN, Hinshaw SP, Conners CK, Klaric J, Abikoff HB, Abramowitz A, Arnold LE, Elliot G, Greenhill LL, Hechtman L, Hoza B, Jensen PS, March JS, Pelham WE, Pfiffner L, Severe J, Swanson J, Vitiello B, Wigal T (2000a) Parenting and family stress treatment outcomes in attention deficit hyperactivity disorder (ADHD): An empirical analysis in the MTA study. *J Abnorm Child Psychol* **28**: 543–553.

Wells KC, Pelham WE, Kotkin RA, Hoza B, Abikoff HB, Abramowitz A, Arnold LE, Cantwell DP, Conners CK, Del Carmen R, Elliott G, Greenhill LL, Hechtman L, Hibbs E, Hinshaw SP, Jensen PS, March JS, Swanson JM, Schiller E (2000b) Psychosocial treatment strategies in the MTA study: Rationale, methods, and critical issues in design and implementation. *J Abnorm Child Psychol* **28**: 483–505.

Wener C (1990) *Developmental Psychopathology from Infancy to Adolescents.* New York: McGraw-Hill.

Worland J (1976) Effects of positive and negative feedback on behavior control in hyperactive and normal boys. *J Abnorm Child Psychol* **4**: 315–326.

Zentall SS (1985a) A context for hyperactivity. In: Gadow KD, ed. *Advances in Learning and Behavioral Disabilities.* Greenwich, CT: JAI Press, pp. 273–343.

Zentall SS (1985b) Stimulus control factors in search performance of hyperactive and non-hyperactive children. *J Learn Disabil* **18**: 480–485.

Zentall SS (1986) Effects of color stimulation on performance and activity of hyperactive and non hyperactive children. *J Educ Psychol* **78**: 159–165.

Zentall SS (1993) Research on the educational implications of attention deficit hyperactivity disorder. *Excep Child* **60**: 143–153.

Zentall SS, Zentall T (1976) Activity and task performance of hyperactive children as a function of environmental stimulation. *J Consult Clin Psychol* **44**: 693–697.

What is attention deficit hyperactivity disorder?
Attention deficit hyperactivity disorder (ADHD) is a term used to describe the condition of children who are inattentive, impulsive, and active at levels higher than expected for their mental and chronological age.

How is ADHD diagnosed?
The three core symptoms used to diagnose ADHD are:
- *Attention problems:* Inattention and distractibility, difficulty in sustaining attention and apparently not listening. Difficulties in organizing and following through instructions. Losing things and forgetfulness.
- *Impulsivity:* Difficulties in waiting for his/her turn, often blurting out answers before questions are completed. Butting into conversations or games.
- *Hyperactivity (restless overactivity):* Running about or climbing excessively, always on the go, fidgeting with hands or feet, or unable to sit still.

Britain, like most of Europe, uses the World Health Organization's International Statistical Classification of Diseases and Related Health Problems (ICD) system. The ICD category defined by the presence of all the three features above is called 'hyperkinetic disorder'. As well as these three features, the condition will have to have been present from an early age and in more than one setting, such as at home and in school. Hyperkinetic disorder occurs in about one child in 100, and in boys more often than girls.

In North America the American Psychiatric Association's Diagnostic and Statistical Manual of Mental Disorders (DSM) is used, where only one of the above criteria – attention problems or impulsivity/hyperactivity – is necessary to fulfil the diagnosis of 'attention deficit hyperactivity disorder'. This occurs in about 4–7% of school-age children.

The North American terminology and the wider diagnostic criteria used for ADHD are now common in the UK. It is recognized that a far greater number of children need help than those with the full set of features indicating hyperkinetic disorder.

It is important to stress that an ADHD *diagnosis* is made on the basis of a *recognizable behaviour pattern*. The *cause* of the behaviour may be complex. But children with the condition can be helped though good parenting, management at school and the controlled use of medication.

The symptoms of ADHD will often begin to diminish as the child or adolescent grows up. It is less common for adults to have ADHD.

Children with ADHD are difficult to bring up. They are liable to develop educational, behavioural and conduct problems or emotional difficulties and to suffer from low self-esteem.

What is the cause?
In the past, professionals tended to blame parents for the behaviour of a child with ADHD. Others have said the condition was due to additives in the food. However, research has not supported the popular view that ADHD is due to eating food additives, preservatives or sugar. Although the symptoms of some children get worse with certain foodstuffs, this is not the main cause of ADHD.

It is now known that ADHD is associated with a minor difference in the chemical tuning of the brain. It is commonly genetic, and many children with ADHD have a parent or close relative with a similar condition.

In rare cases ADHD is associated with pregnancy or birth complications. In a few cases it arises as a direct result of disease or trauma to the central nervous system.

Poor parental management is not thought to be a primary cause of ADHD but can make the symptoms worse.

What difficulties do children with ADHD present in the classroom?
Children with ADHD present many difficulties in the classroom.
- They find it difficult to listen to and take in instructions, are rarely ready to start their work, and often fail to complete a work set.
- They have difficulty concentrating, are easily distracted and are disorganized and forgetful.

- Other behaviours include: calling out, interrupting and butting into conversations inappropriately.
- Hyperactivity may be particularly marked in younger children who may have difficulties in staying in their seat. Some wriggle so much they actually fall out of their seats.
- Older children may appear more restless and fidgety, often fiddling dangerously with equipment.
- Children with ADHD are frequently unpopular with other children because of their unpredictable and irritating behaviour.

Children with ADHD are a challenge for the teacher but can be very rewarding if well managed.

All pupil learning is enhanced by increased attention to task so that the following strategies could well benefit the class as a whole not just the child with ADHD.

Classroom organization

The following *tips* are often found useful:
- Place pupils with ADHD in the least distracting place - not near a window or door.
- Seat children near the front and between good role models in a position where good eye contact can be maintained with the teacher.
- Working in pairs rather than groups and having a separate desk will be easier for the child with ADHD to manage.
- Write the timetable on the board or have it available daily.

Routines
- Clearly defined rules that are few in number and frequently rehearsed help to prompt the child with ADHD.
- Use consistent routines. Model and teach routines, e.g. turn-taking, distributing materials, sharing the equipment.
- Give warnings for beginning and ending of lessons. Children with ADHD have difficulty in re-focusing their attention when changing from one activity to another. Prepare them for the transition.
- Prepare pupils for changes to the timetable if known in advance, e.g. a change of teacher.
- Place particular emphasis on ensuring that all materials/equipment are readily available.
- Keep classroom interruptions to the minimum.

Structuring the learning tasks
- Give clear, concise instructions after establishing eye contact. Ask the pupil to repeat directions back to the teacher.
- Break tasks down into small steps – 'chunking'. Tasks should initially be short, and when mastered, gradually increased in complexity.
- Incorporate short breaks for physical activity into lessons that involve lengthy periods seated.
- Pair written instructions with oral instructions. Use a multi-sensory approach to learning.
- Give regular feedback, as children with ADHD respond to frequent positive reinforcement.
- Provide alternative ways for pupils to present their work, including tape, word processor, using teacher or peer as scribe, and through diagrams and pictures.
- Aid organization through the use of lists, daily task sheets, charts and report cards.
- Use highlighter pens to focus attention on key words and instructions.
- Use cooker timers for work completion, changing time on task, etc.

Strategies for managing behaviour

Remember that the behaviour of the child with ADHD is not intended to irritate teachers or peers. They are unable – not unwilling – to work. These pupils need help in managing their behaviour if they are to take advantage of the learning experiences of the classroom.
- Frequent use of praise and rewards. These should be given immediately. Pupils with ADHD respond better to immediate rather than delayed rewards. Reprimands should be brief and given calmly. They should be very specific and involve a reminder of the required task. Avoid sarcasm, anger and arguments.
- Minor disruptions are best ignored.
- Involve the pupil in his/her management plan. S/he will feel empowered and learn to problem-solve.
- Transition times as well as less structured times such as breaks and meal times should be closely monitored. The child with ADHD will find these difficult.
- Identify specific problem situations and specific behaviour problems (e.g. blurts out answers before questions have been completed; wanders around the classroom).

- Teach children to self-monitor. This is effective in reducing unwanted behaviours and is an important skill for children with ADHD to acquire.
- Praise appropriate behaviour at every opportunity.
- Use choices and distractions to avoid confrontations.
- Be alert to opportunities for incidental social skills training, e.g. joining in a conversation, making requests, paying and receiving compliments.
- Use whole-class rewards to encourage peer support.

General
- Teachers and parents need to work closely together. Use a school–home book or daily report card. A daily report card is a list of individual target behaviours that represent a child's most salient areas of impairment. Teachers set daily goals for each child's impairment targets, and parents provide rewards at home for attaining goals. Use a homework assignment chart that can be signed daily by parents, and supervise writing down of homework assignments.
- Check that the child has no other associated problems such as clumsiness or dyslexia, for which you may need help.
- The school's arrangements for medication should ensure that it is given reliably and with the minimum of fuss. It should be timed to avoid peaks and troughs and 'rebound'. For methylphenidate (Ritalin) this is generally 4 hours after the previous dose.
- Treat each day as a new beginning. Do not dwell on previous failings.

Many of these suggestions will already be in the repertoire of class teachers but will need to be prominent in the management of children with ADHD.

These strategies may be suitable for inclusion in pupils' Individual Educational Plans. More specific advice on behavioural management techniques including contingency management and response–cost reinforcement programmes, should be available from your local Educational Psychology service.

Further information
READING
- *Attention Deficit/Hyperactivity Disorder – a Practical Guide for Teachers.* Paul Cooper and Catherine Ideus. 1996. London: David Fulton.
- *ADD Hyperactivity Handbook for Schools.* Harvey C Parker. 1992. Plantation, FL: Specialty Press.
- *Attention Deficit Hyperactivity Disorder: a Multi-disciplinary Approach.* Henryk Holowenko. 1999. London: Jessica Kingsley.
- *ADD: Practical Activities in School.* Tony Attwood. 1998. City???: First and Best in Education.
- *Das Therapieprogramm für Kinder mit hyperkinetischen und oppositionellen Problemverhalten (THOP).* Manfred Döpfner, Stephanie Schürmann and Jan Frölich. 2002. Weinheim: BeltzPVU.

VIDEO
- Hyperactive Children in the Classroom. University of Southampton Media Services.

The above are obtainable in the UK from ADDISS (see Appendix 1.2 for contact details). ADDISS often run conferences that would be helpful to teachers.

8
PHARMACOTHERAPY IN ADHD

Paramala J Santosh

The neurochemical basis of ADHD is still unclear. The features of ADHD can, however, be relieved by drugs with actions on catecholaminergic neurotransmission, such as methylphenidate, implying an underlying impairment in dopaminergic function (Raskin et al. 1983, Cook et al. 1995) and noradrenergic function (Raskin et al. 1983). Medication can have greatly beneficial effects, but a difficulty with both psychosocial and pharmacological treatments of ADHD is the lack of maintenance of effects once treatment has been discontinued and the failure of generalization to settings in which treatment has not been active. Situations in which symptoms cause the most impairment should be targeted for treatment.

Pharmacotherapeutic strategy
- First-line medication: methylphenidate (immediate release, Concerta, Metadate CD, etc.), dexamphetamine, Adderall (immediate release and XR).
- Second-line medication: atomoxetine, guanfacine, imipramine, nortriptyline, bupropion, pemoline, clonidine.
- Third-line medication: carbamazepine, risperidone, buspirone, venlafaxine, nicotine patches.
- Experimental medication: moclobamide, cholinergic agents.

Indications for medication
Medication is usually necessary when treating hyperkinetic disorder. It is also to be considered if the disorder meets the DSM-IV criteria for ADHD or if psychological treatments have been insufficient alone in managing symptoms. Carefully crafted medication or enhanced monitoring as done in the NIMH Multimodal Treatment Study of Children with ADHD (MTA Cooperative Group 1999) is recommended only in those not responding to routine therapy.

Greater hyperactivity, inattention and clumsiness in the absence of emotional disorder predict greater positive response to methylphenidate (Taylor et al. 1987). However, it has also been shown that symptoms in those with less severe ADHD improve more completely. If hyperactivity is present only in one situation – e.g. just at school or at home – then stresses in that situation should be sought and alleviated as the first line of management. With *school-specific problems*, specific learning disabilities should be sought carefully through assessment by a clinical or educational psychologist. If present, then adjustment of educational techniques and expectations should be given a try before anti-hyperactivity treatments. If hyperactive behaviour is *confined to the home situation*, then the possibility of adverse parenting influences should be considered, leading to a parent training approach. In pervasive and severe cases, without autistic or affective comorbidity, a multimodal treatment approach will be needed. Medication should be initiated with proper monitoring of target symptoms. *Patients without hyperactivity (ADD)* may benefit from and tolerate lower doses of stimulants.

It is important to help people with ADHD and their families to understand the effects of medication and how it should be given. A factsheet is included as Appendix 8.1, and opportunities should be provided for responsive discussion.

Stimulants

Pharmacotherapy with psychostimulants is one of the key elements in the treatment of ADHD. The literature on stimulant medications – methylphenidate, dexamphetamine and pemoline – is voluminous. In most cases a stimulant is the first choice medication. More is known about stimulant use in children than about any other drug. Its onset of action is rapid, the dosage easy to titrate, and positive response often can be predicted from a single dose.

Methylphenidate use has a substantial evidence base: over treatment periods of up to 3 years (Jensen et al. 2005); numerous short-term studies; meta-analysis (McMaster University 1999); and several published clinical guidelines (European Clinical Guidelines for HKD – Taylor et al. 1998, 2004; UK Guidance on the Use of MPH for ADHD in Childhood – NICE 2000; Scottish National Clinical Guideline on Attention Deficit and HKD – SIGN 2001; US guidelines, e.g. AACAP 1997, 2002).

Most hyperactive children improve on stimulants, although actual response rates vary according to the measures used and definition of positive response. A study using a wide range of doses of methylphenidate and dexamphetamine found that 96% of children with ADHD improved behaviourally in response to one or both drugs (Elia et al. 1991). Contrary to common assumptions, stimulants have a wide variety of social effects in addition to improving the core symptoms of inattention, hyperactivity and impulsivity. Stimulant effects on attentional, academic, behavioural and social domains, however, are highly variable between individuals (Rapport et al. 1994).

Methylphenidate (MPH) is usually the first choice, although dexamphetamine may be preferred, for instance if the child has epilepsy, or pemoline in adolescents who have comorbid substance abuse and conduct disorder. The starting dose for MPH is 5 mg (for dexamphetamine, 2.5 mg) twice daily, with the dose being adjusted in the light of response. Dose is usually not calculated based on body weight but rather on individual response. However, the usual range for MPH is 0.2–0.7 mg/kg/dose rounded to the nearest 2.5 or 5 mg; this may need to rise as high as 15 mg three times a day before a response is seen. If very high doses are necessary, it is advised that a specialist be consulted. It is advised that the dosage is given as a three times a day schedule. Dexamphetamine dose is usually one half the dose of MPH, and the dose of pemoline is roughly 1.5 times the total daily dose of MPH.

Dexamphetamine often has a longer duration of action than MPH, permitting less frequent doses, but its disadvantages include greater risk of growth retardation, appetite suppression and compulsive behaviours, and higher potential for abuse by the patient's peers and family. Up to 25% respond positively to one of the drugs but not the other. Therefore, if one stimulant is insufficiently effective, another should be tried before using another drug class.

Magnesium pemoline has the least abuse potential of the stimulants. It may be given once a day, although absorption and metabolism vary widely and some children need two daily doses. It shows effects within the first 1–2 hours after a dose, lasting for 7–8 hours after ingestion (Sallee et al. 1992, Pelham et al. 1995). At current dose recommendations it may be as effective as the other stimulants, the half-life increasing with chronic administration (Sallee et al. 1985). However, the frequency of choreoathetoid movements (Sallee et al. 1989), insomnia, chemical hepatitis (Nehra et al. 1990) and even very rarely fulminant liver failure (Berkovitch et al. 1995) has resulted in pemoline being removed from both the the UK and US markets. If it is used, it should be in a specialist centre, and liver enzymes should be assessed before treatment because the onset of hepatitis is unpredictable and routine laboratory follow-up studies may not be sufficient. Instead patients should be alerted to notify the clinician immediately if nausea, vomiting, lethargy, malaise or jaundice appears, or if abdominal discomfort persists for more than two weeks.

LONG-ACTING STIMULANTS
In the last decade, one of the major advances in paediatric psychopharmacology has been the development of various extended-release delivery systems for stimulant drugs. Long-acting preparations are appealing for children for whom the standard formulations act briefly, for those who experience severe rebound, or for whom administering medication every four hours is inconvenient, stigmatizing or impossible. The most commonly used and systematically studied long-acting stimulants are the OROS MPH preparation (Concerta XL), a capsule containing a mixture of immediate- and delayed-release beads (Equasym XL), Dexedrine Spansule (dexamphetamine), and Adderall (a mixture of amphetamine salts). Extended-release preparations help make dosing more convenient for patient, parents and teachers; may improve efficacy through increasing compliance; may decrease potential for abuse and diversion; and have a favourable safety profile. Recent European guidelines (Banaschewski et al. 2006) suggest that treatment can be initiated using longer-acting stimulants such as Concerta. Concerta can be started as an 18 mg/day dose and increased weekly by 18 mg/day if necessary to a maximum of 54 mg/day.

PRECAUTIONS WITH STIMULANTS
Stimulants are contraindicated in the presence of schizophrenia, hyperthyroidism, cardiac arrhythmias, angina pectoris, glaucoma, or a history of hypersensitivity to drug. Stimulants should be used with caution in those with hypertension, depression, tics (or family history of Tourette syndrome), pervasive developmental disorders, severe mental retardation, or a history of substance use disorder.

SIDE-EFFECTS WITH STIMULANTS
Although the stimulants have an extremely high margin of safety, side-effects are similar for all stimulants and increase linearly with dose. Often waiting a few weeks or decreasing the dose eliminates or reduces common side-effects such as irritability, headaches, abdominal pain and loss of appetite. Mild *appetite suppression* is almost universal and may be addressed by giving medication after breakfast and lunch (Swanson et al. 1983), encouraging a high

calorie snack after dinner, and reducing the dose on weekends and during the summer. Persistent or severe side-effects may require changing drugs. *Rebound effects* consist of increased excitability, activity, talkativeness, irritability and insomnia beginning 4–15 hours after a dose. It may be seen as the last dose of the day wears off or for up to several days after sudden withdrawal of high daily doses of stimulants. This may resemble a worsening of the original symptoms and is encountered frequently by clinicians. Management strategies include increased structure after school, a dose of medication in the afternoon but smaller than the morning and midday doses, use of long-acting formulations, and the addition of clonidine or guanfacine to the regime. *Sleeplessness* is a frequent problem, and it is clinically important to distinguish those children whose insomnia is an unwanted effect of the drug from those children whose insomnia may be due to the recurrence (or worsening) of the behavioural difficulties as the medication effect subsides. For the first group of children the addition of clonidine before bedtime, decreasing the afternoon stimulant dose, or moving it to an earlier time may be sufficient. For the latter group, an evening dose of a stimulant may be helpful (Green 1991). Persistent *stimulant-related dysphoria* may decrease with lowering the dose, but may require switching to a different stimulant or to an antidepressant medication. The use of stimulants for patients with *tics* has been controversial and is discussed later in this chapter. *Growth retardation* (decrease in expected weight and height gain) resulting from stimulant use is small although it may be statistically significant. The magnitude is dose related and appears to be greater with dexamphetamine than with MPH or pemoline (Zeiner 1995). It can be minimized by using drug-free periods, and preliminary data on adolescents show no significant deviation from expected weight and height growth velocities (Vincent et al. 1990). Although in general there are no adverse *cardiovascular effects* of stimulants, black male adolescents may be at a higher risk from mild chronic elevation in blood pressure (Brown and Sexson 1989). There is little evidence that stimulants produce a decrease in the *seizure* threshold (Crumrine et al. 1987) or that *addiction* results from the prescription of stimulants for ADHD. *Self-initiated increase in dose* by emotionally unstable adults with substance use disorders is possible and needs to be suspected in those who repeatedly claim to have lost medication, or in parents who repeatedly insist that higher doses are necessary to control symptoms, when the child is functioning well in other settings. It may be better to use long-acting preparations such as Concerta as this is relatively safe, being very difficult to abuse because of the delivery system. Other drugs that are useful in this setting are atomoxetine and bupropion. MPH can be used in the presence of well-controlled epilepsy. If seizures worsen or emerge during treatment, MPH needs to be changed to dexamphetamine.

MONITORING WITH STIMULANTS
When children are started on stimulants one needs to monitor pulse and blood pressure at each increase and subsequently every 3–6 months. Adverse effects should be monitored by parents, e.g. with the rating scale presented in Appendix 8.2. A detailed scheme of dosage and monitoring is provided in Chapter 11, but will of course need to be adjusted to local circumstances. Weight and height should be charted at least 6 monthly and should be monitored using a growth chart. Tics, depression, irritability, lack of spontaneity, withdrawal

and excessive perseveration should be monitored at each visit. Routine haematological tests are unnecessary.

Non-stimulant medication

The leading drug treatment in ADHD remains the use of central sympathomimetic stimulants. Abundant randomized controlled trials have shown the superiority of this approach to placebo (Santosh and Taylor 2000) and behaviour therapy (MTA Cooperative Group 1999). The stimulants' value has been extended by the introduction of extended-release preparations (Wolraich et al. 2001). They have, however, attracted strong public controversy, and families are sometimes deterred from the treatment by media publicity. Some families encounter adverse effects of the medication and therefore stop it. Some children do not respond at all.

Effective non-stimulant drugs could have advantages. A different mechanism of action could lead to useful effects on subgroups of children, or types of problems that are not helped by current treatments. Drugs without abuse potential might prove more acceptable to prescribers and consumers. Several such drugs are in frequent use, though most are not licensed for the purpose. Atomoxetine is the first non-stimulant drug to be licensed worldwide for use in paediatric and adult ADHD.

Atomoxetine

Atomoxetine (previously termed tomoxetine) works as a selective presynaptic noradrenaline reuptake inhibitor, with little affinity for other noradrenergic receptors or other neurotransporters or receptors. The plasma half-life is usually about 4 hours; an active metabolite, 4-hydroxyatomoxetine, is excreted in urine after glucuronidation. In 5–10% of people, a polymorphism of the cytochrome enzyme P450 2D6 leads to a longer plasma half-life of up to 19 hours.

Atomoxetine is the first non-stimulant medication approved for treating ADHD and is a specific noradrenaline reuptake inhibitor. There is good evidence of its efficacy in ADHD and it is a non-scheduled drug, which has advantages. It is to be used at a dose of 1.2 mg/kg body weight, up to a maximum of 1.8 mg/kg. It can be used as either a once or twice daily dose, and appears reasonably safe. It produces minimal increase in blood pressure, heart rate and gastrointestinal symptoms (nausea and vomiting are possible especially during the early part of treatment). It may be particularly useful in those with comorbid tics or anxiety/depression (studies indicate its effect, but no clear studies test whether it is better than MPH in these circumstances); or in those who have not responded to stimulants (of whom about one-third will respond to atomoxetine). Symptoms have usually started to improve by 3–4 weeks, but the full effect may not be apparent for 6–8 weeks (unlike with stimulants), so parents have to be informed about this possible delay at the start of treatment. Atomoxetine can be initiated at half the required total dose, then increased over the next couple of weeks to the necessary dose in order to decrease the chances of side-effects (especially upper gastrointestinal effects).

So far there are insufficient grounds on which to compare the newer drug with established treatments. The effect sizes reported seem a little smaller than those of MPH, but not necessarily significantly so. Kratochvil et al. (2002) have reported a random allocation, but non-blind, comparison of atomoxetine with methylphenidate: the effect on ADHD ratings and the frequency of adverse effects were similar. (Vomiting and sleepiness were commoner with atomoxetine, but were usually transient.) A poster presentation in 2004 by Jeffery Newcorn and colleagues gave a brief description of a randomized blind comparison, which unfortunately is not yet otherwise published. It indicated that atomoxetine was less effective than OROS-MPH. This trial did, however, exclude children who had previously had a poor response to MPH. This was for sound ethical reasons – it would scarcely have been justifiable to randomize them to a drug known not to help them. But the effect could well have been to bias the comparison in Concerta's favour; and a subgroup analysis of children who had not previously received stimulants (the key group for clinicians choosing the first treatment) yielded no significant differences between the preparations.

The cost of atomoxetine is greater than that of extended-release preparations such as OROS-MPH, so it is not usually the first choice. Its different mode of action, however, gives hope that it will avoid some problems. The level of dopamine as well as noradrenaline is raised in rat prefrontal cortex with atomoxetine, but not (unlike with MPH) in striatum or nucleus accumbens (Bymaster et al. 2002). It could therefore be valuable in cases where tics, pervasive developmental disorder, anxiety or Tourette syndrome are also present and may be worsened by stimulants. It is not a controlled drug, and this will reassure prescribers and families. One should remember, though, that in this population stimulants are more likely to be a protection against the development of substance abuse than a risk for it.

Antidepressants
Antidepressants have been in use for many years. The antidepressants that work in ADHD increase available levels of catecholamines, typically noradrenaline. Although far less studied than stimulants, controlled trials of tricyclic antidepressants in both children and adolescents demonstrate efficacy in the treatment of ADHD (Spencer et al. 1996, Popper 1997). Despite the narrow margin of safety, they may be used as second-line drugs for stimulant non-responsive ADHD, and for those who develop significant depression or other side-effects on stimulants and patients with comorbid tics or Tourette syndrome, anxiety disorder or depression. Their longer duration of action averts the need for a dose at school, and rebound is not a problem. Efficacy in improving cognitive symptoms does not appear as great as for stimulants. Drawbacks include serious potential cardiotoxicity, especially in pre-pubertal children; the danger of accidental or intentional overdose; troublesome sedation and anti-cholinergic side-effects; and possibly declining efficacy over time.

IMIPRAMINE
Imipramine is a tricyclic antidepressant that has been used in ADHD. Many reports, including double-blind placebo-controlled randomized trials, have demonstrated that imipramine is effective in ADHD. In children over 6 years, one should start with 10 mg daily and increase over 10 days to 20 mg up to the age of 8 years; to 20–50 mg up to the age of 14 years; and to 50–80 mg for patients over 14 years.

In adults, start with 25 mg and gradually increase to 150 mg/day maximum. The maintenance dose in adults is 50–150 mg/day. Drawbacks include potential cardiotoxicity, especially in pre-pubertal children; the danger of accidental or intentional overdose; troublesome sedation; anticholinergic side-effects; lowering seizure threshold; and possibly declining efficacy over time. Careful monitoring of therapeutic efficacy, vital signs and ECG at baseline and follow-up is expected. Parents must be reminded to supervise administration of medication and to keep pills in a safe place.

DESIPRAMINE

Desipramine is a noradrenergic tricyclic antidepressant that has been shown to be useful in ADHD. It is a second-line treatment but has significant cardiac side-effects. Desipramine dose should be built up gradually to a maximum of 2.5 mg/kg/day in divided dosage. Pulse, blood pressure and ECG should be monitored at baseline and 3 monthly, and plasma levels may be necessary if anything more than a small dose is used. One should watch for tachyarrythmias, and QTc interval should be monitored. Female patients appear to reach higher blood levels with same weight-adjusted dosage than male patients and also show more side-effects. Desipramine has fewer anticholinergic side-effects than imipramine but it is more cardiotoxic. Divided doses should be prescribed, to produce more stable levels. It has been withdrawn in the UK after reports of unexplained deaths.

BUPROPION

Bupropion (an aminoketone) is a relatively new monocyclic antidepressant that undergoes extensive biotransformation to three metabolites that are pharmacologically active. An increased incidence of side-effects may be associated with increased levels of the metabolite hydroxybupropion. Its actions are primarily noradrenergic and anticholinergic, while antihistaminic and orthostatic–hypotensive effects are negligible. Its major use is as an aid in the cessation of cigarette smoking. Bupropion may decrease hyperactivity and aggression and perhaps improve cognitive performance of children with ADHD and conduct disorder (Conners et al. 1996), and was found to be as effective as MPH in a double-blind, controlled trial (Barrickman et al. 1995). It is administered in two or three divided doses daily, beginning with 50 mg b.i.d. and gradually increasing to a maximum of 250 mg/day in children and 350 mg/day in adolescents. Its most serious side-effect is a decrease in seizure threshold, and it may exacerbate tics. Side-effects may worsen if bupropion is combined with fluoxetine.

VENLAFAXINE

Venlafaxine (a phenylethylamine) inhibits reuptake of both serotonin and noradrenaline, and has no significant affinity for muscarinic, cholinergic, histaminic or alpha-1-adrenergic receptors. It has a relatively short half-life in adults (3–7 hours) and is given in divided doses. Open trials of venlafaxine in adult ADHD suggest that it is useful in treating the core symptoms of ADHD (Hedges et al. 1995).

Alpha-2 adrenergic agonists

GUANFACINE HYDROCHLORIDE

This is a long-acting alpha-2 agonist and has a more favourable side-effect profile than clonidine. It has recently been used as monotherapy for children with ADHD and Tourette syndrome, whose tics become worse with the use of stimulants. It has also been used in combination with a stimulant in the treatment of children with ADHD who cannot tolerate the sedative side-effects of clonidine or in whom clonidine has too short a duration of action leading to rebound effects. As yet only open trials have been published (Chappell et al. 1995, Hunt et al. 1995).

CLONIDINE
Clonidine has been shown in placebo-controlled trials to attenuate hyperactivity and disruptive behaviours (but not inattention) in ADHD children (Connor et al. 1999). Clonidine is initiated at a dose of 25–50 µg at bedtime and the dose is titrated gradually over several weeks up to 150–300 µg per day in three or four divided doses. Pulse and blood pressure should be monitored for bradycardia and hypotension. When discontinuing clonidine, the dose should be tapered rather than stopped suddenly; and erratic compliance with medication increases the risk of adverse cardiovascular events. Families should be cautioned about this, and clonidine should not be prescribed if it cannot be administered reliably. Depression and impairment of glucose tolerance can occur.

Antipsychotics
RISPERIDONE
Risperidone is an atypical neuroleptic, with a combination of dopaminergic and serotonergic actions that are usually prescribed for other indications such as schizophrenia and aggressive behaviour in people with mental retardation. The preliminary evidence suggests that it is effective in controlling aggressive and disruptive behaviour in children with ADHD. Common adverse effects include overeating and obesity; dietary advice should be given before prescription, and growth should be monitored. Prolactin is often raised, and can cause symptoms; blood glucose and lipid metabolism are sometimes altered. Extrapyramidal symptoms (including neuroleptic malignant syndrome) are much less common than when typical neuroleptics are prescribed. The drug's place seems likely to be reserved for severely aggressive problems when behavioural therapy and stimulants have been insufficient.

HALOPERIDOL
Haloperidol should be used only in low dose and unusual circumstances because of lesser effectiveness relative to other drugs, sedation, potential cognitive dulling, and the risks of tardive dyskinesia and neuroleptic malignant syndrome.

Other drugs
Buspirone is a full 5HT1A agonist at the somatodendritic autoreceptor and a partial agonist at the postsynaptic 5HT1A receptors. Buspirone acts on the noradrenergic, serotonergic and dopaminergic receptor systems. An open clinical trial has suggested that it can help to improve hyperactivity, impulsivity and oppositionality (Malhotra and Santosh 1998).

Acetylcholinesterase inhibitors, such as donepezil, have been suggested – especially for the treatment of residual cognitive problems in people who have benefited from other drugs – on the basis of small-scale open trials (Wilens et al. 2002).

Other drugs used in practice include carbamazepine, moclobamide and nicotine receptor agonists.

Combination of a stimulant and a non-stimulant

The problems presented by severe hyperactivity can be very severe, and families may become desperate. Clinicians often feel pressed to prescribe unduly high dosages (for which there is no evidence of value) and combinations of drugs, sometimes to target different aspects of the symptom complex. This can be justifiable in extreme cases, but the concurrent use of inadequately evaluated drugs can create hazards, and call for specialist advice and careful monitoring. The most common combination currently used for ADHD is *a stimulant and clonidine*, although there are no published trials of safety or efficacy. The combination is theoretically appealing due to complementary actions and non-overlapping side-effect profiles. Anecdotal clinical experience supports the usefulness of these two drugs, especially for children with severe ADHD who cannot be managed satisfactorily with stimulant alone. However, there have been recent reports of unexplained deaths in three children who at one time had been taking both MPH and clonidine, but the evidence linking the drugs to the deaths is tenuous at best (Fenichel 1995, Popper 1995, Swanson et al. 1995). Pending clarification, extra caution is advised when treating children with cardiac or cardiovascular disease. When combining clonidine with additional medications or if dosing of medication is inconsistent (Swanson et al. 1995) an alternative strategy might be to substitute dex-amphetamine for MPH or guanfacine for clonidine.

The combination of *imipramine and MPH* has been associated with a syndrome of confusion, affective lability, marked aggression and severe agitation (Grob and Coyle 1986). The combination of imipramine and MPH can increase plasma levels of imipramine and has been associated with a syndrome of confusion, affective lability, marked aggression and severe agitation. As blood levels of desipramine can increase unpredictability with MPH, blood levels may be necessary for monitoring, if used in combination.

Developmental trajectory and medication response

ADHD IN PRESCHOOLERS

Behavioural interventions such as parent training approaches are useful. Stimulants are probably less effective than in school-age children and produce greater side-effects.

ADHD IN SCHOOL-AGE CHILDREN

Medication is superior to behavioural interventions in this age-group. Behavioural interventions are essential when treating comorbidity in ADHD. In children with ADHD, administration of MPH results in more precise timing performance and an enhancement in working memory (Baldwin et al. 2004).

ADHD IN ADOLESCENTS

Non-compliance with medication is a greater problem in treatment of adolescents due to their desire to avoid taking medication during school hours and the increased prevalence of stimulant-related dysphoria. The risk of misuse of stimulants is increased in adolescents; giving or selling medication to peers is more common than abuse by the patients themselves. The drug interactions that could result from undisclosed substance misuse should always be borne in mind. Concerta or atomoxetine are good options in this group. Adolescents with ADHD demonstrate significantly less variability and better driving performance when receiving OROS-MPH q.d. compared to MPH t.i.d., particularly in the evenings (Cox et al. 2004).

ADHD IN ADULTS

It is difficult to develop clinical skills in the management of residual adult manifestations of developmental disorders without clinical experience with their presentation in childhood. Adult patients are increasingly seeking treatment for the symptoms of ADHD, and physicians need practice guidelines. Adult ADHD often presents differently from childhood ADHD. Because adult ADHD can be comorbid with other disorders and has symptoms similar to those of other disorders, it is important to understand differential diagnoses. Physicians should work with patients to provide feedback about their symptoms, to educate them about ADHD, and to set treatment goals. Treatment for ADHD in adults should include a medication trial, restructuring of the patient's environment to make it more compatible with the symptoms of ADHD, and ongoing supportive management to address any residual impairment and to facilitate functional and developmental improvements (Weiss and Weiss 2004). Atomoxetine is the one medication with a licence for use in adults – if they have been treated in childhood (but, confusingly, not if the first presentation is in adult life). Both stimulants and atomoxetine are effective in adults but the effect size is marginally lower than in children.

Medication in the presence of comorbidity

ADHD IN THE PRESENCE OF TOURETTE SYNDROME

As many as 60% of the children with ADHD develop transient, usually subtle, tics when one of the stimulant medications is initiated (Borcherding et al. 1990, Ikowicz et al. 1992). Stimulants should be used with caution when there is a patient or family history of tics. If ADHD symptoms cause functional impairment and other medications are ineffective or have unacceptable side-effects, and if parents are capable of close monitoring, a stimulant may be used even with a history of tics. If tics appear or worsen, the usual response is to observe for a few days or weeks, but if tics remain problematic, dose reduction or a different medication may be tried. Clinical judgement is required to balance the relative impairment from tics and from ADHD symptoms, and in considering efficacy and safety of stimulants versus other medication or psychosocial treatments. For children who already have Tourette syndrome or chronic tics, low to moderate doses of *methylphenidate* often improve attention and behaviour without significantly worsening the tics (Gadow et al. 1992). On the other hand, withdrawal of chronic MPH in children with ADHD and Tourette syndrome may result in a decrease in tic frequency and severity, with an increase when MPH is re-initiated. Some studies have found worsening of tics in 25–30% of patients (Spencer et al. 1996). The few studies available suggest that clonidine is as effective in children with

Tourette syndrome plus ADHD, as in children with ADHD without tics (Leckman et al. 1991). Tricyclic antidepressants (TCAs) such as *desipramine*, *imipramine* and *nortryptiline* appear to reduce ADHD symptoms without affecting the severity of tics (Riddle et al. 1988; Spencer et al. 1993a,b). The usual daily starting dose of TCAs is 25 mg, increasing by 25 mg increments every 1–2 weeks. Most children respond to doses between 25 and 100 mg/day given in once or twice daily doses. Side-effects of low-dose TCAs (25–100 mg/day), are generally minimal, but potential cardiotoxic effects have to be monitored during treatment.

ADHD WITH ANXIETY
Studies conflict on whether response to stimulants is reduced in children and adolescents with comorbid anxiety disorders. Low doses of MPH have been shown to produce an elevation of heart rate in children with ADHD with comorbid anxiety (Tannock et al. 1995). Pliska (1989) found fewer stimulant responders amongst subjects with ADHD and comorbid anxiety, and some had a placebo response as large as the stimulant response itself. Despite some other studies finding that children with comorbid anxiety responded as well as those without anxiety (Livingston et al. 1992, Gadow et al. 1995), it is currently generally accepted that stimulants are not the first-line drugs in this group. Patients with ADHD and comorbid anxiety disorder or depression may actually respond better to TCAs than to stimulants (Kutcher et al. 1992, Spencer et al. 1996). Buspirone may be an appropriate choice in this population.

ADHD WITH MENTAL RETARDATION
Patients with ADHD and comorbid mental retardation may benefit from and tolerate lower doses of stimulants. Among mentally retarded children with ADHD, higher parent ratings of impulsivity and activity, and higher teacher ratings of activity, impulsivity, inattention and conduct problems predict greater positive response to stimulants. Children with an IQ <45 are much less likely to have a clinically significant positive response. These children are at greater risk for side-effects including tics and social withdrawal (Handen et al. 1991, Santosh and Baird 1999).

ADHD WITH CONDUCT DISORDER
No single intervention is effective with severe conduct disorder. Multimodal interventions must target each domain assessed as dysfunctional, and must be suited to the age and ethnicity of the patient. Treatment must be delivered long enough to make a difference. Multiple services delivered in a continuum of care are best suited for treatment of conduct disorder. Although stimulants and other medication are frequently prescribed to preschool children with conduct disorder, there is no convincing support that medication is effective in the short or long term, especially in the absence of ADHD. In all cases of conduct disorder, psychophar-macological treatment alone is insufficient. The best case for medication can be made for management of comorbid ADHD symptoms with stimulants (Hinshaw et al. 1989, Hinshaw 1992). It is diagnostically essential in these youths with multiple comorbid disorders to perform an extensive psychiatric evaluation and review using numerous informants.

If there is a subgroup of adolescents with ADHD who may potentially abuse prescribed psychostimulants, it may be those who also have substance use disorder and conduct disorder. An important treatment consideration is to establish a prior history of response and duration of ADHD treatment, noting whether any previous abuse of medication existed. Although abstinence from all illicit substances prior to psychopharmacological treatment is ideal, this rarely occurs in adolescent outpatients with substance use disorders and conduct disorders. Once serious substance abuse is significantly reduced, by using cognitive behavioural techniques and/or systemic family therapy, one can begin cautious and carefully monitored psychopharmacological treatment of the ADHD. It might be preferable to treat such adolescents with medication that have a lower abuse potential such as Concerta or pemoline (Riggs et al. 1995) or buprapion (Conners et al. 1996). Although TCAs can be effective in treating ADHD, they may be too dangerous in these very impulsive youths, with potential untoward interactions when used with illicit substances and high mortality in overdose.

Effect evaluation

Factor scores from the Attention Problems and Hyperactivity domains of the Achenbach Child Behavior Checklist 6–18 (CBCL/6-18) and Teacher's Report Form (TRF) (Achenbach 2001) and the Conners' scales (Conners 1997, 1998a,b) can be used to monitor after a week of treatment. Both parents and school should be used in target symptom monitoring. Comparison with placebo is powerful but unnecessary.

INTEGRATION OF APPROACHES

The MTA study (MTA Cooperative Group 1999) showed that there are many advantages of adding medication to behaviour therapy but little advantage of adding behaviour therapy to medication. Combined therapy has some benefits especially in controlling aggressive behaviour at home, improving the overall sense of satisfaction of parents and in achieving 'normalization'. However, the routine use of combination treatment is not cost-effective.

Choice of treatment

Although behaviour therapy may be less effective, it may still be offered if opted for by family or child. Multimodal behaviour therapy with parent training, school intervention and cognitive–behavioural therapy is effective, especially in milder cases. The re-analyses of the MTA data suggest that in those with hyperkinetic disorder, medication is clearly superior to behavioural treatment, and so it may be sensible to initiate treatment with stimulants in this subgroup of ADHD as the first-line treatment. In those who are treated with only behavioural therapy, one should move to using stimulants or other medication within 8–12 weeks, if optimal control of symptoms has not been achieved (Santosh et al. 2005).

Attention deficit disorder (ADD) without hyperactivity

Stimulants continue to remain useful in this subtype of the disorder, but lower doses may be required for optimal control. One has to be clear that the impairment is not attributable to global learning difficulty, and that it can be attributable to ADD. Medication improves attentiveness in all subtypes of ADHD, including ADD (Barbaresi et al. 2006).

Adjunctive treatments

Despite medication remaining the mainstay of treatment, other adjunctive treatments may be necessary to optimize outcomes. Training of social competence may be important, especially in those who have poor social skills. Individual psychotherapy may be helpful in managing low self-esteem, and family support, psychoeducation and respite care may be useful. Remedial education may also help in some cases. Appropriate behavioural interventions for comorbid conditions are essential.

Duration of treatment

Treatment trial evidence extends to 36 months, and discontinuation trial evidence shows that need can end. Adult trial evidence shows continued efficacy. It is recommended that a trial discontinuation is undertaken every 12 months. However, long term treatment may be necessary in a subgroup of subjects.

Conclusion

Most children with ADHD who need drug therapy are best served at present by a stimulant and, if that fails, by a trial of a second stimulant. Non-stimulant drugs may prove of particular value when the family fears a stimulant, or includes drug-abusing members; or when adverse reactions (such as anxiety) or complicating factors (such as autism or tics) limit the value of stimulants. Atomoxetine is the best evaluated of the non-controlled drugs and the only one so far to be licensed. When aggressive behaviour is severe, and is associated with mental retardation or autism spectrum disorder, then risperidone is probably the best established alternative; but cautious clinicians are likely first to try a less toxic drug.

REFERENCES

AACAP (1997) AACAP Official Action. Practice parameters for the assessment and treatment of children, adolescents, and adults with attention-deficit/hyperactivity disorder. *J Am Acad Child Adolesc Psychiatry* **36** (Suppl): 85S–121S.

AACAP (2002) AACAP Official Action. Practice parameter for the use of stimulant medications in the treatment of children, adolescents and adults. *J Am Acad Child Adolesc Psychiatry* **41** (Suppl): 26S–49S.

Achenbach T (2001) *Manual for the ASEBA School-Age Forms and Profiles.* Burlington, VT: ASEBA/Research Center for Children, Youth and Families.

Baldwin RL, Chelonis JJ, Flake RA, Edwards MC, Field CR, Meaux JB, Paule MG (2004) Effect of methylphenidate on time perception in children with attention-deficit/hyperactivity disorder. *Exp Clin Psychopharmacol* **12**: 57–64.

Banaschewski T, Coghill D, Santosh P, Zuddas A, Asherson P, Buitelaar J,Danckaerts M, Dopfner M, Faraone SV, Rothenberger A, Sergeant J, Steinhausen HC, Sonuga-Barke EJ, Taylor E. (2006) Long-acting medications for the hyperkinetic disorders : A systematic review and European treatment guideline. *Eur Child Adolesc Psychiatry* [Epub ahead of print.]

Barbaresi WJ, Katusic SK, Colligan RC, Weaver AL, Leibson CL, Jacobsen SJ (2006) Long-term stimulant medication treatment of attention deficit/hyperactivity disorder: results from a population-based study. *J Dev Behav Pediatr* **27**: 1–10.

Barrickman LL, Perry PJ, Allen AJ, Kuperman S, Arndt SV, Herrmann KJ, Schumacher E (1995) Bupropion versus methylphenidate in the treatment of attention deficit hyperactivity disorder. *J Am Acad Child Adolesc Psychiatry* **34**: 649–657.

Berkovitch M, Pope E, Phillips J, Koren G (1995) Pemoline-associated fulminant liver failure: testing the evidence for causation. *Clin Pharmacol Ther* **57**: 696–698.

Borcherding BG, Keysor CS, Rapoport JL, Elia J, Amass J (1990) Motor/vocal tics and compulsive behaviours on stimulant drugs: is there a common vulnerability? *Psychiatry Res* **33**: 83–94.

Brown RT, Sexson SB (1989) Effects of methylphenidate on cardiovascular responses in attention deficit hyperactivity disordered adolescents. *J Adol Health Care* **10**: 179–183.

Bymaster FP, Katner JS, Nelson DL, Hemrick-Luecke SK, Threlkeld PG, Heiligenstein JH, Morin SM, Gehlert DR, Perry KW (2002) Atomoxetine increases extracellular levels of norepinephrine and dopamine in prefrontal cortex of rat: a potential mechanism for efficacy in attention deficit/hyperactivity disorder. *Neuropsychopharmacology* **27**: 699–711.

Chappell PB, Riddle MA, Scahill L, Lynch KA, Schultz R, Arnsten A, Leckman JF, Cohen DJ (1995) Guanfacine treatment of comorbid attention-deficit hyperactivity disorder and Tourette's syndrome: preliminary clinical experience. *J Am Acad Child Adolesc Psychiatry* **34**: 1140–1146.

Conners CK (1997) A new self-report scale for assessment of adolescent psychopathology: Factor structure, reliability, validity, and diagnostic sensitivity. *J Abnor Child Psychol* **25**: 487–497.

Conners CK, Casat CD, Gualtieri CT, Weller E, Reader M, Reiss A, Weller RA, Khayrallah M, Ascher J (1996) Bupropion hydrochloride in attention deficit disorder with hyperactivity. *J Am Acad Child Adolesc Psychiatry* **35**: 1314–1321.

Conners CK, Silarenios G, Parker JD, Epstein JN (1998a) The revised Conners' Parent Rating Scale (CPRS-R): factor structure, reliability, criterion validity. *J Abnor Child Psychol* **26**: 257–268.

Conners CK, Silarenios G, Parker JD, Epstein JN (1998b) Revision and restandardization of the Conners Teacher Rating Scale (CTRS-R): factor structure, reliability, criterion validity. *J Abnor Child Psychol* **26**: 279–291.

Connor DF, Fletcher KE, Swanson JM (1999) A meta-analysis of clonidine for symptoms of attention-deficit hyperactivity disorder. *J Am Acad Child Adolesc Psychiatry* **38**: 1551–1559.

Cook EH, Stein MA, Krasowski MD, Cox NJ, Olkon DM, Kieffer JE, Leventhal BL (1995) Association of attention-deficit disorder and the dopamine transporter gene. *Am J Hum Genet* **56**: 993–998.

Cox DJ, Merkel RL, Penberthy JK, Kovatchev B, Hankin CS (2004) Impact of methylphenidate delivery profiles on driving performance of adolescents with attention-deficit/hyperactivity disorder: a pilot study, *J Am Acad Child Adolesc Psychiatry* **43**: 269–275.

Crumrine PK, Feldman HM, Teodori J, Handen BL, Alvin RM (1987) The use of methylphenidate in children with seizures and attention deficit disorder. *Ann Neurol* **22**: 441–442.

Elia J, Borcherding BG, Rapoport JL, Keysor CS (1991) Methylphenidate and dextroamphetamine treatments of hyperactivity: are there true non-responders? *Psychiatry Res* **36**: 141–155.

Fenichel RR (1995) Combining methylphenidate and clonidine: the role of post-marketing surveillance. *J Child Adolesc Psychopharmacol* **5**: 155–156.

Gadow KD, Nolan EE, Sverd J (1992) Methylphenidate in hyperactive boys with comorbid tic disorder: II. Short-term behavioural effects in school settings. *J Am Acad Child Adolesc Psychiatry* **31**: 462–470.

Gadow KD, Sverd J, Sparfkin J, Nolan EE, Ezor SN (1995) Efficacy of methylphenidate for ADHD in children with tic disorder. *Arch Gen Psychiatry* **52**: 444–455.

Green WH (1991) *Child and Adolescent Clinical Psychopharmacology.* Baltimore: Williams & Wilkins.

Grob CS, Coyle JT (1986) Suspected adverse methylphenidate–imipramine interactions in children. *J Dev Behav Pediatr* **7**: 265–267

Handen BL, Feldman H, Gosling A, Breaux AM, McAuliffe S (1991) Adverse side effects of methylphenidate among mentally retarded children with ADHD. *J Am Acad Child Adolesc Psychiatry* **30**: 241–245.

Hedges D, Reimherr FW, Rogers A, Strong R, Wender PH (1995) An open trial of venlafaxine in adult patients with attention deficit hyperactivity disorder. *Psychopharmacol Bull* **31**: 779–783.

Hinshaw S (1992) Academic underachievement, attention deficits, and aggression: comorbidity and implications. *J Consult Clin Psychol* **60**: 893–903.

Hinshaw S, Buhrmester D, Heller T (1989) Anger control in response to verbal provocation: effects of stimulant medication for boys with ADHD. *J Abnorm Child Psychol* **17**: 393–407.

Hunt RD, Arnsten AFT, Asbell MD (1995) An open trial of guanfacine in the treatment of attention-deficit hyperactivity disorder. *J Am Acad Child Adolesc Psychiatry* **34**: 50–54.

Jensen PS, Garcia JA, Glied S, Crowe M, Foster M, Schlander M, Hinshaw S, Vitiello B, Arnold LE, Elliott G, Hechtman L, Newcorn JH, Pelham WE, Swanson J, Wells K (2005) Cost-effectiveness of ADHD treatments: findings from the multimodal treatment study of children with ADHD. *Am J Psychiatry* **162**: 1628–1636.

Kratochvil CJ, Heiligenstein JH, Dittman R, Spencer TJ, Biederman J, Wernicke J, Newcorn JH, Casat C, Milton

131

D, Michelson D (2002) Atomoxetine and methylphenidate treatment in children with ADHD: a prospective, randomized, open-label trial. *J Am Acad Child Adolesc Psychiatry* **41**: 776–784

Kutcher SP, Reiter S, Gardner DM, Klein RG (1992) The pharmacotherapy of anxiety disorders in children and adolescents. *Psychiatr Clin N Am* **15**: 41–67.

Leckman JF, Hardin MT, Riddle MA, Stevenson J, Ort SI, Cohen DJ (1991) Clonidine treatment of Gilles de la Tourette's syndrome. *Arch Gen Psychiatry* **48**: 324–328.

Malhotra S, Santosh PJ (1998) An open clinical trial of buspirone in children with AD/HD. *J Am Acad Child Adolesc Psychiatry* **37**: 364-371.

McMaster University (1999) *Treatment of Attention-Deficit/Hyperactivity Disorder. Evidence Report/Technology Assessment No. 11. AHRQ Publication No. 00-E005.* Washington, DC: Agency for Health Care Policy and Research (online: http://www.ncbi.nlm.nih.gov/books/bv.fcgi?rid=hstat1.chapter.14677).

MTA Cooperative Group (1999) A 14-month randomized clinical trial of treatment strategies for attention-deficit/hyperactivity disorder. The MTA Cooperative Group. Multimodal Treatment Study of Children with ADHD. *Arch Gen Psychiatry* **56**: 1073–1086.

Nehra A, Mullick F, Ishak KG, Zimmerman HJ (1990) Pemoline-associated hepatic injury. *Gastroenterology* **99**: 1517–1519.

NICE (2000) *Guidance on the Use of Methylphenidate (Ritalin, Equasym) for Attention Deficit/Hyperactivity Disorder (ADHD) in Childhood. Technology Appraisal Guidance No 13.* London: National Institute for Clinical Excellence (online: http://www.cambsmh.nhs.uk/documents/Clinical/Methylph-guidance_ADHD.pdf).

Pelham WE, Swanson JM, Furman MB, Schwindt H (1995) Pemoline effects on children with ADHD: a time-response by dose-response analysis on classroom measures. *J Am Acad Child Adolesc Psychiatry* **34**: 1504–1513.

Pliska SR (1989) Effect of anxiety on cognition, behaviour, and stimulant response in ADHD. *J Am Acad Child Adolesc Psychiatry* **28**: 882–887.

Popper CW (1995) Combining methylphenidate and clonidine: pharmacologic questions and news reports about sudden death. *J Child Adolesc Psychopharmacol* **5**: 157–166.

Popper CW (1997) Antidepressants in the treatment of attention-deficit/hyperactivity disorder. *J Clin Psychiatry* **58** Suppl 14: 14–29.

Rapport MD, Denney C, DuPaul G, Gardner MJ (1994) Attention deficit disorder and methylphenidate: normalization rates, clinical effectiveness, and response prediction in 76 children. *J Am Acad Child Adolesc Psychiatry* **33**: 882–893.

Raskin LA, Shaywitz BA, Anderson GM, Cohen DJ, Teicher MH, Liakis J (1983) Differential effects of selective dopamine, norepinephrine or catecholamine depletion on activity and learning in the developing rat. *Pharmacol Biochem Behav* **19**: 743–749.

Riddle MA, Hardin MT, Cho SC, Woolston JL, Leckman JF (1988) Desipramine treatment of boys with attention-deficit hyperactivity disorder and tics: preliminary clinical experience. *J Am Acad Child Adolesc Psychiatry* **27**: 811–813.

Riggs P, Baker S, Mikulich S, Young S, Crowley T (1995) Depression in substance-dependent delinquents. *J Am Acad Child Adolesc Psychiatry* **34**: 764–771.

Sallee FR, Stiller R, Perel J, Bates T (1985) Oral pemoline kinetics in hyperactive children. *Clin Pharmacol Ther* **37**: 606–609.

Sallee FR, Stiller RL, Perel JM, Everett G (1989) Pemoline-induced abnormal involuntary movements. *J Clin Psychopharmacol* **9**: 125–129.

Sallee FR, Stiller RL, Perel JM (1992) Pharmacodynamics of pemoline in attention deficit disorder with hyperactivity. *J Am Acad Child Adolesc Psychiatry* **31**: 244–251.

Santosh PJ, Baird G (1999) Pharmacotherapy of psychopathology in children and adults with intellectual disabilities. *Lancet* **354**: 233–242.

Santosh PJ, Taylor E (2000) Stimulant drugs. *Eur Child Adolesc Psychiatry* **9** Suppl 1: 127–143

Santosh PJ, Taylor E, Swanson J, Wigal T, Chuang S, Davies M, Greenhill L, Newcorn J, Arnold LE, Jensen P, Vitiello B, Elliott G, Hinshaw S, Hechtman L, Abikoff H, Pelham W, Hoza B, Molina B, Wells K, Epstein J, Posner M (2005) Refining the diagnoses of inattention and overactivity syndromes: A reanalysis of the Multimodal Treatment study of attention deficit hyperactivity disorder (ADHD) based on ICD-10 criteria for hyperkinetic disorder. *Clin Neurosci Res* **5**: 307–314.

SIGN (2001) *Attention Deficit and Hyperkinetic Disorders in Children and Young People. SIGN Publication No. 52.* Edinburgh: Scottish Intercollegiate Guidelines Network (online: http://www.sign.ac.uk/guidelines/fulltext/52/index.html).

Spencer T, Biederman J, Kerman K, Steingard R, Wilens T (1993a) Desipramine treatment of children with attention-deficit hyperactivity disorder and tic disorder or Tourette's syndrome. *J Am Acad Child Adolesc Psychiatry* **32**: 354–360.

Spencer T, Biederman J, Wilens T, Steingard R, Geist D (1993b) Nortriptyline treatment of children with attention-deficit hyperactivity disorder and tic disorder or Tourette's syndrome, *J Am Acad Child Adolesc Psychiatry* **32**: 205–210.

Spencer T, Biederman J, Wilens T, Harding M, O'Donnell D, Griffin S (1996) Pharmacotherapy of attention-deficit hyperactivity disorder across the life cycle. *J Am Acad Child Adolesc Psychiatry* **35**: 409–432.

Swanson JM, Sandman CA, Deutsch C, Baren M (1983) Methylphenidate hydrochloride given with or before breakfast: I. Behavioural, cognitive, and electrophysiologic effects. *Pediatrics* **72**: 49–55.

Swanson JM, Flockhart D, Udrea D, Cantwell D, Connor D, Williams L (1995) Clonidine in the treatment of ADHD: questions about safety and efficacy. *J Child Adolesc Psychopharmacol* **5**: 301–304.

Tannock R, Ickowicz A, Schachar R (1995) Differential effects of methylphenidate on working memory in ADHD children with and without comorbid anxiety. *J Am Acad Child Adolesc Psychiatry* **7**: 886–896.

Taylor E, Schachar R, Thorley G, Wieselberg HM, Everitt B, Rutter M (1987) Which boys respond to stimulant medication? A controlled trial of methylphenidate in boys with disruptive behaviour. *Psychol Med* **17**: 121–143.

Taylor E, Sergeant J, Doepfner M, Gunning B, Overmeyer S, Mobius HJ, Eisert HG (1998) Clinical guidelines for hyperkinetic disorder. European Society for Child and Adolescent Psychiatry. *Eur Child Adolesc Psychiatry* **7**: 184–200.

Taylor E, Dopfner M, Sergeant J, Asherson P, Banaschewski T, Buitelaar J, Coghill D, Danckaerts M, Rothenberger A, Sonuga-Barke E, Steinhausen HC, Zuddas A (2004) European clinical guidelines for hyperkinetic disorder—first upgrade. *Eur Child Adolesc Psychiatry* **13** Suppl 1: 17–30.

Vincent J, Varley CK, Leger P (1990) Effects of methylphenidate on early adolescent growth. *Am J Psychiatry* **147**: 501–502.

Weiss MD, Weiss JR (2004) A guide to the treatment of adults with ADHD. *J Clin Psychiatry* **65** Suppl 3: 27–37.

Wilens TE, Biederman J, Wong J, Spencer TJ, Prince JB (2002) Adjunctive donepezil in attention deficit hyperactivity disorder youth: case series. *J Child Adolesc Psychopharmacol* **10**: 217–222.

Wolraich ML, Greenhill LL, Pelham W, Swanson J, Wilens T, Palumbo D, Atkins M, McBurnett K, Bukstein O, August G (2001) Randomized, controlled trial of OROS methylphenidate once a day in children with attention-deficit/hyperactivity disorder. *Pediatrics* **108**: 883–892

Zeiner P (1995) Body growth and cardiovascular function after extended treatment (1.75 years) with methylphenidate in boys with attention-deficit hyperactivity disorder. *J Child Adolesc Psychopharmacol* **5**: 129–138.

APPENDIX 8.1
USING MEDICATION EFFECTIVELY: A FACTSHEET FOR FAMILIES

Why is medication used in ADHD?
Medication can be the most powerful way of increasing attentiveness and reducing impulsivity and hyperactivity. However, because of the risk of unwanted effects, medication is usually reserved for severely affected children who have failed to benefit from psychological and educational interventions. For those who need it, medication should be used alongside psychological approaches such as attention training and behaviour modification at home and at school.

What types of drugs are used?
The stimulants *methylphenidate (Ritalin)* and *dexamphetamine* are the most commonly used, and are safe and effective preparations for the treatment of ADHD. *Tricyclic antidepressants* can also be used but are less effective than stimulants, have greater side-effects and are occasionally toxic to the heart. Thus, stimulants are the first choice for medication. The main effect of *clonidine*, which is a non-stimulant, is on impulsiveness and overactivity. It is usually given in conjunction with stimulants as, by itself, it has little effect on inattentiveness. *Risperidone* is a major tranquillizer used very rarely and in small doses only for the most severe problems. Its use and effects for children in the long-term have not yet been studied.

How long have these drugs been available?
The use of stimulant medication for ADHD is not new. They were first shown to be effective in 1937. Though the benefits were recognized then, stimulants were not widely used until the late 1950s when the new preparation methylphenidate was first introduced. After 40 years, the safety and effectiveness of methylphenidate have been well researched in scores of trials.

How do they work?
Stimulants act on the part of the brain that controls attention and impulsivity. Their effect is to increase the child's natural ability to concentrate on tasks and to reduce impulsiveness and restlessness.

When stimulants are successful for a child with established ADHD, parents note that their children are calmer, less restless, less impulsive, less demanding and more reflective.

Teachers note that children are more settled and can complete work without supervision. Children may also be more organized, have neater writing, produce more academic work, be better behaved, and be more popular with their peers and socially 'in tune'.

Children notice that they can think more clearly, can concentrate on their work, and are less in trouble at home and at school: "everyone is nicer to me".

Stimulants do not cure ADHD – all they do is help children to improve their attention by inhibiting their impulsivity. This helps them to make the best of their abilities with regard to education, relationships and behaviour until some improvement comes with maturity.

What are the research findings?
The results of numerous trials show that between 60% and 90% of children with ADHD will respond to stimulant medication.

The aim of giving medication to children with ADHD is to maintain or build their confidence, and improve family relationships and their will to learn until age brings a natural resolution.

It is said that stimulants are nonspecific in their action and that they would be of equal benefit to children without ADHD. Certainly, stimulants have an effect on all people, but the degree of response differs. It is possible that those without ADHD might be improved by an imperceptible amount. Children with major problems of attention, impulsivity and hyperactivity show a marked response to this therapy.

Are stimulants suitable for children below 6 years?
Several trials have shown that there are benefits to children in the younger age groups. It is right to be cautious

in medicating preschool children, even though scientific studies have not indicated an age limit below which medication should not be given. Treatment for preschool children should be supervised at a specialist clinic.

What are the side-effects?
THE MYTHS

The use of amphetamines raises anxiety about addiction. Though used in children with ADHD for over half a century, there is no evidence that they are addictive or cause increased risk of later substance abuse when used properly.

Adults use tea and coffee to help them focus their attention. Methylphenidate is safer and has fewer side-effects than the caffeine in a cup of coffee.

In the past, reduced growth was thought to be a side-effect of long-term medication because it caused reduced appetite. Recent studies do not support this idea. Growth catches up so that eventually there is no difference in height and weight between children having medication and those not on medication. Although this is of no great concern, measures of weight and height of children receiving medication are still recorded.

EASILY MANAGED SIDE-EFFECTS
Suppression of appetite

This is not a problem when the drug is taken just before or with a meal, as the food arrives in the stomach before the appetite is lost. Thus children should have a good breakfast. Most children will have a reduced appetite at lunchtime and can catch up on their eating in the evening. 'Grazing' is common.

If a child eats too little, stopping the afternoon dose generally allows for catch-up nutrition with a larger and later evening meal. Medication 'holidays' at weekends and during school holidays also aid weight gain.

Wakefulness

Wakefulness is rarely a troublesome side-effect in the correctly treated child. The untreated child with ADHD finds it hard to settle down to sleep, and medication frequently enables the child to calm down before bedtime. Sometimes giving half the normal dose two hours before bed is helpful. If medication makes this worse, this problem can be easily resolved by reducing the last dose of the day and paying particular attention to the behavioural management of bedtime.

OTHER EFFECTS
Emotional lability

Some children become withdrawn, over-focused, tearful and miserable. This occurs in one in ten of the children treated and tends to happen at the start of medication or when the dose is increased. It is particularly a problem when medication is introduced in an inflexible, clumsy way and is poorly monitored.

Most emotional problems resolve if the dosage is halved. It is usually possible to increase very gradually to the previous dose. Remaining problems will disappear within 4 hours of stopping medication.

Rebound behaviour

This can be a problem when the effects of medication start to wear off, particularly when this coincides with the end of the school day. A behavioural 'blow out' can be overcome by adding a small dose at the time the previous dose is wearing off.

The possibility of tics

There is an identified association between ADHD and tic disorders. These are unrelated to the use of methylphenidate medication in most children. If, however, a child already suffers from Tourette syndrome, methylphenidate may make tics worse. Other medication can then be used instead. However, quite often tics improve on methylphenidate so that it is certainly worth a trial.

How long should my child continue on medication?
Medication is continued for as long as parents see significant benefits. For some, this will take 6 months, for others 2 years, and for some, until school leaving or longer.

Medication 'holidays', or breaks, can be useful to see if the problem behaviours return. Some parents prefer their children to be medication-free during weekends and holiday periods. Parents should not, however, feel guilty about their children being on medication 'full time': the quality of their family life is important. If necessary, these medicines can be stopped suddenly without any need to ease off gradually.

Increasingly, some adults are being recognized as suffering from ADHD since childhood and are being prescribed medication.

Summary
ADHD is characterized by inattention, poor impulse control and overactivity. It is the extreme end of a spectrum of behaviour. Most children come to professional attention in their first few years at school.

Stimulant medication is safe and parents are in charge of its continued prescription. Parents can decide to stop medication at any time if they have concerns about its effectiveness or side-effects.

Types of medication
METHYLPHENIDATE
Also known as:
- Ritalin, available as 10 mg tablets.
- Equasym, available as 5 mg, 10 mg, 20 mg tablets
- Ritalin SR, available as 20 mg tablets.

How does it act?
Methylphenidate (MPH) is a central nervous system stimulant with greater effects on mental than motor activities. The effects are thought to be due to cortical stimulation and stimulation of the basal ganglia and other parts of the brain that control attention and impulsiveness.

What is the effect?
Improvement in the core symptoms of ADHD – attention and concentration are improved; restless overactivity and fidgeting are reduced; the child is less impulsive.

What are the possible side-effects?
- Very common: reduced appetite
  Ensure the child has a good breakfast
  Allow for a prolonged evening meal – 'grazing'
- Common: difficulties in settling to sleep
  Decide on the cause: if MPH is given too late, reduce the last dose
  If the child is unsettled, consider adding a small dose two hours before bedtime
- Emotionality: the child may become subdued, tearful, over-focused, have vague nausea and abdominal pain.
  This may happen early in treatment and often disappears spontaneously. Reduce or stop medication; restart and increase very slowly.
- Rare: problems in visual accommodation and blurred vision.
  See optometrist, consult prescribing doctor.
- Tics: MPH may make tics worse in a child with severe tics or Tourette syndrome.
  Other medication may be considered first.
  This is dose-dependent in Tourette syndrome and is easily reversible when the medication is stopped.
- Epilepsy: MPH reduces the seizure threshold and theoretically may increase the possibility of fits.
  Current thinking is that the risk of destabilizing epilepsy with MPH has been overstated unless seizure control is unstable.
- Very rare: hallucinations, clinically significant raised blood pressure or heart rate.
  Stop medication, consult prescribing doctor.

What is the dosage?
This may vary from child to child. It will be adjusted according to the beneficial effect on the child and any side-effects.

Generally for 6- to 9-year-olds, we start with 5 mg MPH twice daily (morning and lunch time). We increase at weekly intervals by 5 mg until the desired effect is reached, up to 45 mg. A third dose may also be added, particularly for children whose problems are worse in the afternoon and for those who need to do homework.

How long does the effect last?
MPH starts to work after 20–30 minutes, peaks at 1½–2 hours and lasts about 3–4 hours. It has almost entirely 'washed out' by 5 hours.

This means that MPH is very safe and it is easy to adjust the dose. But it also means that timing of the dose is important to avoid ups and downs (rebounds).

Longer-acting preparations

Sustained-release Ritalin contains the medication in a wax matrix that slowly releases the MPH during the day. Studies show that in some children effects on concentration may be apparent 9 hours later. It is important that the tablet should not be chewed but swallowed whole.

One 20 mg tablet of Ritalin SR is equivalent to two doses of 10 mg of regular MPH. Ritalin SR has been less widely researched than standard Ritalin but clinical experience suggests that it suits only some children. It may have a slow onset of action, so that regular Ritalin will need to be prescribed as well as for the morning dose.

Sometimes there are major difficulties for a child taking medication at school. Ritalin SR may then be helpful if the difficulties cannot be managed by problem-solving and negotiation.

Ritalin SR is not licensed in the UK and is not stocked routinely. Any pharmacy will need to obtain it from a company with an import licence.

Concerta XL uses an osmotic delivery system to release MPH. It has an overcoat that delivers part of the total dose immediately. The rest of the MPH is released slowly to provide a smooth concentration profile providing efficacy for approximately 12 hours.

Concerta is as effective as standard immediate-release Ritalin and has the same safety profile. Parents generally prefer it. As a new preparation of MPH, Concerta has been the subject of only limited research and is not yet licensed for use in the UK.

Drug interactions

MPH interacts with some anticonvulsant drugs, phenylbutazone and tricyclic antidepressants. It is also likely to interact with some herbal preparations such as St John's Wort.

Caffeine-containing drinks such as cola and coffee may cause increased nervousness, jitteriness and insomnia.

Other comments

MPH is the first-line medication for most children with ADHD. It is found to be slightly more effective generally than dexamphetamine. But there are some children for whom dexamphetamine works better.

A trial of medication for one month is usually monitored for side-effects and for improvement in symptoms.

DEXAMPHETAMINE

Also known as:

• Dexedrine, available as 5 mg tablets.

How does it act?

Dexamphetamine (DEX) is a sympathomimetic amine which has central stimulant and appetite-reducing properties. It has a similar action to methylphenidate.

What is the effect?

Like MPH, DEX improves the core symptoms of ADHD. Attention and concentration are improved; restless overactivity and fidgeting are reduced; the child is less impulsive.

What are the possible side-effects?

As with MPH, most side-effects are mild and pass off after a short time.

DEX reduces the likelihood of having seizures and is therefore the choice if the child has poorly controlled epilepsy.

What is the dosage?

DEX is more potent than MPH. The dosage is half that of MPH, starting with 2.5 mg twice daily.

How long does the effect last?

DEX starts to work after 20 minutes and lasts approximately 5 hours. The dose is repeated every 4–5 hours during the day.

Drug interactions
Sympathomimetic amines interact with a range of drugs including antidepressants, anticonvulsants and some anaesthetics. Caffeine-containing drinks such as cola and coffee may lead to increased nervousness, jitteriness and insomnia.

IMIPRAMINE
Also known as:
• Tofranil, available as 25 mg tablets and as syrup 25 mg/5 ml.

How does it act?
Imipramine is a tricyclic antidepressant (TCA) similar to other TCAs such as amitriptyline, desipramine, clomipramine and nortriptyline. They are thought to increase the availability of neurotransmitters, especially serotonin and noradrenaline.
    Their action in ADHD is probably different from their antidepressant action.

What is their effect?
TCAs reduce the three core symptoms of ADHD. They are useful instead of stimulants (MPH or DEX) when severe tics are present; when stimulants have not been effective; when emotional disturbance is made worse by stimulants; and when there is a possibility of misuse of stimulants.

What are the possible side-effects?
• Common and short-lived: sedation, dry mouth, difficulty passing urine, constipation, blurred vision, nausea, anxiety and headaches.
• Rare: Increased likelihood of seizures. Therefore they need to be used carefully in epilepsy.
• An increase in dental caries in long-term use suggests regular dental check-ups are necessary.
• Elated mood in susceptible children.
• Rare but very serious effects: cardio-toxicity, with a few cases of sudden death.
• They are very toxic in overdoses.

What is the dosage?
2.5 mg/kg daily divided into 2 or 3 doses. Children over 6 years should start with 10 mg daily, increasing over a period of 10 days to 20 mg (to 8 years), to 20–50 mg (to 14 years), and to 50–80 mg (over 14 years).
    The effect on ADHD is achieved quickly and at a lower dosage than the effect on depression.

Drug interactions
The addition of any other sedative drug or alcohol will cause sleepiness, dizziness. The blood level of TCAs will markedly and unpredictably rise if MPH is given simultaneously.
    A gap of at least 14 days should occur after any monoamine oxidase inhibitor has been taken to avoid possible hypertensive crises.
    There is an increased risk of cardiac arrhythmia if antipsychotic drugs are taken.

Special instructions
In addition to the usual monitoring, baseline electrocardiographs (ECGs) should be carried out before treatment and if dosage is increased. Medication should be stopped if the heart rate is more that 130/min or if the ECG is abnormal.
    Because of the potential toxicity, imipramine is regarded as a second-line treatment for ADHD.
    If it is decided to stop medication, this should be carried out gradually, usually over 4 weeks.
    Imipramine is useful when stimulants make tics much worse; when stimulants have not been effective; or when emotional disturbance has become worse with stimulants; and when there is a possibility of misuse of stimulants.

CLONIDINE
Also known as:
• Catapres, available as 100 μg and 300 μg tablets also available as liquid.
• Dixarit, available as 25 μg tablets.

How does it act?
Clonidine is an antihypertensive drug used to treat high blood pressure. It has recently been found to be effective for treating children with ADHD.

It is a first-line treatment for children with tics.

What is its effect?
Clonidine's main effect is on impulsiveness and overactivity. It is often given with stimulant medication as it has little effect on inattention. It is less effective generally on ADHD symptoms than imipramine.

What are the possible side-effects?
Some children may be sleepy with it at first and when the dose is increased. They may have a dry mouth and dry eyes (a problem for contact lens wearers).
- Rare but serious: low blood pressure and cardiac arrhythmias may occur. A serious rebound increase in blood pressure may occur if the Clonidine is stopped suddenly. A rebound of tics may also occur.
- Other side-effects: include headaches, dizziness, constipation, feeling high, nightmares, fluid retention, rashes, feeling sick, slow pulse, hands unusually sensitive to cold.

What is the dosage?
To avoid problems with blood pressure, the dosage is built up gradually over 2–4 weeks and the effect evaluated after 6 weeks on the full dosage of 3–5 μg/kg/day divided into two doses at breakfast and bedtime.

Usually start with 25 μg at night, increasing by 25 μg to 100–200 μg, if tolerated.

Drug interactions
Other drugs used to treat hypertension will make dizziness and faintness more likely. Tricyclic antidepressants antagonize effects of the clonidine so that the dose may need to be increased.

Special instructions
- Clonidine is used as a third-line treatment for ADHD, particularly when tic disorders are present or there is extreme hyperactivity and emotional swings.
- Blood pressure, pulse and ECG should be measured at baseline and for monitoring.
- Combination therapy with stimulant medication needs close specialist monitoring.
- A trial of clonidine is usually evaluated after 6 weeks on the full dosage.

RISPERIDONE
Also known as:
- Risperdal, available as a solution 1 mg/1ml, and as tablets: 2 mg, 3 mg, 4 mg and 6 mg.

How does it act?
Risperidone, like the other major tranquillizers, acts by blocking dopamine transmission in the brain. It targets the limbic system and therefore produces fewer side-effects than the other tranquillizers. It also has an antagonistic effect on serotonin, adrenergic and histaminergic receptors.

What is its effect?
It has been found helpful in treating children with ADHD whose symptoms have not been well controlled by other medication.

It is less effective than stimulants for improving concentration.

It is likely to be particularly useful in children with autistic spectrum disorders.

What are the possible side-effects?
- Minor effects: agitation, anxiety, poor concentration, headaches, dizziness, runny nose (*many of these effects will wear off as your child's body adjusts to the drug*); also dry mouth, constipation, difficulty in passing urine, blurred vision.
- Major problem: weight gain – often severe.
- Occasional effect: swelling of breasts and secretion of milk (in boys as well as girls).
- Serious effects: gradual onset of stiffness and tremor (parkinsonism); rapid onset of rhythmic movements particularly in tongue and face (tardive dyskinesia).

- Rare: low white blood count, seizures.
- Rare major effect: neuroleptic malignant syndrome (raised temperature, muscle rigidity, changing level of consciousness, raised heart rate and unstable blood pressure).

How is it given?
In liquid form, risperidone is measured out by a syringe and may be given in juice.

On day one a single dose of 0.25 mg is given; on day two, 0.25 mg can be given twice daily; after this the dose can be increased by 0.25 mg every 3–5 days as instructed by your doctor to 1 mg twice daily.

Drug interactions
There is an increased risk of cardiac arrhythmia when given with antidepressants.

Care is needed for children taking anticonvulsants – risperidone can make seizures more common yet increase the blood level of anticonvulsants.

Whilst most of the side-effects are mild and pass off, some are severe and worrying.

If your child develops any unwanted movements or stiffness, STOP the medication immediately and consult your doctor.

Special instructions
- Baseline full blood count and liver function tests should be carried out and repeated every 3–6 months.
- Blood pressure and weight should be measured regularly.
- The use of risperidone should still be thought of as experimental and used in specialist clinics only.
- For most children with ADHD, the risks of using risperidone are greater than the possible usefulness.

APPENDIX 8.2
SIDE-EFFECTS RATING SCALE

Name: . . . .   Date: . . . .

Person completing this form: . . . .

Behaviour	No Problem										Serious Problems
Difficulty getting off to sleep	0	1	2	3	4	5	6	7	8	9	10
Difficulty in staying asleep	0	1	2	3	4	5	6	7	8	9	10
Nightmares	0	1	2	3	4	5	6	7	8	9	10
Loss of appetite	0	1	2	3	4	5	6	7	8	9	10
Stomach aches	0	1	2	3	4	5	6	7	8	9	10
Headaches	0	1	2	3	4	5	6	7	8	9	10
Tics	0	1	2	3	4	5	6	7	8	9	10
Nervous movements	0	1	2	3	4	5	6	7	8	9	10
Feeling dizzy	0	1	2	3	4	5	6	7	8	9	10
Feeling sick	0	1	2	3	4	5	6	7	8	9	10
Feeling drowsy	0	1	2	3	4	5	6	7	8	9	10
Feeling irritable	0	1	2	3	4	5	6	7	8	9	10
Feeling unhappy	0	1	2	3	4	5	6	7	8	9	10
Crying a lot	0	1	2	3	4	5	6	7	8	9	10
Loss of interest in others	0	1	2	3	4	5	6	7	8	9	10
Daydreaming	0	1	2	3	4	5	6	7	8	9	10
How easy is he/she to manage?	0	1	2	3	4	5	6	7	8	9	10

Any other different behaviour:

Current medication:

9
BEHAVIOURAL AND COGNITIVE APPROACHES

Maxine Sinclair

"It is stressed that no intervention strategies to date, whether employed singularly or in combination, have proved clinically sufficient and durable for the troubling and troublesome problems of these youngsters, thus necessitating the continuing search for integrated components – cognitive, behavioural and pharmacologic – that will constitute an adequate treatment package."

Hinshaw and Erhardt (1991)

The cardinal triad of inattention, impulsivity and hyperactivity that characterizes attention deficit hyperactivity disorder frequently co-occurs with one or more comorbid conditions and/or one or more secondary functional impairments. Epidemiological studies consistently report significant comorbidity with the greatest overlap associated with oppositional defiant disorder (35–60%), conduct disorder (30–50%), anxiety (25–40%) and specific learning disabilities (10–26%) (Tannock 1998). Secondary symptoms often include academic underachievement, interpersonal relationship difficulties, peer rejection and interpersonal aggression. Primary and secondary symptoms manifest in different combinations to provoke impairments in the domains of functioning critical to mastering the major tasks of childhood (McArdle et al. 1997). Treatment regimes need to be broadly based if they are to be effective in producing enduring benefits across core symptoms, functional domains and environmental settings.

Treatment options for ADHD are empirically and behaviourally based rather than aetiologically derived. The main established treatment strategies for ADHD are pharmacotherapy, behavioural therapy and cognitive behavioural therapy (CBT). Of these, central nervous system stimulant medication and behaviour therapy have proven the most effective. CBT on its own has proved rather disappointing (for reviews, see Abikoff 1987, Hinshaw and Erhardt 1991), but when combined with behavioural reinforcement has provided demonstrable benefits for children with aggressive and antisocial behaviour patterns (Kazdin et al. 1987a,b).

Medication is often the treatment of choice, and indeed a plethora of contemporary research exists that denotes the superiority of stimulant medication in effecting improvements in both primary and secondary symptoms of ADHD. The ability of medication alone to alter the long-term course for the better is harder to demonstrate. Additional limitations to medication as sole therapy include the significant minority of patients who fail to who respond or experience an adverse reaction. The beneficial effects of medication are restricted to the active life of the drug, and the extreme ends of the day are often difficult periods for children with ADHD and their families. Equally important is the acceptability of medication as a viable treatment option to the young person and their family. There is an increasing tendency to make autonomous decisions as the child progresses into adolescence, and non-compliance with medication is quite common, as the child rejects situations that signal difference from his or her social group. Behavioural therapy and CBT are not without their own limitations: they do not usually normalize the child by themselves, and the magnitude of improvement is often not as large as medication. Benefits appear to be confined to the duration of the active administration of behavioural strategy, and failure to achieve good fidelity to treatment is associated with a less favourable outcome. Psychosocial therapies have their own dissenters. The strategies are more effortful than medication options and some children and/or their families are either not able to commit themselves to this treatment option or reject its validity.

Current consensus, encouragingly, endorses informed parental choice.

Rationale for behaviour therapy

A popular neuropsychological paradigm is that ADHD represents a significant impairment in the ability to inhibit or delay a behavioural response (Barkley 1997a,b). Inhibition as a conditioning deficit posits that ADHD results from an imbalance between two opposing neuropsychological systems, a behavioural inhibition system (BIS) and a behavioural activation system (BAS), which Gray (1982) proposed to be the controls for responses to signals of punishment and reward. The BIS is activated in contexts of punishment, non-reward or novelty and results in the withholding of a response, while the BAS is triggered by signals of reward resulting in behavioural activation. Individuals with ADHD are thought to have an underactive BIS and so are less likely to inhibit responses when these are associated with punishment, non-reward or novelty. That is, they are less responsive to conditioned stimuli (Quay 1977).

Direct contingency management

Direct contingency management is premised on the principles of operant/instrumental conditioning. Actions are increased or strengthened, and thus shaped, by consequences that are rewarding (positive reinforcement) or that lead to the avoidance of, or escape from, punishment (negative reinforcement). Actions are reduced or eliminated by punitive sanctions (loss of privileges, fines) that follow, contingently, their unwanted performance. Equally important is that the child's behaviour itself can act as an operant thereby shaping the behaviours of others and setting up negative feedback loops.

It may appear to be counterintuitive to propose a psychological treatment format that is anchored in operant conditioning techniques when the theory postulates that ADHD children are less responsive to conditioned stimuli. However, it is not the case that they do not respond, rather they respond less well than non-ADHD peers. Consequently they need larger and more powerful consequences (Barkley 2000) and should receive more prompts, cues and reinforcements than non-ADHD peers. The idea is to increase the likelihood that the child will orient to the parameters that are necessary for goal-directed behaviour, and so increase the probability of BIS activation.

Direct contingency management studies usually employ single-case designs implemented in institutions (e.g. inpatient ward or residential school). They are generally more intensive than therapies conducted in the home and can command greater treatment fidelity as they are usually administered by paraprofessionals or clinicians rather than teachers or parents. The experimental control obtained under these conditions is difficult to replicate in the home setting, but they produce behavioural improvements that are often larger than those obtained with CBT. Effect size is often comparable to low-dose medication alone; and in combination with low-dose medication can produce effects nearly identical to those produced by high-dose medication alone (Carlson et al. 1992).

Clinical behaviour therapies have typically used between-group designs and involve parent training and teacher consultation as the behavioural strategy. The methodology generates statistically and clinically significant improvements but these are usually not as large as with direct contingency management or medication alone. Normalization is rarely achieved although aggressive behaviours in the classroom have been normalized by behaviour therapy alone (Abikoff and Gittleman 1984).

General principles
At least four levels of intervention need to be implemented in concert to produce robust change (Evans et al. 1998):
1. Alter the immediate consequences of the undesirable behaviour
2. Reduce the probability of the behaviour occurring by rearranging the environment in order to eliminate so-called 'setting events' (i.e. events that trigger a response)
3. Facilitate (teaching, reinforcing and shaping) the emergence of alternative skills; a variety of systematic reward and response cost procedures should be an integral component of any schedule
4. Design long-term prevention through imparting new patterns of behaviour.

Each of these tasks may be served by either one or a combination of the major types of learning: operant and classical conditioning, observational (modelling) and cognitive learning.

The two most commonly used behavioural interventions are:
1. Creating and maintaining a well-structured/'prosthetic' environment to compensate for poor stimulus control
2. Parent training.

Prosthetic environments
Since children with ADHD lack stimulus control, environments need to be constructed that exert external control. These strategies address the immediate antecedents in a child's environment (home, school or community) that predict or trigger the behaviour. Common triggers include instructional demand, withholding of a desired object or activity, and withdrawal of parental attention. A functional assessment interview and direct observation are used to identify 'setting events' and 'maintaining events' (the consequence to the child that reinforces or increases the probability of behavioural repetition). The information is used to develop hypotheses about the function of the behaviour, and these form the foundations of the intervention. Strategies are developed aimed at reducing/eliminating setting events by identifying appropriate supports (people, technology, information) or skill

development needed by the child to circumvent these difficulties. Effective strategies are those that are easily adapted to the family context and which effectively and efficiently reduce challenging behaviours and do not themselves produce secondary stressors. Immediate and frequent positive reinforcers valued by the child positively reinforce desirable behaviours. Undesirable behaviours are penalized, penalties ranging from ignoring of behaviours if mild to loss of privileges or a fine. Insufficiently structured environments can enhance ADHD symptoms (Prinz and Miller 1994) and children with ADHD appear to function better in structured environments.

PARENT TRAINING

Parent training is based on social learning theory and uses a didactic approach. Its use is predicated on research evidence that indicates that parents of ADHD children display a more negative and controlling style of parenting with their ADHD children than parents of comparison children (Barkley 1985, 1990). When ADHD behaviour is brought under better control with stimulant medication, the parents' negativity and control reciprocally diminish (Humphries et al. 1978, Barkley and Cunningham 1979, Barkley 1989). The acute shift in parental style induced by medication does not preclude the possibility that the child's negative behaviours may have been shaped by reciprocal reinforcement of the parent–child interaction. Negative parenting has been demonstrated to predict noncompliance in the classroom and playground, poor academic achievement, and laboratory stealing (Dornbusch et al. 1987, Anderson et al. 1994). Although hostile parenting is not thought to have an aetiological role in hyperactivity, it appears to play a substantial role in the development, escalation and maintenance of oppositional and antisocial behaviours (Rutter et al. 1998). These antisocial traits appear to mediate increased risk for later substance abuse, criminality and antisocial spectrum disorders in adulthood (Klein and Mannuzza 1991, Hinshaw 1994).

Barkley (1997a,b) theorizes that impairment in self-regulation such as emotion is one of the consequences of a deficient inhibitory process. Children with ADHD show greater prepotent emotional reactivity (i.e. a dominant and habitual emotional response that may or may not be appropriate to the stimulus/provocation) to 'charged' events and less capacity to regulate emotion/arousal states. We can postulate that these prepotent responses will be derived from an ADHD child–parent relationship that is often characterized by reciprocally elevated levels of negative interactions, angry conflicts and less positive and facilitative behaviour towards each other. Dodge (1991) proposed a similar hypothesis to account for reactive aggression. He postulated that parenting behaviour that result in poor attachment between parents and child, for example through a lack of warmth and caregiving behaviour towards the child, may in turn foster feelings of insecurity, vulnerability, and eventually hostility and aggression in social relationships. Thus the experience of warmth and caregiving from parents/carers should diminish the risk of later violence associated with reactive ag-gression. Furman and Wehner (1994) proposed that a lack of parental warmth and caregiving and the resulting poor parent-child attachment shape, at least to some extent, the child's negative expectations about their and others' roles and behaviour. In reactively aggressive boys, these negative expectations may reinforce the boys' already existing hostile and aggressive behaviour patterns. Whilst their evidence was not conclusive, Melnick and

Hinshaw (2000) found that of the factors they examined, parental coaching/modeling and emotion-related behaviours during conflict were most highly associated with their child's emotion regulation abilities.

Home-based intervention seeks to sever this association by enhancing the problem-solving capacity of the child and his/her family. The aim of this component is to lower the emotional climate of the home – that is, to reduce angry, hostile and critical responses from both parents and child – while maintaining reasonable expectations for the child's performance. Through the provision of formal education about the nature of the child's condition, and strategies for managing challenging behaviour more effectively, family members become support structures for the young person. Appendix 9.1 provides the outline for a home-based approach, described as 'Management without Medication'.

Typically, parent training involves educational, assessment, strategy generation and implementation stages. These are demonstrated using role-play and modelling techniques by the clinician to modify or teach new parenting skills. The parents are encouraged to practice the new strategies and record and monitor outcome. In this way they are taught to be scientific practitioners. Behavioural methods are taught to assess and analyse behavioural difficulties that will be used to inform subsequent behavioural modification plans. Goals for intervention are established through the development of realistic and achievable rules that will be shared with the child. Appropriate behaviour is reinforced with praise and other more tangible rewards that are intrinsically reinforcing for the child. Mildly punitive strategies are reserved for less adaptive behaviours, and in keeping with Barkley's (2000) position parents are advised of the judicious use of sanctions combined with more frequent positive rewards.

The intervention period is usually 8–12 sessions; there are a number of published parent training programmes (Webster-Stratton 1990, 1992a,b, 1998, Webster-Stratton et al. 2004; Barkley 1997a,b), common features of which include:
- Psychoeducation – ADHD and social learning theory
- Behaviour management principles and ABC (antecedent–behaviour–consequence) relationships
- Attending (acknowledging and responding to) adaptive behaviours
- Rewards – immediate, novel and valued by child
- Rewarding and ignoring: rationale and practice
- Using positive skills and Premack principles [whereby any behaviour by the subject that happens reliably and preferentially can be used as a reinforcer for a desired behaviour that occurs less reliably – e.g. most children like to watch television and it is something they will do willingly without any interference from their parents, so parents can use this behaviour to encourage/condition their child to complete a task such as homework by rewarding completion with watching television] to practice attending and increase adaptive behaviours
- Giving effective commands – short, specific; and the importance of consistency within and between parents
- Establishing behaviour rules, and attending and rewarding compliant behaviours
- Constructionist strategies – e.g. token economy, attention

- Reductionist strategies – e.g. ignoring, time out, response-cost, logical consequences
- Problem solving
- Parenting cognitions (thoughts/assumptions about their child and his/her behaviour).

Coercion theory (Patterson 1982) predicts that changes in the parental disciplinary practices (e.g. increased consistency and supervision, decreased harshness) and in parent–child interaction (e.g. reductions in negative reinforcement patterns) should effect behavioural improvement in externalizing domains. Research indicates that these programmes are effective in improving the parents' child management skills, enhancing parental self-confidence, and reducing family stress and oppositional behaviour (Barkley et al. 1992) but do not reduce the core symptoms of ADHD as effectively as stimulant medication or enhance the effectiveness of stimulant medication. The body of literature indicating improvements in parent–child interactions following medication alone (Barkley and Cunningham 1979; Barkley 1985, 1988, 1989) documents decreases in negative mother–child interactions when children are treated with stimulant medication, but there is less consistent evidence showing increases in maternal positive behaviour. By comparison, behavioural interventions have not only demonstrated significant decreases in parental negative behaviour and directiveness towards their child but also significant increases in parental positive behaviour and parent reinforcement of prosocial child behaviour (Barkley et al. 1992).

Cognitive–behavioural therapy

RATIONALE

In the 1970s it was argued that traditional behaviour therapy's reliance on operant and classical conditioning failed to accurately predict or explain complex human behaviour. The critics suggested that behaviour therapy needed to expand to include underlying cognition. Michenbaum (1971) in a consideration of externalizing behaviours posited that the internalization of self-statements is the basis of self-control and is fundamental to the normal development of the process of behavioural regulation. Accordingly, processes that interrupt the generation of self-statements are viewed as significant in contributing factors to childhood behavioural problems. As noted above, the direct and cascaded effect of a deficient behavioural inhibition system leads to secondary impairments in executive neuropsychological abilities that are dependent upon behavioural inhibition for their effective execution. These include self-regulation and internal speech processes central to the development and maintenance of self-control. The basic premise is that children with ADHD lack the skills necessary to regulate their behaviour, and this deficiency is hypothesized to account for difficulties in regulating attentive, impulsive and interpersonal behaviours. CBT was predicated as addressing this deficient verbal mediation and inadequate regulation of behaviour (Michenbaum and Goodman 1971) by teaching conscious and effortful control strategies that improve response inhibition. The expectation is that the enhancement and internalization of self-regulating cognitive skills should provide the young person with the means for more appropriate behavioural regulation and facilitate academic functioning.

A number of different treatment procedures and approaches fall under the cognitive–behavioural intervention rubric, including self-instructional training, cognitive modelling, self-monitoring, self-reinforcement, and cognitive and interpersonal problem solving.

CBT interventions for ADHD children are based on a self-instructional approach. The child is taught self-instruction, and internal dialogue procedures that incorporate problem-solving strategies including plan formulation and error coping. The aim of CBT is to teach self-control strategies to redress the deficiencies in self-regulatory processes.

Typical self-management techniques include:
- Collaborative
- Encouragement of planned, self-regulated behaviour
- Enhancement of strategy use in unstructured, peer-oriented settings in which adults are typically unable to prompt, monitor or reward.

Interventions include:
- Stop–Think–Do
- Reinforced self-evaluation
- Anger management
- Social skills
- CBT for affective comorbid conditions
- Cognitive behavioural problem solving.

STOP–THINK–DO

This is usually an individually administered intervention, based on work by Camp et al. (1977), Shure and Spivack (1978), Barkley (1990) and Braswell and Blomquist (1991). The aim is to teach children problem solving strategies using a number of cognitive–behavioural training techniques:
- Problem exploration
- Generating solution strategies
- Self-monitoring and self-guidance while executing the plan
- Self-evaluation of chosen solution.

The programmes consist of approximately eight sessions comprising theoretical rationale and practical exercises (role play, modelling, etc.). The child and/or parents are taught to use (or teach and reinforce strategy adoption) in the home.

REINFORCED SELF-EVALUATION

Based on the work of Drabman et al. (1973) and Turkewitz et al. (1975), this intervention utilizes self-monitoring/self-evaluation anger control strategies. The aim is not to replace reinforcement-based social learning principles but rather to enhance them via verbal mediation and problem solving. The intervention is based on the premise that the child can be motivated to monitor and assess his/her behaviour with accuracy, and this self-evaluation is reinforced by contingent rewards. Programmes consist primarily of three stages:
1. Children learn to appraise, with accuracy, adult ratings of social behaviour
2. They associate accurate self-appraisal with token reinforcement that can be traded for tangible rewards
3. Ratings are set above which accurate appraisal is associated with token reinforcement.

Having operationalized the behavioural goal of the intervention, children are taught and practise self-monitoring and self-evaluation skills during a range of individual and/or group activities. Through modelling of both good and bad examples of this behaviour, the therapist ensures that the child understands the topography of the desired actions. Next a simple rating scale is developed with the child, to be used by both therapist and child to evaluate the child's behaviour during subsequent activities. The therapist and child compare their respective ratings, and the child is encouraged to recall with behavioural specificity the positive and negative aspects of his/her behaviour that underpin these scores. If the child over-inflates positive aspects of his/her behaviour the therapist should take care to reinforce evidence of any appropriate behaviours while seeking to assist the child's recall of those aspects of his/her behaviour that may have led to a less favourable overall evaluation. The child is positively reinforced for accurate self-evaluation. Once accurate self-monitoring and self-evaluation has been mastered, behavioural ratings are selected at and above which the child will receive positive reinforcement. The child's ability to accurately match the adult's rating can earn greater rewards.

Reinforced self-evaluation can be used to increase prosocial behaviour and decrease the frequency of antisocial behaviour.

The technique can be taught to parents and teachers with the goal of enhancing generalization of self-evaluative skills.

ANGER MANAGEMENT
These rehearsal-based interventions emphasize:
- Children's recognition of internal cues of impending anger
- Cognitive–behavioural strategies for redirecting anger
- Rehearsal of these procedures under progressively more realistic provocations from peers.

The programme begins with education about anger and ADHD at a level appropriate to the child's cognitive abilities. Training then proceeds to identification of the external and internal cues that signal incipient anger. A prerequisite to successful anger management is the reading of such cues as an indication of the need to employ self-control strategies. Then alternatives to eliciting aggressive responses are explored:
- Stop to examine possible motives of the provocateur(s)
- Teach, rehearse and practice alternative cognitive and behavioural responses to provocation that will compete with incipient retaliation
- Reinforcement of the use of adaptive anger management strategies.

Hinshaw et al. (1984) argue that the most essential process in effecting change is the graduated rehearsal of the chosen strategy with increasingly realistic provocation by adults and the child's peer group. Without this guided and reinforced practice, the cognitive strategies do not translate into self-controlled behaviour.

Hinshaw et al. (1998) report that there is little evidence on which to recommend self-instructionally based cognitive interventions for children with ADHD; but cognitive behavioural procedures that integrate problem-solving approaches with reinforcement appear to have some benefits in mildly effected ADHD children. They hypothesize that aggressive ADHD youngsters may well be refractory not only to CBT procedures but to nearly all current interventions, and that their needs are best met employing long-term, integrated treatment with maximum power.

SOCIAL SKILLS

A variety of socially inappropriate behaviours seem directly associated with the core features of ADHD. These include interrupting or intruding on the conversation of others, failing to notice or attend to important social cues, and poor frustration tolerance. Others may represent additional neurological deficits in social information processing (Crick and Dodge 1994). Social difficulties in children with ADHD are highly prevalent and frequently lead to peer rejection. Although the evidence for the efficacy of social skills training is less consistent than for behavioural interventions, there is an accumulating body of evidence indicating benefits when associated with behavioural contingency management.

Common features of social skills training include:
- Introducing yourself
- Giving and receiving positive feedback
- Sharing
- Compromising
- Coping with provocation
- Joining a conversation
- Problem solving
- Saying "no"
- Following directions
- Constructive complaining.

Each area usually merits individual attention. The session usually starts with a definition of the target behaviour and the child is encouraged to draw upon his/her own experience to identify potentially problematic functioning. The generation and evaluation of alternative behaviours follow this. Both automatic ways of behaving and hypothesized alternatives are explored using role play, with an emphasis on evaluating the consequences to the child of a chosen course of action. The child is encouraged to identify possible obstacles to using more adaptive behaviours, and these in turn are analysed and solutions are sought to over-come them. Through role play, children are encouraged to rehearse their chosen strategy both within and outside the session. Practice is assumed to facilitate competition between old automatic ways of responding and new laying down of alternatives. Parents and/or teachers are ideal co-therapists as they can provide the context to contingent behavioural management.

As with any other psychological intervention, invariant stages of therapy are:
1. Set goal for child
2. Set behavioural target for the child
3. Ensure targets reflect both severity of the deficit and the child's ability to achieve targets, which should be reasonable and achievable
4. Positively reinforce successful achievement
5. Encourage the child to set incrementally larger targets until the goal is achieved.

Researchers have found that children with ADHD are often knowledgeable about the process of prosocial behaviour and that they rarely exhibit skill deficits. However, in their everyday discourses and interactions they are rarely able to implement this knowledge. Even when social skills training produces improvements in social functioning it does not typically normalize the peer relationships of ADHD children (Pelham and Milich 1984, Krehbiel and Milich 1986); this may be the consequence of the salience of reputation in children's peer groups. Social skills training administered within the child's social context may go some way to alleviating this obstacle.

CBT FOR AFFECTIVE COMORBID CONDITIONS

There is an extensive literature demonstrating the effectiveness of CBT in ameliorating anxiety and depression. The techniques apply also to children who have ADHD, but need to be given with simplicity in explanations appropriate to people with poor listening skills.

COGNITIVE–BEHAVIOURAL PROBLEM SOLVING

Used in conjunction with parent training, this treatment focuses on the cognitive processes and deficits that are considered to mediate maladaptive interpersonal behaviour (Kazdin and Braswell 1985). Research has shown that altering cognitive processes can alter child behaviour at home and school (Kendall and Braswell 1982, Lochman et al. 1984, Arbuthnot and Gordon 1986). Parent training alone is unlikely to alter these processes within the child or the parent. The sessions focus on teaching the parent and the child problem-solving steps that can be used to manage interpersonal situations and to train requisite skills for generating new solutions, developing means–ends and consequential thinking, and taking the perspective and recognizing the feelings of others.

Parent and child are taught the art of win-win negotiation and contract making that can be used to form the basis of behavioural contracts.

Future research

COMPLIANCE THERAPY

A neglected issue in the treatment of children with ADHD is adherence to the therapeutic regimen. Compliance is an important issue because of its expected relationship with long-term outcome. In the treatment of ADHD, poor compliance has been suggested as a possible explanation for poor long-term treatment outcome (Firestone 1982, Brown et al. 1985). Children generally dislike the medication, which is often prescribed over long periods, two risk factors that are generally associated with lower compliance rates in all clinical populations (Epstein and Cluss 1982). Firestone (1982) found that approximately 20% of his patients had discontinued medication by the fourth month and that only 55% were still taking prescribed medication by the tenth month. Similarly, Firestone and Witt (1982) found that only 49% of the families who had agreed to a 4-month behavioural therapy intervention completed the programme. Brown et al. (1987) found that non-compliance with behavioural therapy was not as great as non-compliance with medication in families with a child with ADHD. One might assume that with increased knowledge about this developmental condition, current compliance rates may be a little more favourable.

It would seem that an important use of CBT would be the one it was originally intended for, that is as a mediational strategy to extend the benefits that accrue to more traditional interventions of behavioural therapy and pharmacotherapy. Given the relationship between good medication compliance or behavioural strategy fidelity and short-term outcome, the

151

next stage may include devising and testing CBT interventions to improve the acceptability of both medication and behavioural intervention to ADHD youngsters and their families.

REFERENCES

Abikoff H (1987) An evaluation of cognitive behavior therapy for hyperactive children. In: Lahey BB, Kazdin AE, eds. *Advances in Clinical Child Psychology, vol. 10.* New York: Plenum Press, pp. 171–216.

Abikoff H, Gittelman R (1984) Does behavior therapy normalize the classroom behavior of hyperactive children? *Arch Gen Psychiatry* **41**: 449–454.

Anderson CA, Hinshaw SP, Simmel C (1994) Mother–child interactions in ADHD and comparison boys. *J Abnorm Child Psychol* **22**: 247–265.

Arbuthnot J, Gordon DA (1986) Behavioural and cognitive effects of a moral reasoning intervention for high-risk behaviour disordered adolescents. *J Consult Clin Psychol* **54**: 208–216.

Barkley RA (1985) The social interaction of hyperactive children: Behavioural changes, drug effects and situational variation. In: McMahon R, Peters R, eds. *Childhood Disorders: Behavioral–Developmental Approaches.* New York. Brunner/Mazel, pp. 218–243.

Barkley RA (1988) The effects of methylphenidate on the interactions of preschool ADHD children with their mothers. *J Am Acad Child Adolesc Psychiatry* **27**: 336–341.

Barkley RA (1989) Hyperactive girls and boys: Stimulant drug effects on mother–child interactions. *J Child Psychol Psychiatry* **30**: 379–390.

Barkley RA (1990) *Attention Deficit Hyperactivity Disorder: A Handbook for Diagnosis and Treatment.* New York: Guilford Press.

Barkley RA (1997a) *Defiant Children: A Clinician's Manual for Assessment and Parent Training, 2nd edn.* New York: Guilford Press.

Barkley RA (1997b) *Managing the Defiant Child: a Guide to Parent Training.* New York: Guilford Press.

Barkley RA (2000) *Taking Charge of ADHD: The Complete Authoritative Guide for Parents.* New York: Guilford Press.

Barkley RA, Cunningham CE (1979) The effects of Ritalin on the mother–child interactions of hyperactive children. *Arch Gen Psychiatry* **36**: 201–208.

Barkley RA Guevremont DC, Anastopoulos AD, Fletcher KE (1992) Comparison of three family therapy programs for treating family conflicts in adolescents with attention deficit hyperactivity disorder. *J Consult Clin Psychol* **60**: 450–462.

Barkley RA, Shelton TL, Crosswait C, Moorehouse M, Fletcher K, Barrett S, Jenkins L, Metevia L (2000) Multi-method psycho-educational intervention for preschool children with disruptive behavior: preliminary results at post-treatment. *J Child Psychol Psychiatry* **41**: 319–332.

Braswell L, Blomquist ML (1991) *Cognitive Behaviour Therapy with ADHD Children:Child, Family and School Interventions.* New York: Guilford Press.

Brown RT, Borden KA, Clingerman SR (1985) Adherence to methylphenidate therapy in a psychiatric population: a preliminary investigation. *Psychopharmacol Bull* **21**: 28–36.

Brown RT, Borden KA, Wynne MA, Spunt AL, Clingerman SR (1987) Compliance with pharmocological and cognitive treatments for attention deficit disorder. *J Am Acad Child Adolesc Psychiatry* **26**: 521–526.

Camp BW, Blom GE, Herbert F, van Doorninck WJ (1977) "Think Aloud": a program for developing self-control in young aggressive boys. *J Abnorm Child Psychol* **5**: 157–169.

Carlson GA, Pelham WE, Milich R, Dixon J (1992) Single and combined effects of methyphenidate and behavioral therapy in classroom performance of children with attention deficit hyperactivity disorder. *J Abnorm Child Psychol* **20**: 213–232.

Crick NR, Dodge KA (1994) A review and reformulation of social information processing mechanisms in children's social adjustment. *Psychol Bull* **115**: 74–101.

Dodge KA (1991) The structure and function of reactive and proactive aggression. In: Pepler DJ, Rubins KN, eds. *The Development and Treatment of Childhood Aggression.* Hillsdale, NJ: Erlbaum, pp. 201–216.

Dornbusch JM, Ritter PL, Llederman P, Roberts D, Fraleigh M (1987) The relationship of parenting style to adolescent school performance. *Child Dev* **58**: 1244–1257.

Drabman R, Spitalnik R, O'Leary KD (1973) Teaching self-control to disruptive children. *J Abnorm Psychol* **82**: 10–16.

Epstein LH, Cluss PA (1982) A behavioural medicine perspective on long-term medical regimens. *J Consult*

Clin Psychol **50**: 950–971.

Evans C, Margison F, Barkham M (1998) The contribution of reliable and clinically significant change methods to evidence based mental health. *Evid Based Ment Health* **1**: 70–72.

Firestone P (1982) Factors associated with children's adherence to stimulant medication. *Am J Orthopsychiatry* **52**: 447–457.

Firestone P, Witt J (1982) Characteristics of families completing and prematurely discontinuing a behavioral parent-training program. *J Paediatr Psychol* **7**: 209–222.

Furman W, Wehner EA (1994) Romantic views: Toward a theory of adolescent romantic relationships. In: Montemayor R, Adams GR, Gullota GP, eds. *Advances in Adolescent Development, vol. 6: Relationships During Adolescence.* Beverly Hills, CA: Sage, pp. 168–195.

Gray JA (1982) *The Neuropsychology of Anxiety. An Inquiry into the Function of the Septo-hippocampal System.* New York: Oxford University Press.

Hinshaw SP (1994) *Attention Deficit and Hyperactivity in Children.* Thousand Oaks, CA: Sage.

Hinshaw SP, Erhardt D (1991) Attention deficit-hyperactivity disorder. In: Kendall PC, ed. *Child and Adolescent Therapy: Cognitive Behavioural Procedures.* New York: Guilford Press, pp. 98–128.

Hinshaw SP, Henker B, Whalen CK (1984) Self-control in hyperactive boys in anger-inducing situations: Effects of cognitive–behaviour training and of methylphenidate. *J Abnorm Child Psychol* **12**: 55–77.

Hinshaw SP, Klein RG, Abikoff H (1998) Childhood attention deficit hyperactivity disorder: Nonpharmalogical and combination treatments. In: Nathan PE, Gorman JM, eds. *Treatments that Work.* Oxford: Oxford University Press, pp. 26–41.

Humphries T, Kinsbourne M, Swanson J (1978) Stimulant effects on cooperation and social interaction between hyperactive children and their mothers. *J Child Psychol Psychiatry* **19**: 13–22.

Kazdin PC, Braswell L (1985) *Cognitive–Behavioral Therapy for Impulsive Children.* New York: Guilford Press.

Kazdin AE, Esveldt-Dawson K, French NH, Unis AS (1987a) Effects of parent management training and problem-solving skills training combined in the treatment of antisocial child behavior. *J Am Acad Child Adolesc Psychiatry* **26**: 416–424.

Kazdin AE, Esveldt-Dawson K, French NH, Unis AS (1987b) Problem-solving skills training and relationship therapy in the treatment of antisocial child behavior. *J Consult Clin Psychol* **55**: 76–85.

Kendall PC, Braswell L (1982) Cognitive behavioral self-control therapy for children: a component analysis. *J Consult Clin Psychol* **50**: 672–689.

Klein RG, Mannuzza S (1991) Long-term outcome of hyperactive children: a review. *J Am Acad Child Adolesc Psychiatry* **30**: 383–387.

Krehbiel G, Milich R (1986) Issues in the assessment and treatment of socially rejected children. In: Printz RJ, ed. *Advances in Behavioral Assessment of Children and Families, vol. 2.* Greenwich, CT: JAI Press, pp. 249–271.

Lochman JE, Burch PR, Curry JF, Lampron LB (1984) Treatment and generalization effects of cognitive–behavioural and goal-setting interventions with aggressive boys. *J Consult Clin Psychol* **52**: 915–916.

McArdle P, O'Brien G, Kolvin I (1997) Is there a comorbid link between hyperactivity and emotional psycho-pathology? *Eur Child Adolesc Psychiatry* **6**: 142–150.

Melnick SM, Hinshaw SP (2000) Emotion regulation and parenting in AD/HD and comparison boys: linkages with social behaviors and peer preference. *J Abnorm Psychol* **28**: 73–86.

Michenbaum DH (1971) Training impulsive children to talk to themselves. A means of developing self-control. *J Abnorm Psychol* **77**: 115–126.

Michenbaum DH, Goodman J (1971) Training impulsive children to talk to themselves: A means to developing self-control. *J Abnorm Psychol* **77**: 115–126.

Patterson GR (1982) *Coercive Family Process.* Eugene, OR: Castalia Press.

Pelham WE, Milich R (1984) Peer relationships in hyperactive children. *J Learn Disabil* **17**: 560–567.

Prinz RJ, Miller GE (1994) Family-based treatment for antisocial behavior: experimental influences of dropout and engagement. *J Consult Clin Psychol* **62**: 645–650.

Quay HC (1988) The behavioral reward and inhibition systems in childhood behavior disorders. In: Bloomingdale LM, ed. *Attention Deficit Disorder, vol. 3. New Research in Attention, Treatment and Psychopharmacology.* New York: Pergamon Press, pp. 176–186.

Rutter M, Giller H, Hagell A (1998) *Antisocial Behaviour by Young People.* Cambridge: Cambridge University Press.

Shure MB, Spivak G (1978) *Problem-solving Techniques in Child Rearing.* San Francisco: Jossey-Bass.

153

Tannock R (1998) Attention-deficit hyperactivity disorder: Advances in cognitive, neurobiological, and genetic research. *J Child Psychol Psychiatry* **39**: 65–99.

Webster-Stratton C (1990) *How to Promote Children's Social and Emotional Competence.* London: Sage.

Webster-Stratton C (1992a) The parents, teachers and children videotape series. Seattle: Seth Enterprises.

Webster-Stratton C (1992b) *The Incredible Years. A Trouble-Shooting Guide for Parents of Children Aged 3–8.* Toronto: Umbrella Press.

Webster-Stratton C (1998) Preventing conduct problems in head start children: strengthening parenting competencies. *J Consult Clin Psychol* **66**: 715–730.

Webster-Stratton C, Reid M, Hammond M (2004) Treating children with early-onset conduct problems: intervention outcomes for parent, child, and teacher training. *J Clin Child Adolesc Psychol* **33**: 105–124.

APPENDIX 9.1
MANAGEMENT WITHOUT MEDICATION

For younger children – Summary
Reward immediately the behaviour you want by:
    Praise – tell them why you are pleased
    Smiles, hugs and cuddles
    Favourite activities
    Small presents
Decrease unwanted behaviours by:
    Not giving in
    Ignoring bad behaviour – if behaviour cannot be ignored because it is dangerous or destructive you may
    have to say no, and restrain and remove him/her
    But *avoid shouting, constant criticism, making idle threats, showing you're cross, smacking*
Decide on rules and:
    Give clear instructions
Teach wanted behaviour by:
    Guiding
    Taking one step at a time
    Learning from others
    Watching your child
Keep trying – nobody's perfect
Look after yourself   find ways of keeping calm

Living with a child with ADHD is very stressful for all the family – parents, brothers and sisters.

Parents often find themselves becoming increasingly negative and angry with their child who does not respond to normal parenting. The level of tension in all the family rises, with the mother feeling it most.

The first step in reducing the tension is often in realizing that the child's problem is not your fault. It is not his/her fault either. Because of the differences in chemical tuning of his/her brain, s/he has difficulties in listening, following instructions, managing his/her behaviour, etc., and is unable, not unwilling, to behave normally.

You may find that members of your family are critical of your parenting – "That child needs a good smack!" – but often children with ADHD have been shouted at and smacked for years – has it worked?

Parents can become super parents by learning to use specially effective parenting techniques with their children. ADHD is not caused by poor parent management, but problem behaviours can certainly be improved by special management techniques.

For most parents the first method of coping with children with ADHD is through behavioural management. The techniques of behavioural management are used by professionals and are particularly useful for teachers who come into contact with children with ADHD.

What is behavioural management?

Behavioural management involves giving children clear rules, consistently enforced in a calm atmosphere. Praise is plentiful, immediate, and is supplemented by a clear reward system.

For mild forms of ADHD, behavioural management alone may be sufficient. Even for children who respond extremely well to medication, behavioural strategies can be useful during 'medication holidays'. When behavioural management is used with medication, the dose of medication needed is usually less.

When children have severe ADHD that is complicated by oppositional behaviour and conduct problems, medication has an effect on the core symptoms of attention problems, impulsivity and hyperactivity. But reducing oppositional behaviour, conduct problems and antisocial behaviour can only be achieved by behavioural management.

Sometimes parents will need intensive help from professionals if problems with oppositional behaviour are very severe.

Some parents will find the following guidance sufficient without additional professional help.

For younger children (up to about age 9 years)

TEACHING YOUR CHILD THE BEHAVIOUR YOU WANT

- Children will repeat behaviours if they are rewarded for that behaviour. This is called *reinforcing* the wanted behaviour.
- The behaviour you want may be sitting or playing quietly, tidying up toys, or sharing a game with a sister or brother. We sometimes don't even notice quiet behaviour.
- Use When–Then instructions: "When you have put your toys away, then you can have a story."

INCREASING THE BEHAVIOUR YOU WANT

- *Reinforce* the wanted behaviour:
    by praise
    by smiles, hugs and cuddles
    by a favourite activity – reading a story, a special programme on TV, a visit to the park
    by a small present – crayons, stickers
    by points or stars on a chart.
- You can also *reinforce behaviour in words:*
    "I am so pleased with you because . . ."
    "That was marvellous when you . . ."
    "I like it when you . . ."
    "You did that all by yourself, well done!"
    "Because you were so helpful we can . . ."
- *Catch a child being good and praise.*

Remember – positive reinforcement encourages your child to try harder.

Remember – praising makes parents feel good too: nagging or threatening makes parents feel upset and may reinforce unwanted behaviour.

DECREASING THE BEHAVIOUR YOU DON'T WANT

- Don't encourage children to repeat unwanted behaviour by the reward of giving in. If you don't want them to scream for sweets, ignore their screams and they will learn that you mean what you say. If you give in after 10 or 15 minutes, they will learn that if they scream for that length of time you will give in. So you must carry it through – do not give in.
- Giving in (even for a quiet life) or shouting at the child is likely to reinforce the unwanted behaviour.
- Do not scold but use *simple natural consequences* for everday situations. For example: if water is splashed out of the bath, the bath ends; or, if the child refuses to eat dinner, there will be no ice cream or sweets.

Praise the behaviour you want.

Ignore the behaviour you don't want.

HOW DO YOU WANT YOUR CHILD TO BEHAVE?

- Decide on the *House Rules* (e.g. bedtime routine, meal-time patterns).
- *Routine* makes a child feel secure. S/he needs to know what is acceptable and what is not. All adults in the household need to *agree* about the rules.
- Giving conflicting instructions confuses the child.
- *Give instructions clearly and consistently.*
- Are you sure your child knows what you want?
- Children with ADHD find listening difficult. Make *eye contact* with the child. Give short, clear instructions – wait five seconds for the child to comply – and then praise.
- Use a firm tone of voice and be positive – say "Please clear up after you've finished" not "Don't leave a mess". This may be more demanding and draining for exhausted parents than just saying "Don't . . .", but it is also much more effective in achieving the behaviour you want.
- If your child is in the middle of doing something, rather than abruptly interrupting, give a prompt: "In five minutes it will be bedtime."
- Teach new wanted behaviour by *guiding* – showing and helping, allowing the child to do it when s/he can.
- Encourage him/her to *practise* the new behaviour. Do this one step at a time – breaking down more difficult tasks so that the child can learn one stage at a time.

- *Catch your child being good* – when your child is doing something you want, it is an opportunity to praise.
- *Model* the behaviour you want at all times. In other words, if you want them to be polite, always be polite yourself to them, to everyone. If you don't want them to get into fights or behave aggressively, avoid using smacks or strong language for discipline.

STRATEGIES FOR AVOIDING TROUBLE
- *Play:* Try to improve the relationship with your child by playing with him/her. Instead of giving directions, teaching and asking questions, *attend* to what your child is doing. You can do this by giving a running commentary on what is happening:
    —Describing your child's play: "You're putting the car into the garage."
    —Describing his/her desired behaviour: "You're playing quietly by yourself."
    —Describing his/her likely moods and thoughts: "You're trying really hard to build that model."
  You may find this strange or uncomfortable at first but you will find your child beginning to settle and play longer and less aimlessly.
- *Planning ahead* is an important strategy for avoiding trouble. For example, long phone calls to friends can be made after your child is in bed. Alternatively, practise with your child what s/he can do to be quiet when the telephone rings during the day.
    Another time of trouble may be when feeding the baby. Your older child may need an interesting activity or may be taught to do something to help. Remember to praise him/her for being helpful.
- *Problem solving:* You can develop a problem-solving approach with your child from an early age.
    —First, *define* the problem; for example, the baby keeps taking his/her toys.
    —Second, the child is encouraged to think of as *many solutions* as possible to the problems, however silly (for example, hit the baby, take baby's toy, run away) and more sensible ones (offer baby another toy instead).
    —Help him/her look at the *pros and cons* of each solution (e.g. "If you hit him he may hit you back!").
    —Then *choose* the best option, try it out and see if it works.

For older children (circa 9 years and over)
The types of problems the child and parents experience are different but the principles of management are the same:
    The ABC analysis of behaviour is based on the observation that Behaviour is influenced by Antecedents (what happened before) and Consequences (what happened after) the behaviour.

For older children – Summary
- *Keep calm*
- Set clear rules and boundaries and stick to them
- Have a routine and plan ahead
- Reinforce frequently, clearly and immediately
- Say why you are pleased
- Use natural negative consequences
- Keep calm
- Listen to your tone of voice and balance praise and criticism
- Manage your child's social life - short visits for friends
- Avoid video-games except as a reward
- Look after brothers and sisters
- Look after yourself and your partner
- *Keep calm*
Good Luck!

Antecedents (before) – Behaviour – Consequences (after)

GETTING THE ANTECEDENTS RIGHT
- Short, clear instructions delivered in a positive tone - make sure you have eye contact first.
- Use helpful prompts:
    Lists – in the kitchen, in the bathroom, checklists of what is needed each day at school inside school bag.

157

Charts – (see below) listing tasks to be completed.

Kitchen timers are useful for timing homework, tooth-brushing, television and time out. They can be invaluable in reducing bickering over time-keeping, and children love to race them.

- Identify problem behaviours: was there any regular antecedent (for example, arguments over lost socks in the morning) that might be changed (as by getting clothes ready the night before)?

IMPROVING THE CONSEQUENCES

Reinforcing the behaviour you want

- Using a chart can be very helpful in providing clear visual evidence of the tasks completed.

  You may want to give pocket-money or privileges in response to the tasks completed.

  Remember – start at a very low level (what the child can achieve now) and build up slowly. If you expect too much too quickly you may lose heart.

  Calm, positive persistence wins.

  Always remember to *praise* as well as reinforce in other ways.

  Children with ADHD need reinforcement that is more frequent, more immediate and clear.
- Using a *token* or *point system* linked to a chart can both highlight the tasks achieved and also be linked to a response–cost system (see below) for unwanted behaviours.
- Give praise that is *linked* to the behaviour you are praising. "That's fantastic – all your homework completed tonight!" and praise in front of others.
- Try *Grandma's rule:* first you work then you play.

  For children who are difficult to reward – use as a reward what the child spends most of his/her free time doing. This could be playing on the computer or even lying in bed.

Example: David's Chart

	Mon	Tues	Wed	Thurs	Fri	Sat	Sun
Out of bed by 7.30	√	√	√				
Washed, dressed and breakfast by 8.10	√	√	√				
Ready to leave with school bag packed by 8.20		√	√				
Start homework at 5pm	√	√	√				
Homework completed and checked by 6.30	√	√	√				
Clothes ready, bag packed for next day	√	√	√				
Bath and in bed by 9pm	√	√	√				
Lights out at 9.15	√	√	√				
P for all tasks completed:		P	P				

TARIFF: Star awarded for all tasks ticked

For each star = small reward

Bonus if 7 stars in a row

The tariff can be varied according to the needs of the child. For example, at first there could be separate stars for mornings and evenings. Sequences of behaviour can gradually be established by starting with a high reward for one day and gradually increasing the consecutive days to earn a reward: One star earns a reward on 3 occasions, then two stars on consecutive days (2 in a row) earns a reward on 3 occasions (repeat 3 times), then 3 stars in a row can be repeated and so on.

REDUCING UNWANTED BEHAVIOUR

- Extinguish – do not reinforce in any way. Do not tell off, shout, argue or nag.

  For example, answering back can be dealt with very effectively by the parent avoiding responding in any way.

  Unfortunately many parents find this difficult as they think, "I can't let him get away with this. I can't let him have the last word."

  Ignoring sounds easy but is a hard skill for parents to manage. Ignoring means no eye contact, not speaking to the child, and no physical contact with the child. Ignoring is appropriate for non-dangerous behaviour such as tantrums and answering back. Strategies for dealing with dangerous behaviours are generally dealt with by problem-solving.

- Use *natural consequences* wherever possible.

    For example, if a child is not ready on time s/he will miss a treat.
- *Response cost* can be a powerful way of reminding a child of behaviour to avoid – by deducting points or pocket money.

    Because of their problems, children with ADHD earn fewer rewards than other children. They find it difficult to be motivated by rewards that they think they can never obtain.

    Therefore, the child is given the reward (pocket money or points) at the beginning and must work to keep the reward.

    For example, to reduce swearing, pocket money is put in a jar on a shelf visible to the child. While the child does as asked, the money is theirs. Every time s/he swears, a small amount of money is removed from the jar.
- *Time-out* is shorthand for *time-out from positive reinforcement*. It means removing the child from the fun in the family and all the rewards that were reinforcing the undesirable behaviour, including you telling him/her off.

    It can be difficult for parents to keep quiet themselves. It can be helpful to remind yourself by a slogan – "zip your mouth" or "button your lips".

    It is important that the child knows exactly what behaviour led to time-out. S/he is removed to a place that is unstimulating and boring (the hall or a chair facing a wall and not his/her bedroom) for a previously agreed reason (tantrum, hitting) and not for a minor misdemeanor which is better ignored.

    The time should be short (one minute for each year of age) and the child must be quiet for the last minute and stay for as long as it takes until s/he is quiet for a whole minute. The first few times this may take 40 minutes or more: soon this will reduce to a few minutes only.

    Time-out gives you a break to calm down. Time-out can be difficult to carry out but is frequently useful in interrupting stressful cycles of conflict. It is important to use it calmly and to welcome the child back when s/he is behaving reasonably again.
- *Remember* children with ADHD have good days and bad days. Variable behaviour and mood are typical of ADHD.
- Keep *calm* and do not allow the situation to escalate – walk away from trouble.
- Find ways of coping with your own stress. Use the bathroom to escape quickly for a moment. Learn to relax and look after yourself.

PROBLEM SOLVING

Many children with ADHD have particular difficulties in managing to pause to problem-solve and may often react in a knee-jerk, panicky style. They can often be helped to go through a problem-solving routine:
1. Slow down, what's the problem?
2. What are my choices?
3. What would happen with this choice? How might I feel?
4. Now how do I carry out the best choice?
5. How did that choice work? Should I make another choice next time?

SOCIAL SKILLS TRAINING

Use every opportunity to teach children how to behave. You may also find that your local school or clinic has groups which help. They are likely to train children in improving their skills with others, in making requests, giving and receiving compliments, making and keeping friends. They are likely to use role-play, video-feedback and lots of rehearsal and practice.

You may find that in addition to these strategies your child will need medication.

Often combining medication with behavioural management strategies produces the best outcome overall. Parents frequently find that on medication their child finds it easier to learn to fit in with the family, to get on better with friends and to learn better at school.

10
ADHD AND SLEEP DISORDERS

Paul Gringras, Adam Jaffe and Stephen Sheldon

Early clinical observations suggesting links between night-time sleep problems and day-time behaviours and cognition in children were described by Osler reporting on children with chronic tonsillitis and sleep difficulties in 1892: "The expression is dull, heavy, and apathetic. . . In long-standing cases the child is very stupid-looking, responds slowly to questions, and may be sullen and cross. . . The influence upon the mental development is striking." (Osler, quoted in Carroll and Loughlin 1995a.)

Sleep research has demonstrated that children, like adults, need an adequate amount of good quality sleep, and without this a decline in daytime cognitive abilities and an increase in problem behaviours results. Depriving children of sleep increases daytime sleepiness (Ishihara 1999), impairs verbal creativity and abstract thinking, and can affect cognitive and academic performance (Fallone et al. 2001). Even the loss of just one hour's sleep per night has a demonstrable effect on children's academic functioning and daytime behaviour (Sadeh et al. 2003).

Many of the behavioural and cognitive problems produced by inadequate amounts or quality of sleep overlap with those described in attention deficit hyperactivity disorder (ADHD) (Klorman et al. 1999, Steenari et al. 2003). Steenari and coworkers studied the effects of sleep quantity and quality on a battery of auditory and visual working memory tasks in 60 non-clinical school-age children. Sleep parameters and neuropsychological abilities were measured objectively with actigraphy and computer presented test paradigms. The study found lower sleep efficiency and longer sleep latency were associated with a higher percentage of incorrect response in working memory tasks. Similar specific working memory deficits have also been identified in ADHD (Klorman et al. 1999). The same group employed similar study methodology to examine the effects of sleep quantity and quality on parent and teacher perceived behaviours. They found decreased quantity of sleep time was significantly associated with externalizing symptoms such as aggressive and delinquent behaviour and attention and social problems (Aronen et al. 2000, Steenari et al. 2003).

Parents of children with ADHD report a greatly increased rate of sleep problems when compared with siblings (Ring et al. 1998) or controls (Stein 1999), although parental reports are not confirmed by objective measurements (Ball and Lavigne 1995, Corkum et al. 2001). Objective tests of daytime sleepiness have shown that despite their hyperactive behaviours, children with ADHD are sleepier during the day than siblings or controls (Lecendreux et al. 2000). These findings suggest that theoretically, improvements in those components of attention that accompany wakefulness, including executive functioning, alerting and orienting deficits could result in an overall improvement in ADHD symptomatology. These sleep problems, associated with ADHD have been well described for many years and were indeed part of the initial diagnostic criteria for ADHD in DSM-III (APA 1980).

Debates about associations and causality have led to polarized opinions. At one extreme has been the belief, held by a number of sleep medicine practitioners, that conditions resulting in chronic sleep disruption may actually cause ADHD: "25% of all children with ADHD . . . could have their ADHD eliminated if their habitual snoring and any associated SRBD [sleep-related breathing disorder] were effectively treated" (Chervin et al. 1997). At the other extreme is the belief that sleep disorders in ADHD are merely a peripheral manifestation in children who are difficult to control and who may suffer sleep problems associated with stimulant use.

Evidence from the literature

For the purposes of this chapter we searched Medline and Embase using the keywords: attention deficit hyperactivity disorder, sleep disorder, behaviour disorder, obstructive sleep apnoea syndrome, restless leg syndrome, and periodic limb movement disorder, with limits applied to the age range from infancy to 16 years, humans, and English journals. Searches were taken no further back than 1995 as a previous literature review (Corkum et al. 1998) covered earlier references. Papers were cross-referenced and we also searched relevant bibliographies. As in the earlier review, we found varying case definitions, varying methods of case ascertainment and different outcome measures, which would have made any formal type of meta-analysis impossible. Factors including age, sex and socio-economic status are important confounders, yet few studies had corrected for these.

Primary sleep disorders associated with ADHD

Sleep Onset Insomnia and Sleep Phase Delay Syndrome

The most common sleep disorder associated with ADHD is sleep onset insomnia (Barkley et al. 1990a). Varying definitions exist, but in general studies seek a prolonged sleep latency (time to fall asleep after settling in bed), assuming a chronologically reasonable expected bedtime. Although many factors are known to cause sleep onset insomnia, children with ADHD show evidence of a true sleep phase delay syndrome as evidenced by delayed sleep onset, delayed dim light melatonin onset and delayed wake-up time (Van der Heijden et al. 2005). Though this area remains complex and studies require validation in larger populations, the evidence points towards an intrinsic endogenous circadian pacemaker disorder in the subset of children with ADHD and sleep onset insomnia. Given that sleep rhythms rely to a large extent on the rhythms of endogenous melatonin production, trials of exogenous melatonin seem logical and are further discussed in the Intervention section towards the end of this chapter.

Obstructive Sleep Apnoea Syndrome and ADHD

Following Osler's original observations, the possible role of obstructive sleep apnoea syndrome (OSAS) in causing sleep disruption and ADHD-like symptoms continues to be enthusiastically explored. Attractive biological hypotheses have been advanced, speculating that persistent nocturnal hypoxia may damage vulnerable brain areas(Beebe and Gozal 2002).

TABLE 10.1
Obstructive sleep apnoea syndrome*

Clinical features
- Occasional or frequent nocturnal awakenings may occur
- The parents may note snoring, brief respiratory pauses, and gasps
- Snoring is characteristic but not diagnostic and may be more subtle than the snoring of adults
- Sleep-related enuresis and nocturnal profuse sweating are common associated features
- As a result of nocturnal sleep fragmentation, varying degrees of daytime sleepiness may occur (Sheldon et al. 1997)
- Polysomnography (PSG) with recordings of chest and abdominal movements, airflow at nose and mouth, and ideally oesophageal manometry is again the 'gold standard' objective test (Section on Pediatric Pulmonology 2002), although less invasive measures for OSAS are being actively pursued

Polysomnographic diagnosis
- Adult definitions for many sleep disorders are not equally applicable in childhood
- In polysomnographic terms, in general, an apnoea index ≥1 event per hour is sufficient for diagnosis
- An apnoea + hypopnoea index ≥5 events per hour of sleep without oxygen desaturation; ≥2 episodes of obstructive apnoea and/or hypopnoea associated with at least a 2% arterial oxygen desaturation; ≥1 episodes of obstructive apnoea and/or hypopnoea associated with at least a 3% fall in oxygen saturation; and/or periods of hypercapnia and/or desaturation during sleep associated with snoring, periodic paradoxical respiratory effort, and with either frequent arousals from sleep or markedly negative oesophageal pressure swings

*Schechter (2002).

OSAS is on a broad spectrum of sleep-disordered breathing and is relatively common, estimated to affect 1–3% of children (Schechter 2002). Peak prevalence is in the preschool and early elementary school-aged years, similar to that described for ADHD.

Accurate diagnosis unfortunately requires costly objective analysis using polysomnographic testing; although there are questionnaire-derived OSAS scoring systems, they fail to distinguish primary snoring of no pathological significance from true OSAS (Carroll and Loughlin 1995b) (Table 10.1). For this reason, all studies using subjective measures of SRBD must be interpreted with caution. This important limitation is seen in many questionnaire-based surveys, which seem to indicate associations between symptoms of SRBD and behaviours suggestive of ADHD (Chervin et al. 1997, O'Brien et al. 2003a). In fact, most of the 'cases' will simply have primary snoring, of no pathological significance. Furthermore, snoring and symptoms of obstructive sleep apnoea are related to obesity (Wing et al. 2003) – a proxy marker for social class which is an important confounder.

When objective tests for sleep-related breathing problems including OSAS are employed, no one index of respiratory disturbance accounts for more than a negligible proportion of hyperactivity symptoms (Chervin and Archbold 2001). The only exception to this robust finding is when subjects with OSAS also have periodic limb movements during the night. In these subjects the rate of periodic limb movements in one study showed a linear association with hyperactivity symptoms (Chervin et al. 2002).

PERIODIC LIMB MOVEMENT DISORDER AND ADHD
Periodic limb movement disorder (PLMD) of sleep is defined as the occurrence of periodic

TABLE 10.2
Periodic limb movement disorder (PLMD)*

Clinical features
- The history may reveal frequent awakenings and unrefreshing sleep
- Numerous partial arousals occur and significantly disrupt sleep architecture and continuity
- There are repetitive and stereotypical movements of one or both legs. The arms may also be involved
- Parents may express concerns about these periodic jerking movements. More commonly, patients are unaware of the partial or brief arousals and complaints centre on symptoms of excessive daytime sleepiness (Sheldon et al. 1997)
- Parent questionnaires exist and have a variable diagnostic yield with low sensitivity and specificity (Chervin and Archbold 2001)
- There is a strong genetic component, and in one study of children with ADHD and PLMD 32% of parents with affected children also reported symptoms of PLMD (Picchietti et al. 1999)
- Polysomnography (PSG) with tibialis anterior EMG is again the 'gold standard' objective test, although actigraphy (portable movement detectors and recorders that quantify body movements) is a less accurate, but cheaper method that has been used
- Severity of PLMD may be further explored by noting which movements are associated with arousals during PSG

Polysomnographic diagnosis
- In the case of PLMD, ≥5 EMG-recorded events per hour of sleep is typically considered abnormal
- However, there is a dearth of normative data in Tanner 1 (prepubertal) children, and the significance of PLMD with and without arousals in children remains uncertain

*Sheldon et al. (1997).

episodes of repetitive and highly stereotyped limb movements during sleep. It occurs in around 8% of children (Crabtree et al. 2003) (Table 10.2). A number of studies have shown hyperactivity symptoms are highly correlated with the presence of 5 or more periodic limb movements (PLMs) per hour (Chervin et al. 2002). Even after adjusting for sleepiness, restless sleep in general or use of stimulants, studies have demonstrated a dose-dependent relationship between PLM scores and inattention/hyperactivity scores (Chervin et al. 2002). As in adult studies of PLMD, it appears to be specifically those PLMs associated with arousals that are clinically important and separate the PLMD children with and without high ADHD scores. One group has suggested that the number of arousals during sleep is more directly linked with hyperactivity than the periodicity of PLMs (Crabtree et al. 2003).

Effective treatments for PLMD in adults exist, and Walters et al. (2000) reported on the positive impact of dopaminergic therapy in children with PLMD in sleep and ADHD. In a small uncontrolled study of dopaminergic therapies for children with PLMS and ADHD, PLMS and associated arousals were significantly reduced, and objective measures of visual memory and attention all improved. Such promising reports need urgent replication in larger and well-controlled studies. The use of dopaminergic agents is all the more interesting as animal models have proposed early derangements to dopamine pathways as a consequence of early hypoxia as a possible mechanism for ADHD (Cortese et al. 2005).

DISTURBANCES OF SLEEP ARCHITECTURE
The specific PMLD/ADHD group seem to have a lower REM sleep percentage and less

frequent spontaneous arousals when compared to matched controls. It has previously been suggested that although there are REM changes in ADHD, these are likely to be non-pathological (Corkum et al. 1998). There is still debate on this issue, with recent studies identifying increases in REM sleep latency and decreases in total REM sleep percentage in children with ADHD. Other studies have identified a more restless sleep, shifting more often between sleep stages, with deep and REM sleep more discontinuous (Gruber et al. 2000). Such sleep may be non-restorative, which could produce chronic sleep deprivation.

Extrinsic factors
BEHAVIOUR, COMORBIDITY AND MEDICATION EFFECTS
It is equally important to consider possible causes of poor sleep in ADHD that occur in response to external factors, or factors unrelated to any particular intrinsic physiological sleep disorder. Behavioural sleep disorders (BSDs) include limit-setting sleep disorder (with significant bedtime resistance) and sleep-onset association disorder (presenting with frequent or prolonged night wakening).

Owens et al. (1998) showed in a group of children with established OSAS that has that factors other than indices of respiratory disturbance may cause sleep problems. From a group of 100 children with confirmed OSAS they found that one-quarter showed significant behavioural problems (primarily bedtime resistance) in addition to OSAS. Corkum et al. (1999) highlighted the potential contribution of comorbid psychiatric disorders and stimulant medication to sleep problems. They found dysomnias (bedtime resistance, sleep-onset problems, difficulty arising) were related to confounding factors such as oppositional defiant disorder and stimulant use rather than ADHD. A further study used a well-defined cohort of children with ADHD established after comprehensive assessments and administered standard sleep questionnaires (Mick et al. 2000). In agreement with Corkum's findings, they found that an initial association between ADHD and sleep problems disappeared when psychiatric comorbidity and pharmacotherapy were controlled for. In particular treatment, with stimulants and comorbidity with anxiety and behaviour disorders were significantly associated with sleep disorders.

Although these last two studies underline the importance of a full psychiatric interview, and consideration of all possible comorbidities and medication, unfortunately their reliance on subjective parent interview sleep data limits any generalization of their findings to intrinsic sleep disorders such as OSAS and PLMD, which both require objective measurement.

EFFECTS OF ADHD MEDICATIONS ON SLEEP
Stimulants
In general, most pharmacological studies have shown that stimulants such as methylphenidate used in ADHD can have deleterious effects on sleep, usually prolonging sleep latency (time to fall asleep) (Barkley et al. 1990). However, a recent observational study found that the use of stimulant medication in children with ADHD was not associated with differences in subjective sleep quality or objective sleep measures, in comparison with children with ADHD not taking any medication (O'Brien et al. 2003b). Clinicians continue to report a subset of children with ADHD who seem to settle and fall asleep much easier if they have

received an evening dose of melatonin. The possibility that methyphenidate itself might in some way affect circadian rhythms remains an interesting, if as yet theoretical possibility.

Atomoxetine
This selective noradrenaline reuptake inhibitor based treatment for ADHD appears to have less influence than methyphenidate on sleep-onset insomnia. When the two were compared in a recent study, objective outcome measures showed a mean increase in sleep latency for stimulants compared with no increase for atomoxetine (Sangal et al. 2006).

Clonidine
Although well established as a potentially useful medication for ADHD, the role of clonidine in promoting sleep has always been less certain. Clonidine is a noradrenaline alpha-2-receptor agonist, which has been considered to act mainly on the autoreceptors of presynaptic noradrenergic neurons to reduce their release of noradrenaline. Noradrenaline is thought to act to increase percentages of REM sleep. Clinical experience has often shown that the initial benefits on sleep seem to wear off after a 'honeymoon period', and that higher doses are required with more adverse effects and less benefits. Overnight polysomnograms on children who happen to be taking clonidine have shown varying effects of clonidine on REM sleep. This finding has been more recently elucidated by elegant work from Japan that has shown showed clear dose-related effects of clonidine on sleep (Miyazaki et al. 2004). At low doses (25 µg) REM sleep was increased, with a corresponding decrease in non-REM sleep during the second third of the night. Higher-dose clonidine (150 µg) in contrast significantly decreased REM and increased non-REM sleep on drug nights compared to baseline nights in the entire night.

Modafanil
Although modafinil exhibits a small degree of dopaminergic action by blocking the dopamine transporter, the major effect of modafinil may be attributable to neuronal activity in the hypothalamus, particularly pertaining to the recently discovered peptides hypocretin 1 and 2 (also known as orexin A and B). Modafanil has been licensed for the treatment of excessive daytime sleepiness associated with narcolepsy and OSAS. Its mode of action is still uncertain, and although effects on noradrenergic uptake and dopamine transporter blockade have been suggested, the major effect of modafinil may be attributable to neuronal activity in the hypothalamus, relevant to the recently discovered hypocretin peptides. Theoretically, modafinil could be beneficial in improving those components of attention that accompany wakefulness including executive functioning, alerting and orienting. A small randomized placebo-controlled study of 22 children showed significant improvements in the Test of Variables of Attention, and the Conners Rating Scales over a 6-week period (Rugino and Samsock 2003). The small numbers in this study make accurate estimations of effect size difficult, and a dose ranging and 'head-to-head' comparison with methyphenidate is still required.

Side-effects appear minimal, and it remains to be seen whether this medication will be useful in the management of ADHD per se, or perhaps in a subgroup of children whose daytime symptoms are significantly exacerbated by disturbances in sleep quality or quantity.

Longitudinal studies

Prospective cohort studies should begin to clarify issues around ADHD and sleep associations, confounders and causality. However, we were able to find only one longitudinal study in which a group of children with severe sleep problems in infancy and a control group were followed for 5 years (Thunstrom 2002). A community sample of 2518 infants aged 6–18 months was approached; 83% responded but then drop-outs were high. A case group of those children aged 6–12 months who fulfilled specific criteria for severe and chronic sleep problems (n=27) was compared with a control group of equal size, matched for age and gender. At the age of 5.5 years, seven of the children in the sleep problem group met the criteria for ADHD based on an in-depth assessment by a multidisciplinary team. None of the control children qualified for the diagnosis. Causality, however, remains elusive, as the 'sleep problem group' may of course also share a genetic or physiological predisposition to ADHD (which was not diagnosed at 6 months when the sleep disorders were ascertained).

Intervention studies: Sleep hygiene and melatonin

Despite the wealth of robust controlled trials addressing the daytime treatment of ADHD, it is only more recently that this methodology has been applied to studies of interventions for sleep problems. Given the range of sleep problems associated with ADHD, the studies have simplified matters by focusing on subgroups, mainly with sleep onset insomnia.

Good sleep hygiene has long been the mantra at the outset of treating all sleep disorders. Despite the suggestion that sleep onset insomnia is more related to a phase delay than to poor parenting, there is now research evidence to back up the clinical experience of sleep hygiene helping. Basic, sensible sleep hygiene in a study of 27 children with sleep onset insomnia and ADHD achieved a significant reduction in insomnia for 5 of the children, with an effect size of 0.67 (Weiss et al. 2006).

Melatonin is a logical treatment for sleep onset insomnia, particularly if one believes there is an underlying circadian rhythm disorder. Its clinical use in children with ADHD and sleep problems is long established, but evidence from controlled trials is lacking. Weiss et al. (2006) enrolled the 22 children from their study whose insomnia refractory to sleep hygiene to a double-blind, randomized, cross-over trial of melatonin vs placebo. Using 5 mg of melatonin administered 20 minutes before bedtime, they achieved a significant 16 minute reduction in sleep latency with an effect size of 0.6. The effect of combined sleep hygiene and melatonin from baseline to 90 days post-trial was an impressive 1.7, with this group of children falling asleep on average one hour earlier than at the trial outset.

Conclusions

Methodological problems still hamper interpretation of many studies of sleep and ADHD. Studies are further complicated by the simple fact that ADHD is a disorder of heterogenous aetiology with widely varying comorbidities. For those children with ADHD who also have sleep problems, the identification of different sleep disorder subgroups appears to hold the most promise both in the research area and when planning clinical interventions.

The evidence is compelling that a group of children with ADHD have a true circadian rhythm disorder. The impact of melatonin treatment when targeted at this group appears dramatic in early controlled trials. There is some evidence for an association between OSAS and ADHD but it is weak, and with little to support earlier claims of causality. Nevertheless, sleep-related breathing problems clearly worsen daytime behaviours and cognition in children and need prompt recognition and treatment. PLMD seems to be more strongly associated with ADHD, but recent studies suggest that it is the PLMD associated with arousals that is most strongly linked with symptoms of hyperactivity. The association of REM sleep disruptions, PLMD and ADHD raises yet further questions about confounding factors and directions of causality.

Until others have replicated Thunstrom's findings, there is little apart from speculation to support any proposed causal link. Thus, whilst sleep deprivation or fragmentation with frequent arousals may worsen daytime behaviours, so may the presence of ADHD with oppositional behaviours cause problems around bedtime, affect total sleep duration, and perhaps cause PLMD and arousals that are in some way related to the pathophysiology of ADHD in some children.

CLINICAL IMPLICATIONS
In practical terms perhaps the most important message is that ADHD and sleep-related disorders are common, treatable, and will frequently coexist. Lack of training and services for paediatric sleep disorders (Stores 2001) mean that it is more likely that a sleep disorder will be missed in a child with ADHD than the converse. In the UK and parts of Europe there is often a striking lack of any multidisciplinary approach to paediatric sleep medicine, which is so essential. Effective treatments for most sleep disorders exist and, in addition to resolving sleep problems, may improve daytime behavioural and cognitive problems. There is growing research support for the clinical combination of sleep hygiene and melatonin in children with ADHD and sleep onset insomnia.

Any child with significant symptoms of inattention, hyperactivity and impulsivity should be fully evaluated for a clinical diagnosis of ADHD as discussed in previous chapters. During such an assessment, questionnaires screening for sleep problems should also be routinely used. [Chervin et al. (2003) have described test properties of a questionnaire focusing solely on OSAS and PLMD that involves 20 yes/no questions, and omits the daytime behavioural questions that would already be established during an assessment for ADHD.] Given the shortfalls associated with relying on sleep screening questionnaires alone, the individual clinicians will have to decide – based on resources as well as results (Schechter 2002) – when to progress to referral for more objective investigations.

REFERENCES

APA (1980) *Diagnostic and Statistical Manual of Mental Disorders, 3rd edn (DSM-III)*. Washington, DC: American Psychiatric Association.
Aronen ET, Paavonen E, Fjallberg M, Soininen M, Torronen J (2000) Sleep and psychiatric symptoms in school-age children. *J Child Adolesc Psychopharmacol* **39**: 502–508.
Ball J, Lavigne G (1995) Sleep patterns among ADHD children. *Clin Psychol Rev* **15**: 681–691.

Barkley RA, McMurray MB, Edelbrock CS, Robbins K (1990) Side effects of methylphenidate in children with attention deficit hyperactivity disorder: a systemic, placebo-controlled evaluation. *Pediatrics* **86**: 184–192.

Beebe DW, Gozal D (2002) Obstructive sleep apnea and the prefrontal cortex: towards a comprehensive model linking nocturnal upper airway obstruction to daytime cognitive and behavioral deficits. *J Sleep Res* **11**: 1–16.

Carroll JL, Loughlin GM (1995a) Obstructive sleep apnea syndrome in infants and children: clinical features and pathophysiology. Ferber R, Kryger M, eds. *Principles and Practice of Sleep Medicine in the Child.* Philadelphia: WB Saunders, pp. 163–191.

Carroll JL, Loughlin GM (1995b) Obstructive sleep apnea syndrome in infants and children: diagnosis and management. In: Ferber R, Kryger M, eds. *Principles and Practice of Sleep Medicine in the Child.* Philadelphia: WB Saunders, pp. 193–214.

Chervin RD, Archbold KH (2001) Hyperactivity and polysomnographic findings in children evaluated for sleep-disordered breathing. *Sleep* **24**: 313–320.

Chervin RD, Dillon JE, Bassetti C, Ganoczy DA, Pituch KJ (1997) Symptoms of sleep disorders, inattention, and hyperactivity in children. *Sleep* **20**: 1185–1192.

Chervin RD, Archbold KH, Dillon JE, Pituch KJ, Panahi P, Dahl RE, Guilleminault C (2002) Associations between symptoms of inattention, hyperactivity, restless legs, and periodic leg movements. *Sleep* **25**: 213–218.

Chervin RD, Dillon JE, Archbold KH, Kristen H, Ruzicka DL (2003) Conduct problems and symptoms of sleep disorders in children. *J Am Acad Child Adolesc Psychiatry* **42**: 201–208.

Corkum P, Tannock R, Moldofsky H (1998) Sleep disturbances in children with attention-deficit/hyperactivity disorder. *J Am Acad Child Adolesc Psychiatry* **37**: 637–646.

Corkum P, Moldofsky H, Hogg-Johnson S, Humphries T, Tannock R (1999) Sleep problems in children with attention-deficit/hyperactivity disorder: impact of subtype, comorbidity, and stimulant medication. *J Am Acad Child Adolesc Psychiatry* **38**: 1285–1293.

Corkum P, Tannock R, Moldofsky H, Hogg-Johnson S, Humphries T (2001) Actigraphy and parental ratings of sleep in children with attention-deficit/hyperactivity disorder (ADHD). *Sleep* **24**: 303–312.

Cortese S, Konofal E, Lecendreux M, Arnulf I, Mouren MC, Darra F, Dalla Bernardina B (2005) Restless legs syndrome and attention-deficit/hyperactivity disorder: a review of the literature. *Sleep* **28**: 1007–1013.

Crabtree VM, Ivanenko A, O'Brien LM, Gozal D (2003) Periodic limb movement disorder of sleep in children. *J Sleep Res* **12**: 73–81.

Fallone G, Acebo C, Arnedt JT, Seifer R, Carskadon MA (2001) Effects of acute sleep restriction on behavior, sustained attention, and response inhibition in children. *Percept Mot Skills* **93**: 213–229.

Gruber R, Sadeh A, Raviv A (2000) Instability of sleep patterns in children with attention-deficit/hyperactivity disorder. *J Am Acad Child Adolesc Psychiatry* **39**: 495–501.

Ishihara K (1999) The effect of 2-h sleep reduction by a delayed bedtime on daytime sleepiness. *Psychiatry Clin Neurosci* **53**: 113–115.

Klorman R, Hazel-Fernandez LA, Shaywitz SE (1999) Executive functioning deficits in attention-deficit/hyperactivity disorder are independent of oppositional defiant or reading disorder. *J Am Acad Child Adolesc Psychiatry* **38**: 1148–1155.

Lecendreux M, Konofal E, Bouvard M, Falissard B, Mouren-Simeoni MC (2000) Sleep and alertness in children with ADHD. *J Child Psychol Psychiatry* **41**: 803–812.

Mick E, Biederman J, Jetton J, Faraone SV (2000) Sleep disturbances associated with attention deficit hyperactivity disorder: the impact of psychiatric comorbidity and pharmacotherapy. *J Child Adolesc Psychopharmacol* **10**: 223–231.

Miyazaki S, Uchida S, Mukai J, Nishihara K (2004) Clonidine effects on all-night human sleep: Opposite action of low- and medium-dose clonidine on human NREM–REM sleep proportion. *Psychiatry Clin Neurosci* **59**: 138–144.

O'Brien LM, Holbrook CR, Mervis CB, Klaus CJ, Bruner JL, Raffield TJ, Rutherford J, Mehl RC, Wang M, Tuell A, Hume BC, Gozal D (2003a) Sleep and neurobehavioral characteristics of 5- to 7-year-old children with parentally reported symptoms of attention-deficit/hyperactivity disorder. *Pediatrics* **111**: 554–563.

O'Brien LM, Ivanenko A, Crabtree VM, Holbrook CR, Bruner JL, Klaus CJ, Gozal D (2003b) The effect of stimulants on sleep characteristics in children with attention deficit/hyperactivity disorder. *Sleep Med* **4**: 309–316.

Osler W (1892) Chronic tonsillitis. In: *The Principles and Practice of Medicine.* New York: Appleton, pp. 335–339.

Owens JA, Opipari L, Nobile C, Spirito A (1998) Sleep and daytime behavior in children with obstructive sleep apnea and behavioral sleep disorders. *Pediatrics* **102**: 1178–1184.

Picchietti DL, Underwood DJ, Farris WA, Walters AS, Shah MM, Dahl RE, Trubnick LJ, Bertocci MA, Wagner M, Hening WA (1999) Further studies on periodic limb movement disorder and restless legs syndrome in children with attention-deficit hyperactivity disorder. *Mov Disord* **14**: 1000–1007.

Ring A, Stein D, Barak Y, Teicher A, Hadjez J, Elizur A, Weizman A (1998) Sleep disturbances in children with attention-deficit/hyperactivity disorder: a comparative study with healthy siblings. *J Learn.Disabil* **31**: 572–578.

Rugino TA, Samsock TC (2003) Modafinil in children with attention-deficit hyperactivity disorder. *Paediatr Neurol* **29**: 136–142.

Sadeh A, Gruber R, Raviv A (2003) The effects of sleep restriction and extension on school-age children: what a difference an hour makes. *Child Dev* **74**: 444–455.

Sangal B, Owens J, Allen A, Sutton V, Feng W, Schuh K, Kelsey D (2006) Effects of atomoxetine and methylphenidate on children with attention deficit hyperactivity disorder. *Sleep* (in press).

Schechter MS; Section on Pediatric Pulmonology, Subcommittee on Obstructive Sleep Apnea Syndrome (2002) Technical report: diagnosis and management of childhood obstructive sleep apnea syndrome. *Pediatrics* **109**: e69.

Section on Pediatric Pulmonology (2002) Clinical practice guideline: diagnosis and management of childhood obstructive sleep apnea syndrome. *Pediatrics* **109**: 704–712.

Sheldon SH, Spire JP, Levy HB (1997). Pediatric sleep medicine: differential diagnosis. In: *Pediatric Sleep Medicine*. Philadelphia: WB Saunders, pp. 185–214.

Steenari MR, Vuontela V, Paavonen EJ, Carlson S, Fjallberg M, Aronen E (2003) Working memory and sleep in 6- to 13-year-old schoolchildren. *J Am Acad Child Adolesc Psychiatry* **42**: 85–92.

Stein MA (1999) Unravelling sleep problems in treated and untreated children with ADHD. *J Child Adolesc Psychopharmacol* **9**: 157–168.

Stores GA (2001) *Clinical Guide to Sleep Disorders in Children and Adolescents.* Cambridge: Cambridge University Press.

Thunstrom M (2002) Severe sleep problems in infancy associated with subsequent development of attention-deficit/hyperactivity disorder at 5.5 years of age. *Acta Paediatr* **91**: 584–592.

Van der Heijden KB, Smits MG, Van Someren EJ, Gunning WB (2005) Idiopathic chronic sleep onset insomnia in attention-deficit/hyperactivity disorder: a circadian rhythm sleep disorder. *Chronobiol Int* **22**: 559–570.

Walters AS, Mandelbaum DE, Lewin DS, Kugler S, England SJ, Miller M (2000) Dopaminergic therapy in children with restless legs/periodic limb movements in sleep and ADHD. Dopaminergic Therapy Study Group. *Pediatr Neurol* **22**: 182–186.

Weiss MD, Wasdell MB, Bomben MM, Rea KJ, Freeman RD (2006) Sleep hygiene and melatonin treatment for children and adolescents with ADHD and initial insomnia. *J Am Acad Child Adolesc Psychiatry* **45**: 512–519.

Wing YK, Hui SH, Pak WM, Ho CK, Cheung A, Li AM, Fok TF (2003) A controlled study of sleep related disordered breathing in obese children. *Arch Dis Child* **88**: 1043–1047.

11
ASPECTS OF MEDICAL MANAGEMENT

Eric Taylor and Peter Hill

The specific therapies for ADHD have been considered in Chapters 7, 8, 9 and 10. Figure 11.1 summarizes a general plan of approach to intervention. The scientific rationale has been outlined in successive consensus papers (Taylor et al. 1998, 2004; Banaschewski et al. 2006).

The process begins with education and advice. Sometimes this is all that is required. Some families are seeking primarily a diagnosis – or, more broadly, a diagnostic formulation. Very often they want reassurance that the child's behaviour is not the fault of the parents. Very often families are much readier to modify their interactions when the advice is in a framework of specific measures to deal with a specific problem, than when it has been perceived as instruction on how to reach an ordinary standard.

Checklist on basic information
- Information about condition to parents [Appendix 1.1 (p. 21) gives a simple factsheet].
- Advice to family on further sources of information [Appendix 1.2 (p. 23) gives such a list for the UK, which may be a useful framework for other countries too].
- Information about condition to child (best given orally or via the kidshealth.org website).
- Letter to school (head/class teacher, SENCO, educational psychologist as appropriate) if consent has been given [Appendix 7.1 (p. 115) is a leaflet for schools about ADHD].
- Letter to referrer setting out the case formulation and treatment plan
    —Copy of this to general practitioner if not referrer
    —Copy of this to school doctor
    —Copy of this to parents and child is usually good practice, if they have agreed.

Basic handling framework
Before proceeding to specific therapies, it should be clear that parents have been advised about, or already show:
- Appropriate expectations
- Structuring of their child's day
- The value of household rules, e.g. in reducing confrontations.

Basic handling practices
Parents should be instructed in:
- Positive parental attending to child. The goals here are that parents can play, or have

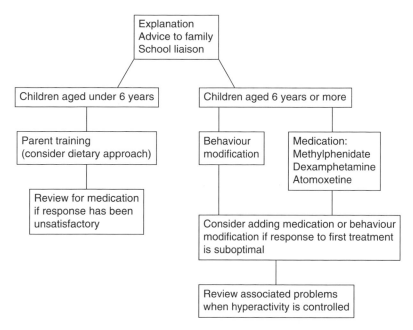

Fig. 11.1. Summary of a general approach to the initial stages of treatment for ADHD.

other positive interactions with their child; show him or her that they have noticed desired behaviour, whether prompted or not; and use praise and affection for their child's achievements
- Effective communication with child (ensuring child's attention is secured, keeping instructions brief and clear, checking child has understood)
- Contingency management (e.g. reward schemes with star charts or points schemes; using parental praise for compliance/achievement).

It should also be established that problems in school have been appropriately recognized and that there is a plan for handling them.

If these basic frameworks and practices have not been achieved, then a cost-effective action will probably be a parenting support group or a visit to the school. These are usually provided within a generic service, e.g. by a mental health worker in primary care. Specialist referral, however, will be needed if the situation is more urgent or if this first-line approach is insufficient.

Services will vary in the extent to which specific therapies are given in clinics that specialize in ADHD. Advantages of a specialist clinic include greater expertise in the skills of delivering treatment, and the opportunity of creating a service organization that promotes long-term follow-up, liaison with voluntary sector and other agencies, and a group atmosphere for young people with similar problems.

One potential problem for a specialist clinic is achieving appropriate referrals to it, or appropriate selection criteria if cases are taken from referrals to a generic service. One good way is to educate referrers. Appendix 11.1 reproduces recent WHO advice for action to be taken in primary care; this could be incorporated into referral guidelines or made available on a clinic's website.

Specific therapies

After the process of assessment, formulation and education, a decision is required about the treatment with which to start. In practice the choice is usually between a stimulant medication, atomoxetine, behaviour therapy, and perhaps (for some younger children) a dietary approach.

The choice should not be made automatically or inflexibly but in line with the best interests of the individual child. Options should be explained and the family involved in the choice. The issues will be set out separately for children before and after their sixth birthday, although this choice of age is somewhat arbitrary.

FOR CHILDREN AGED 6 YEARS OR OLDER

Medication is well evaluated and known to be the most powerful treatment in terms of effect size. Not all cases will need it, not all families will accept it, and not all children will be suitable for it. Psychological intervention may prove sufficient.

Re-analysis of data from the MTA trial has suggested that a subgroup, consisting of those children with ADHD who also meet the restrictive criteria for hyperkinetic disorder, are particularly likely to need medication (Santosh et al. 2006). In that group, a medication approach was much more effective than intensive behaviourally oriented psychosocial treatment. This superiority applied not only to the core symptoms of inattentiveness and restlessness but also to social adjustment and symptoms of anxiety. In hyperkinetic disorder, medication should be presented to families as the preferred treatment. When families decline medication, it should be kept open for discussion if other approaches fail.

In milder cases of ADHD, especially in those children who only just meet criteria, the advantages of medication over behaviour therapy are less clear. The choice for families is less constrained, and when behaviour therapy is available many families will elect it. Nevertheless, when psychological intervention is insufficient in alleviating symptoms and promoting academic and social progress, then a trial of medication will be indicated.

FOR CHILDREN AGED 5 YEARS OR YOUNGER

More detailed consideration of the options before school age is provided in Chapter 12. The current evidence favours parent-training procedures. Evidence about medication is scanty (a large controlled trial is in progress), but experience suggests that children aged 4 or more are often helped. Different countries vary substantially in their licensing arrangements, but in both the UK and USA methylphenidate (MPH) is currently licensed only down to the age of 6 years, and dexamphetamine (DEX) down to 3 years; this age differential results only from historical accident and does not indicate any superiority for DEX in young children.

There is some evidence for the effectiveness of an individually constructed elimination diet (Carter et al. 1993). This is based on the principle of cutting out all foods apart from a very small number, testing for the effect of this elimination, and – if a positive effect is found – adding further foods singly and gradually, observing for adverse reactions. Foods so identified will then be removed from the child's eventual diet. This is the 'few foods' approach to constructing an elimination diet. The advice of a paediatric dietitian is recommended, and care should be taken that a child is not established long-term on a very restrictive diet. The use of elimination diets is not, of course, confined to children under 6. Older children's diets, however, are less securely under the control of the parents, and fidelity to the diet becomes harder to maintain, so dietary approaches have correspondingly less to offer.

For children of all ages, a wide variety of complementary approaches has been promoted. We do not think there is adequate evidence for other diets such as the Feingold or gluten-free diets, or those that include supplementation of minerals, megavitamins or herbs. There is no firm scientific evidence for the effectiveness on core ADHD symptoms of homeopathy, psychoanalytic psychotherapy, naturopathy, or cranial osteopathy, though we are aware of individuals, parents and professionals, who express enthusiasm for one or another of these. Accordingly we do not include such interventions in our approach.

Omega-3 fatty acids have, at the time of writing, a more promising case. They are present in fish oils and there are several proprietary preparations. Trial evidence has not shown much benefit, if any, for children with ADHD. A trial of reasonable quality was based on clumsy children; while their clumsiness did not improve, there was a larger improvement than with placebo on rating scale measures of unwanted behaviour, including hyperactivity (Richardson and Montgomery 2005). A substantial trial in young offenders in an institution showed a reduction in violent incidents when a mixture of fish oil, vitamins and minerals was given, by comparison with a group treated with placebo (Gesch et al. 2002). These are not grounds for prescribing the treatment, but families wishing to try it could be supported with appropriate monitoring, using similar measures to those for medication. The chief disadvantage is the cost.

Giving medication

The next sections give detailed advice. This should of course be modified by local circumstances. It is intended to provide a framework that could be audited and to indicate to commissioners the level of practice that is expected and should be purchased. Resources do not always allow evidence-based protocols to be followed, but if that is so it should be explicit.

CHOICE OF STARTING MEDICATION

Which stimulant?

Reviews by NICE have found no difference in efficacy between MPH and DEX, or between immediate- and extended-release MPH, although the evidence is not conclusive. Cost-effectiveness is therefore largely determined by the price of the drugs. In current practice, DEX is substantially the cheapest; but in our view this is outweighed by its presence in the illegal drug scene and by the lack of good evidence on safety. Excluding DEX, the next most cost-effective is immediate-release MPH, and we think this remains the drug of first choice for the majority of patients.

Immediate release or long-acting medication?

Drugs with longer action are considerably more costly. Their efficacy may not be greater, nor their adverse effects less, but they have other advantages – especially, that they do not have to be taken at school. The school does not have the expense and risk of maintaining good dispensing, and the child does not have the stigma of being seen to take a pill (see Chapter 8). The judgement needs to be made individually for each child, in the light of their circumstances, about whether these factors outweigh cost and indicate an extended-release preparation from the start.

Extended-release preparations of stimulants include Concerta XL (action lasts up to 12 hours) and Equasym XL (action about 8 hours). Adderall[1] is very restricted in its availability outside North America; Ritalin LA[2] is in the licensing process in Europe; Ritalin SR is an older preparation based on wax matrix. Atomoxetine (Strattera) is licensed in many countries, including several European ones.

The comparative merits of the extended-release preparations have been hotly disputed and are reviewed in Chapter 8. The factors influencing the decision are:

- Cost-effectiveness (implying that extended-release MPH is preferable to atomoxetine)
- Length of action: atomoxetine usually has an action through the day and night, and this is often very welcome to families who may struggle in mornings and evenings
- Previous history of response: atomoxetine helps some children who are not helped by MPH, and vice versa
- Adverse effects: the balance of adverse effects varies, with insomnia, anorexia, interference with growth (and occasionally tics or agitation) being prominent for the stimulants, while atomoxetine is more likely to be associated with nausea and sedation
- Potential for diversion and misuse: this is not high for MPH, but does exist, and may lead to a preference for a non-stimulant in a household containing members who abuse drugs
- Child and family wishes.

Accordingly, we think that both atomoxetine and extended-release preparations of MPH should be available.

If treatment is starting with a long-acting preparation, then cost-effectiveness considerations[3] suggest starting with extended-release MPH and proceeding to atomoxetine if the former is unhelpful.

If immediate-release MPH has already failed, or produced unacceptable adverse effects, then it is more logical to proceed to atomoxetine.

Of the available extended-release MPH preparations, Concerta XL has the advantage

---

[1] Adderall is composed of four amphetamine salts: amphetamine aspartate, amphetamine sulphate, dexamphetamine saccharate, and dexamphetamine sulphate (this last is the active ingredient of Dexedrine). These four component salts are metabolized at different rates.It is sold in either an immediate-release tablet or an extended-release capsule, marketed as Adderall XR.

[2] Ritalin LA comprises immediate-release and sustained-release beads using the proprietary SODAS drug delivery system.

[3] Since these are determined by price, and price will vary from time to time and place to place, the prescriber is advised to check these generalizations against current circumstances.

of lower cost and longer action; but see below ('Titration With Extended-Release Methylphenidate') for other considerations in the choice.

PREMEDICATION ASSESSMENT
Check that:
• Full diagnostic assessment confirms hyperkinetic disorder or ADHD
• Parents (and child if competent) accept medication as a contribution to management
• School will cooperate in administration of medication and monitoring its effect. The beneficial effects are more likely to be seen in the classroom than at home, but it is undesirable to allow children to take their own drugs unsupervised. The use of long-acting preparations may avoid the need for school to administer, but monitoring by teachers is still needed)
• There is no history of previous hypersensitivity to MPH
• Child has normal heart and blood pressure on physical examination (abnormal results are not an absolute contraindication; if medication is essential then MPH may be the safest, but it would be wise to obtain an opinion from a paediatric cardiologist)
• Child is seizure-free or has treated epilepsy with infrequent seizures. (The risk of destabilizing epilepsy with MPH has been overstated, and small-scale reports suggest that it does not worsen well-controlled epilepsy. In poorly controlled cases, the evidence is not clear. The convention in such cases is to use DEX in the first instance, and indeed DEX is a weak anticonvulsant in its own right)
• Child does not have Tourette syndrome. This is not necessarily a contraindication but consider trying clonidine first. Simple tics are not a contraindication. Tics characteristically fluctuate spontaneously in their intensity, so a temporary worsening after stimulants are started does not necessarily mean that the stimulant has worsened them
• Child does not have pervasive developmental disorder. Unpredictable effects mean that medication is best carried out by, or in consultation with, a specialist centre
• Household does not contain substance misusers. Misuse by the patient is very unlikely indeed, but siblings or parents may misuse for weight loss, examination success or mood stimulation. MPH can be sold for (small) profit to the unsophisticated.

If these checks indicate that there is a concern:
• Specialist opinion is needed; refer if child is not already under the care of a child psychiatrist or paediatrician with a special interest
• Consider obtaining assistance of paediatric dietician and implementing an elimination diet, initially using either a food diary or a few-foods ('oligoantigenic') approach to identify foodstuffs that worsen behaviour. This is more feasible in younger children, but if it has not been previously tried, and the family can handle the considerable demands of reorganizing the diet, then it may be worth attempting. Monitor using frequent measures as for medication.

OBTAIN BASELINES
• Weigh and measure height, plotting on growth chart
• Parent and teacher rating scales, e.g. Conners (short CRS or CRS-R; Conners 1997), •

Strengths and Difficulties Questionnaire (SDQ; Goodman 1997), or SNAP-IV (Swanson et al. 2001)

• Parent and teacher side-effects questionnaires (see Appendix 8.2, p. 141)
• Record the blood pressure and pulse rate, and enquire about any history of heart disease, or family history. If there is a family history of arrhythmias or sudden death, then ECG is advised before treatment to check for the possibility of congenital Q-T prolongation or other abnormality.

START TITRATION OF METHYLPHENIDATE

Individuals' dose requirements vary considerably, and the best approach is usually to start with a small dose and work upwards, with monitoring of clinical response and adverse effects, including school reports. The frequency of monitoring and dosage adjustment will depend on the amount of professional time available. The best results described are those from the MTA trial (MTA Cooperative Group 1999a), in which the dose was changed and response was checked every day. This is seldom feasible in routine practice, and weekly checks are enough for a reasonably rapid titration. Even weekly checks, however, are sometimes hard to achieve; a single-handed practitioner with a not especially cooperative school may have to settle for less often. If the checks are less frequent than 4-weekly, however, it is likely that the impetus of monitoring will be lost. The schedule below therefore expects checks every week during the initial phase of dose establishment, but allows for the interval to be up to 4 weeks. School reports are crucial and worth waiting for. The effect is greater at school than at home, so the optimal dose by parent reports may lead to over-treatment at school.

It is usually best to aim for maximum coverage during the daytime, starting at 5 mg in the morning, 5 mg at midday, and 5 mg in mid-afternoon. Whether to include weekends and holidays is discretionary.

Monitor with regular questionnaires from parents and school. The precise timing will depend on school terms; aim for weekly report in the first stages of treatment, and then as in the checklist below. The following need to be established:
(1) Symptomatic and behavioural gain
(2) Performance improvement (academic, peer group)
(3) Adverse effects.

Personal reviews are also needed periodically because some adverse effects – such as lack of spontaneity, depression, excessive perseveration, and the advent of tics or (very uncommonly) dystonias – may not be adequately reported and need to be detected by personal observation.

After 1–4 weeks (depending on availability of teacher questionnaires), review personally or by telephone and enquire about beneficial and adverse effects. If there is room for improvement, increase the dose to 10 mg in the morning, 10 mg at midday, and 5 mg in mid-afternoon. If a single-dose regime is being used, increase dose to 10 mg in the morning [a 5 mg scored tablet preparation (Equasym) allows fine tuning since a 2.5 mg dose increment becomes reliable; quartering 10 mg tablets is not reliable]. Continue to monitor at home and school with questionnaires.

After approximately *a further 1–4 weeks* (that is, 2–8 weeks from baseline), review personally, and enquire about beneficial and adverse effects, and examine physically including pulse rate, blood pressure, and growth in height and weight (with plotting on growth chart). If there is room for improvement, increase dose to 15 mg in the morning, 15 mg at midday, and 5–10 mg in mid-afternoon. Modify the dose timings in the light of response. A single dose regime should provide clear evidence of benefit or not by now. Try to move to three times daily. Continue to monitor at home and school with questionnaires. Ask specifically if child is dazed or perseverating (a dose-related side-effect).

After approximately *2 further weeks* (that is, 4–10 weeks from baseline), consider:

(1) Whether a sufficiently good effect has been obtained in health and educational gain terms. A 'good' effect, for a child who does not show other problems, is that all the symptoms of ADHD are no worse than 'mild'. In complex cases, clinical judgement should determine whether the outcome is good enough

(2) If there is room for improvement, and if adverse effects are not troublesome, and if the child weighs more than 25 kg, consider an increase to 20 mg morning, 20 mg midday, 5–10 mg mid-afternoon; and thereafter, if appropriate, to a maximum of 0.7 mg/kg for each of three doses

(3) Review whether any adverse effects are tolerable (and reduce dose if necessary). Enquire about desired and undesired effects at school and home. Determine which of the doses gave the best combination of control of hyperactivity and freedom from adverse effects; if that was satisfactory, continue

(4) If not satisfactory, stop MPH and change to an extended-release preparation, atomoxetine or DEX (see below).

CHECKLIST FOR REVIEW

After the initial establishment of a suitable regime, review at 3 months and then at 6-monthly (or, in stable cases, annual) intervals with:

• Parents' rating
• Teachers' rating
• Side-effects (parents' report)
• Side-effects (teachers' report)
• Personal review, with mental state and physical examination.

Observe effects of unintentional withdrawal of medication, making an active attempt to assess whether to continue. If there has been no unintentional withdrawal, discontinue approximately every 12–24 months to test the continuing requirement.

Physical monitoring should be approximately 3-monthly, weighing and measuring height, recording them on growth chart, and checking pulse and blood pressure. This aspect of monitoring does not require specialist input and will often be done, together with the prescribing, in primary care. Blood tests are not routinely necessary (*pace* the manufacturers' recommendations, for which we have been able to find no evidence).

TITRATION WITH EXTENDED-RELEASE METHYLPHENIDATE

The same principles hold, but the dosage schedule is simplified. In the case of Concerta

XL tablets we recommend starting with one daily tablet of 18 mg, and increasing after 1 week to 36 mg, and after another to 54 mg. The aim is to reach either a good response, or adverse effects, or a ceiling of 2 mg/kg/day or 72 mg/day – whichever of these endpoints comes first.

Concerta XL is said to have an action lasting about 12 hours; Equasym XL and Ritalin LA about 8 hours. The choice may therefore depend on the evening actions; loss of control in the evenings will indicate the longer-acting drug; insomnia may suggest the shorter-acting one. The drugs vary in their ratio of immediate-release to delayed-release MPH: Concerta has the lowest ratio, about 23% being immediate-release; Equasym about 30%, Ritalin LA about 50%. The choice may therefore depend on the need for a bigger response early in the day (e.g. depending on the school timetable). There is, however, a range of individual variation in response. Equasym XL is somewhat more expensive (in the UK at least at the time of writing) but has the advantage that the capsules can be opened and the contents sprinkled on food. This helps some children who have difficulty swallowing; but the opportunity to administer it surreptitiously should not be taken because of the harmful effects of stealth on trust.

Extended-release preparations are supposed to be given instead of immediate-release, not in addition. The preparations have been developed to give a good profile of action across the day, and were originally intended to reduce the risk of tolerance developing during the day. Nevertheless, the range of individual variation suggests that some children may be helped by an additional small dose (e.g. 5 mg) of immediate-release; either in the morning to assist with control at the beginning of the day, or in the evening to prevent an unsettling loss of action (which may manifest either in disruptive behaviour or in initial insomnia).

TITRATION WITH ATOMOXETINE

The dose is fixed, at 1.2 mg/kg/day. Start for a week with a test dose of 0.5 mg/kg daily in the morning and then proceed to the full dosage (in a single morning dose) if well tolerated. Allow 6 weeks to judge the effect. Slow metabolizers may develop adverse effects at lower doses, and dosage increase should then proceed more cautiously. Adverse effects of sedation, nausea or weight loss should be watched for; they may be reduced by dividing the dose into two, one in the morning and one in the evening.[1] A twice-daily dose may also be needed to obtain 24-hour control. The checklist for administering rating scales is as for MPH. If the response at 6 weeks is suboptimal, consider an increase to 1.8 mg/kg if there have been no adverse effects.

TITRATION WITH DEXAMPHETAMINE

This follows the same principles of basic conditions, baseline, and monitoring.
- *Baseline* measurements
- *1–4 weeks* – DEX 2.5 mg morning, 2.5 mg midday, 2.5 mg mid-afternoon
- *1–4 further weeks* – if room for improvement, DEX 5 mg morning, 5 mg midday, 2.5 mg mid-afternoon (can omit if insomnia)

---

[1] Current pricing is by the tablet, whatever its strength, so splitting the dose doubles the cost

- *2–4 further weeks* – if room for improvement, DEX 7.5 mg morning, 7.5 mg midday, 2.5–5 mg mid-afternoon (can omit if insomnia).

If no benefit is obtained from DEX, or if side-effects are unacceptable, withdraw over a few days and proceed to atomoxetine (if not previously given) or a second-line drug (see below).

Managing adverse effects of stimulants

The commonest adverse effects, usually elicited by questioning, are: insomnia, appetite disturbance, stomach aches, headaches, and sensation of dizziness. Most of these adverse effects are dose related and transient and can be managed symptomatically.

INSOMNIA

Insomnia has often been present before medication; sleep hygiene and behavioural approaches should be employed. Chapter 10 outlines a suitable approach. It should be remembered that while MPH is capable of producing sleeplessness, it can also reduce insomnia by easing children's transition into sleep. Both reducing the dose and giving a later dose can be tried as a response to sleep difficulties.

Sedation in the evening is sometimes justified, but there is no professional consensus on how and when to use it, and we recommend it only when the symptomatic measures have failed. If the cardiovascular system is normal, one can add clonidine 50–250 μg as an evening dose, utilizing the drowsiness that is often an unwanted effect in daytime use. (Increase dose with caution; ECG monitoring recommended; advise against sudden discontinuation.) Melatonin is particularly useful in correcting the situation where a child has fallen into the habit of late bedtime and late rising. It is short-acting; the dose is 2–10 mg; but most preparations lack the strict quality controls applied to drugs in the pharmacopoeia, so the amount being received can be unpredictable. Alternative night sedations include an antihistamine (promethazine, trimeprazine, diphenhydramine), or trazodone at bedtime (dose according to age and weight).

POOR GROWTH

Poor growth in height or weight can occur and is probably due to appetite suppression. The child may need an altered balance of food during the day, with encouragement to a good breakfast (before the medication has taken effect) and permission for 'grazing' in the evenings – which parents often resist, but can result in an adequate food intake being maintained. Insomnia is sometimes due to hunger, so food should be accessible to the child in the evenings. Reduction of dosage may be necessary to maintain eating, or a switch from a stimulant to atomoxetine may remove the problem. When a growth problem is significant, then a 6-week holiday from the drug usually allows a catch-up growth. If it does, the holidays can be repeated; if it does not, then fuller physical evaluation is needed in case growth failure has a different cause.

Some practitioners add risperidone to the treatment regime to increase appetite. The hazards of risperidone, however, seem to us to be too great to recommend this as an indication for the drug in any but extreme situations.

179

TABLE 11.1
Drug interactions

Drug for hyperactivity	Concomitant drugs	Possible interactions
Methylphenidate	Monoamine oxidase inhibitors	Hypertensive crisis
	Tricyclic antidepressant	Level of tricyclic can be increased
	Anticonvulsant	Levels of phenytoin and phenobarbitone increased
	Inhaled anaesthetic	Hypertension – discontinue methylphenidate beforehand
	Clonidine	Uncertain – see below
	Antipsychotics	Hypertensive effect of stimulants can be increased – monitor
Atomoxetine	Monoamine oxidase inhibitors (MAOIs)	Hypertensive crisis – avoid MAOIs for 2 weeks after atomoxetine discontinued
Clonidine	Antihypertensives	Hypotension
	Anaesthetics	Hypotension
	Beta-blockers	Risk of hypertension when clonidine withdrawn (withdraw beta-blockers first)
	Methylphenidate	Cases of sudden death reported, but quite unclear whether the drug combination was responsible, and a trial has supported using the combination (Hazell and Stuart 2003)
Risperidone	Anaesthetics	Hypotension
	Cardiac antiarrhythmics	Prolongation of Q-T; arrhythmias
	Fluoxetine	Risperidone plasma level increased
	Anticonvulsants (incl. carbamazepine and valproate)	Anticonvulsant effect reduced
	Sedatives	Sedative effects potentiated
	Clonidine	Hypotension theoretically possible
	Stimulants	See 'Methylphenidate' above

NB: This is not a complete list but a selection of those likely to be encountered: check with package inserts or formularies.

HEADACHE, STOMACH ACHE

Abdominal pain or headache may persist beyond the first few weeks and be distressing, indicating a need to change medication.

INTERACTIONS WITH OTHER DRUGS

Possible interactions should always be considered when combining anti-hyperactivity drugs or when other medication is being received. Table 11.1 provides a selective listing of some of the most significant interactions to consider.

If first-line medications fail

A lack of response to stimulant medication may stem from many causes; management is summarized in Figure 11.2.

The commonest reason is probably a failure to take the medicine. Children often find medication unwelcome and stigmatizing. Adolescents often may experience it as coercion

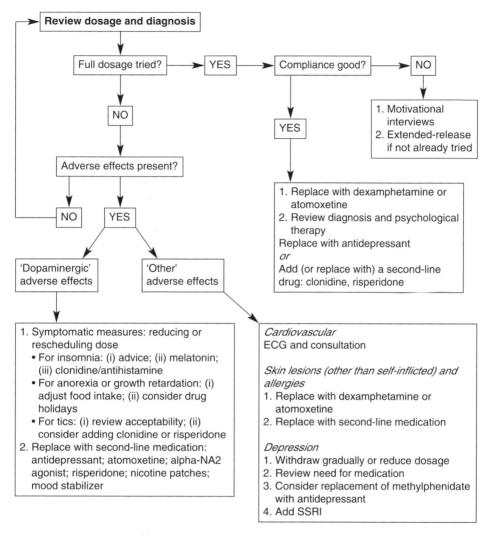

Fig. 11.2. When first-line treatments fail.

by adult authority. Both issues are best tackled by developing the young person into an intelligent user. Education should be directed to the child at least as much as to family and school. If the prescriber listens to their concerns and adjusts medication accordingly, then the patients can become partners in therapy. It is sometimes useful to get them to involve a trusted adult or friend to help in self-monitoring. Lack of insight is characteristic, and can lead to children underestimating the impact of medication.

Another reason for non-compliance – unwelcome comments and attention from teachers and peers – can often be avoided by using an extended-release preparation to avoid the need for repeated daytime doses. When adverse effects have led to limited compliance, then symptomatic management (see above) or dose reduction will usually suffice. When it does not, then second-line drugs are indicated.

One common mistake is to abandon stimulants (or atomoxetine) prematurely in favour of second-line drugs. Some children need doses at the bottom of the range, others at the top, and fine-tuning dosage with monitoring by rating scales will increase the response rate. Only after this process should one judge that the disorder is refractory to first-line therapy. Full review is then indicated.

It may be that further knowledge of the case will lead to recognition of another problem, such as pervasive developmental disorder or Tourette syndrome, or a comorbid condition such as an anxiety disorder. If so, then more selective drugs without dopaminergic actions (including atomoxetine) are a logical choice. Antidepressants such as imipramine or bupropion have reasonable trial evidence for superiority to placebo; and others such as venlafaxine and moclobemide have anecdotal evidence in support. Even more selective drugs may be able to control ADHD without adverse effects. Guanfacine, an alpha-2 noradrenergic agonist, has been valuable in open trials.

Mood stabilizers such as valproate should be considered when a bipolar element is present. Neuroleptic drugs can also reduce hyperactivity, probably through different mechanisms. Haloperidol is the best-studied neuroleptic in controlled trials, but it is unacceptably toxic. Risperidone seems to be the most valuable in practice. Its metabolic effects, however, mean that it should be a drug of late resort. It is most often used for the combination of gross overactivity with aggression, and especially with children in the spectrum of autism.

TITRATION WITH IMIPRAMINE
- *Baseline* measurements
- *2 weeks* – 50 mg daily dose (single or divided). Regular monitoring as before, with parent and teacher symptom questionnaires but not side-effect questionnaires
- *2 further weeks* – 75 mg daily dose (single or divided). This seems to us to be a sensible upper limit. Some, but not all, studies suggest that there may be further improvement with higher doses. With this in mind it may be appropriate to increase up to a total dose of 150 mg/day. With doses over 50 mg/day the risk of cardiac dysrhythmia increases and it is necessary to monitor with ECGs monthly. Regular monitoring as before, with questionnaires.

If appraisal is satisfactory, follow-up is as for stimulants. The checklist for administering rating scales is as for MPH.

In the longer term, scientific study has not yet indicated for how long treatment should be prolonged. However, we do know that some disability often persists into adult life and that medication is still effective in adult life (see Chapter 14). Furthermore, discontinuation studies have shown that some (but not all) children are still receiving benefit even after years of treatment and revert to uncontrolled hyperactivity if placebo is substituted for their usual medication. It is therefore clear that medication should often be thought of as long-term.

Some children stop as soon as they are able to decide for themselves, or as soon as they have completed public examinations; this may reflect a failure of education and counseling, in that they have perceived the treatment as something imposed upon them rather than as an aspect of management in which they are actively engaged. Continuing contact with a clinic is desirable, so that they can progressively gather knowledge about their condition and responsibility for its management. They can, for instance, monitor their own progress, using a rating scale whose items they have formulated for themselves in discussion with clinicians. This fits well with a policy of periodic discontinuation of medication – e.g. for a period of 2 weeks every 2 years – to assess continuing need.

Inferences from treatment response

Response to medication is not helpful in confirming or refuting a diagnosis of ADHD. Lack of response – as considered above – can be due to many factors besides the diagnosis being wrong. Change with medication does not confirm the diagnosis, because most people (children and adults alike) will show a qualitatively similar reaction to medication whether they have ADHD or not.

Nevertheless, the response can be very helpful for the broader formulation of the case. Once hyperactive behaviour is reduced, it becomes much clearer whether impairment of function was due to the hyperactivity itself or had another cause. Accordingly, when in doubt whether hyperactivity is in itself a key impairment for a child, it can be useful to have a low threshold for the decision to make a trial of medication, but a higher threshold for the judgement of whether medication has an overall value to the child in improving function – and therefore whether it should be continued in the longer term.

A good response to medication can also be helpful in clarifying which associated features in a complex presentation need intervention in their own right.

Hyperactivity as a part of complex presentations

Previous chapters have emphasized how common it is for hyperactive behaviour to be associated with other types of problem, and Chapter 6 has described the need both for differential diagnosis and for recognizing coexistent problems. The clinical analysis that follows from this turns on three key questions: whether the classic ADHD pattern of inattentiveness and impulsive restlessness is present (as opposed to another pattern of over-activity, disruptiveness or educational failure); what other components are present; and how the association has come about in the individual case. There are several reasons for ADHD being associated with other disorders: these are summarized in Table 11.2.

The apparently simple question, "What is the diagnosis?" is often an unhelpful way of approaching complex clinical problems. ICD-10 (WHO 1993) uses an extensive set of ex-clusion criteria to achieve a single psychiatric diagnosis as often as possible. DSM-IV (APA 1994) allows – even encourages – multiple psychiatric diagnoses, but still includes some exclusion criteria. There is an implicit hierarchy, in which (for example) the presence of autism makes it unnecessary to diagnose lower-order problems such as ADHD, or ADHD makes it unnecessary to diagnose an oppositional disorder. There are several assumptions buried in this, and they may not be true. In practical terms, it can divert the formulation of a case away from recognizing multiple components.

183

TABLE 11.2

TABLE 11.2
Reasons for associations between hyperactivity and other problems

Disorder	Criterion overlap	One problem	Complication	Shared risks	Combination is separate disorder	Other
Oppositional/ conduct	No	No	Often	No	Possible	Rating bias
Anxiety	A little	Dyscontrol	Occasional	Likely but unknown	Unlikely	Misdiagnosis
Autism	No	No	No	Probable	Unlikely	Masking
Bipolar	Yes	Unclear	No	Unknown	Unlikely	Misdiagnosis

Sometimes clinicians are even more stringent than the diagnostic schemes in applying exclusion criteria. Some may, for instance, consider that an individual child does not have ADHD because he or she has another disorder such as fragile X syndrome or epilepsy – and one result can be that ADHD treatment is not given. There is an assumption here, that ADHD is an explanatory diagnosis competing with the other neurological condition – and this is unjustified. Previous chapters have emphasized that the diagnosis of ADHD is a description, not an explanation. It exists on a separate axis from brain pathology.

A similar common error is to exclude the diagnosis of ADHD because an attachment disorder or a post-traumatic disorder is thought to be present. Again, this is to confuse de-scription with cause. ADHD may result from long-lasting early neglect (see Chapter 1) as well as from physical challenges to brain development. Predictive studies of which children respond to medication have emphasized that the symptom pattern, not the underlying cause, is the key determinant (e.g. Taylor et al. 1987). The presence of affected family members suggesting genetic susceptibility does not predict outcome; neither do histories of early neglect or physical abuse. The effect of medication seems to be on the brain processes underlying behaviour change, however they came about.

IS THE ADHD PATTERN OF INATTENTIVENESS AND IMPULSIVE RESTLESSNESS PRESENT?

This is the point at which the disorganized pattern of hyperactivity needs to be distinguished from similar patterns, such as the grandiose expansiveness of mania; the intentional breaking of legitimate rules (as in non-hyperactive conduct disorder); the tension and preoccupation that can characterize anxiety states; the driven (and often stereotyped) overactivity in cata-tonic states; or the ritualized activity of some children in the spectrum of autism. Chapter 6 goes into more detail. In all these conditions, typical ADHD can be present as well, and when it is it can be treated, but extended observation may be needed to establish that is indeed the classic pattern of inattentiveness and impulsiveness rather than one of the other forms of overactivity.

Table 11.3 shows features associated with typical forms of each condition; the disorders are conceptualized as separate dimensions of disturbance that often coexist.

TABLE 11.3
Features associated with conditions other than ADHD that also feature hyperactivity

	Stereotyped activity	Grandiosity, euphoria	Emotional lability	Persistent depression or worry	Impulsive	Lack of focus on task	Rapid activity change
HKD*			+		+	+	+
Autism	+						
Catatonia	+						
Anxiety				+		+	
Mania		+	+		+		+
Tourette	+		+		+		

*HKD = hyperkinetic disorder.

If the hyperkinetic pattern is present and impairing, then it is usually appropriate to treat it even in the presence of other types of disorder. Caution in the use of stimulants may be necessary, as considered in the next section, and enhanced monitoring is often required, but associated disorders are seldom absolute contraindications.

WHAT ARE THE OTHER COMPONENTS?
The initial assessment of coexistent problems (Chapter 6) needs to be reviewed when hyperactivity has been reduced by successful treatment. Some problems may have resolved: defiant and antisocial behaviour may no longer be a problem, either because they have already been targets of behaviour therapy or because medication has reduced their frequency and intensity. Other problems may be more prominent, because medication has made them worse (as can sometimes happen for tics or stereotypies) or because they have been unmasked by the reduction in hyperactivity. Sometimes, for instance, the social impairment of children in the spectrum of autism is only obvious when their hyperactivity is reduced to the point where sustained interactions with other children become feasible and can therefore be assessed.

Other problems again may be untouched even when hyperactivity is well controlled. Sometimes, for example, the child is more attentive in class but there is no corresponding increase in learning; this may be the cue to re-evaluate academic potential with psychometric testing (especially if this was previously unreliable because of lack of engagement in tasks or great scatter of scores). It is in this sense that the response to medication can be a real help in formulating the case. In other respects, treatment response is unreliable as a guide to diagnosis. Lack of response does not in itself show that the diagnosis of ADHD was wrong, and response does not mean it was correct, for the actions of drugs are multiple and affect those without ADHD as well as those who show it. A good response cannot be taken to infer that a neurological disease is present, because in current knowledge the response is not conditioned by the underlying causes.

COEXISTENCE OF NEURODEVELOPMENTAL DISORDERS
These conditions – such as pervasive developmental disorders, general and specific learning

problems, tics and Tourette syndrome – have many features in common. They start in the first years of life, they tend to persist over time, they show strong genetic influences, and they are more common in males than in females (with the exception of Rett syndrome, in which the underlying genetic change is usually lethal in males). Each is more common in the presence of the others.

Autism

Children with autism will require the assessment and management of that condition as well as of the hyperactivity. If overactive behaviour is of the stereotyped rather than the disorganized type, then stimulants are unlikely to be useful and atomoxetine has not yet been shown to be valuable. Clinical practice in this situation is often to try antidepressants (e.g. imipramine, sertraline) and to be prepared to proceed to a dopamine antagonist (e.g. risperidone) if the benefits outweigh the hazards. If the impulsive/inattentive pattern is present, then a stimulant or atomoxetine is usually the first choice of medication; but adverse effects are quite common, and a low initial dose (e.g. MPH 2.5 mg b.i.d.) is advised. If the benefits do not outweigh the problems, then medication policy is usually to try second-line drugs (such as clonidine, imipramine, sertraline, valproate and risperidone) as described in Chapter 8. The idea is then to choose the regime that gives the best results: this is often no medication at all. Monitoring should include ECG for tricyclic antidepressants (at each dose increase and then 3-monthly), and metabolic monitoring for atypical neuroleptics – including fasting blood glucose, prolactin and lipids – if the dose is above a low level (equivalent to 2 mg/day of risperidone). These monitoring recommendations are controversial and not backed by good evidence; they correspond to the major hazards of medication, but the prevalence of such reactions and therefore the cost-effectiveness of monitoring regimes are unknown. Many children and families will not agree to regular blood tests. In that event, it is reasonable to continue with treatment after explaining the risks.

Tics

Children with multiple tics or the full Tourette syndrome need care in management. Assessment can be complex (see Chapter 6), and drugs with dopaminergic actions carry the hazard of making tics worse. This hazard should not, however, be exaggerated. The course of Tourette syndrome is typically fluctuating, and so a worsening of tics can sometimes be misattributed to the medication.

Drug treatment should begin with a clear decision about the intended purpose. Is it to control ADHD, to reduce tics, or both? In practice the tics themselves are often not a target for treatment with drugs. They are stigmatizing rather than damaging, and many children are best served by a matter-of-fact acceptance and a robust attitude to taunting by others. A minor increase in tic frequency may well be an acceptable price for good control of hyperactivity with medicine.

For cases in which ADHD is the target, the initial choice of medication is considered in Chapter 8. The pros and cons need discussing with the child and parents (or guardians). Our current practice is usually to start with cautiously increasing doses of MPH, adding clonidine if necessary. Atomoxetine is theoretically appropriate; at the time of writing we do not have the trial evidence or sufficient clinical experience to be able to advocate it securely, but this uncertainty may well change in the near future. Nicotine patches have been helpful for some children (a 5, 10 or 15 mg patch is applied for 8–10 hours each day), but the value is often limited by nausea and malaise.

Intellectual impairment

General intellectual impairment, as evidenced by a low IQ, is often associated with hyperactive behaviour, especially the inattentive component. This is sometimes because insufficient allowance is made for the fact that a child with developmental delay will be functioning at a lower level of attentional ability and self-control than a child of greater maturity. There is no generally established doctrine about how to make this judgement. A useful clinical rule of thumb is to determine the probable mental age of the child, consider what would be expected, in the control of attention activity and impulse, for a normal child whose chronological age is equivalent to that mental age, and make judgements of abnormality accordingly. The problems of children with the dual diagnosis of mental retardation and ADHD are complex, and have received little attention in the research or clinical literature. An extended account is therefore provided in Chapter 13.

Specific learning disabilities can also be encountered. These can take many different forms and there is no unique pattern of psychological test disturbance. Problems of working memory and attention are so frequent in hyperkinetic disorder that they do not call for an alternative diagnosis, and they may be solely responsible for poor academic learning. However, they cannot always be assumed to be the sole cause. Specific problems in reading, numerical ability and the expression of thoughts on paper can also be found. A child with academic problems should therefore receive a psychologist's assessment with psychometric tests, because the educational interventions needed may be wider than the correction of attention and memory (see Chapter 4). The presence of specific academic difficulties, however, does not alter the indications for treatment of the ADHD itself, nor the ways in which treatment is given.

OPPOSITIONAL, CONDUCT AND ANXIETY DISORDERS

The Multimodal Treatment Study has indicated that medication is still indicated in these associated conditions, but that the addition of behavioural therapy is often desirable (MTA Cooperative Group 1999b). They are discussed in more detail in Chapter 6, and their drug treatment in Chapter 8.

COEXISTENCE OF MENTAL ILLNESS OR DISEASES OF THE BRAIN

Schizophrenia should be seen as a contraindication to stimulants, even when there is a previous history of ADHD. MPH can provoke and intensify psychotic symptoms; indeed, it is sometimes used diagnostically for this action. A more common and more difficult situation arises when the child does not show schizophrenia, but is at risk for it, either because of a strong family history or because of quasi-delusional thinking or hallucinations that coexist with developmental delays. Scientific evidence is not available to guide practice; our experience is that stimulants can be beneficial, and our judgement is that the best prevention of schizophrenia in high-risk subjects is to achieve the best possible current social adjustment – so that stimulants to control ADHD are a legitimate intervention. Second opinions and specialist advice are advised.

Developmental coordination disorder
This is very common in ADHD, and may affect as many as half of the children with the severe form that we are calling 'hyperkinetic disorder'. Within groups of children with ADHD, motor problems may cluster together with symptoms of inattentiveness, and this has led some clinical researchers to propose a subdivision of ADHD, 'Deficits in attention, motor control and perception' (DAMP). It is possible that the underlying neurocognitive problems are similar to some of those found experimentally in ADHD; poor timing and poorly sustained response readiness could underlie both. However, until research clarifies whether a valid subtype is present, and what its relation is to motor problems in children without ADHD, the ICD-10 approach is to recognize developmental coordination disorder when it is present and to classify it on a different axis, of specific disturbances of development. This avoids the trap of incoordination being used as diagnostic evidence for the presence of hyperkinetic disorder. These motor problems, even if transient, may have a considerable impact on development by impairing socially valued activities such as sport. The main clinical implication is to suggest the need for help for the incoordination – e.g. remedial physical education, occupational therapy or physiotherapy. It does not condition the treatment of the ADHD.

Epilepsy
ADHD is found in more than a third of children with epilepsy (e.g. Dunn et al. 2003). There are several possible reasons for this, and all of them may be encountered in individual cases. First, there is a group of causes that can be seen as mediated by abnormal brain mechanisms. The genetic and environmental factors that are risk factors for epilepsy may also determine the presence of ADHD. More directly, subclinical seizures can in themselves impair concentration. Clinically this can be difficult to detect: an absence seizure may be hard to distinguish from a micro-lapse of attention, and simultaneous behavioural and EEG recording is often necessary to make the distinction. Nevertheless, it is plain that for children with poorly controlled epilepsy, seizure activity can in itself produce an impairment of attention that is improved by treatment with antiepileptic drugs.

Less directly, seizures can have a general impact upon broader mental function. A good example would be the association of frequent EEG spike-and-wave activity during sleep with behavioural disturbance in the daytime.

An underlying neurological disease may account for both epilepsy and ADHD. An epileptic focus, say in the frontal lobe, may be reflecting underlying structural damage that would also be capable of producing ADHD symptoms even if epilepsy were not a consequence.

A more indirect route involving brain mechanisms is that the toxic effects of anticonvulsant drugs may in themselves produce symptoms of ADHD. Furthermore, non-compliance with medication may be a result of ADHD and therefore lead to poorer seizure control and an apparent association between severity of epilepsy and ADHD symptomatology.

All these possibilities need to be considered in the individual case, as they will guide management. As well as these brain mechanisms, a number of extracerebral mechanisms can account for associations between ADHD and epilepsy in individual cases. The presence of ADHD probably restricts the access to other kinds of intervention. Parents may be less able to take their children to diagnostic services or less able to achieve satisfactory compliance with medication. Reduced access to treatment may therefore mean that the association between the presence of seizures and the presence of ADHD reflects the failure to adequately control either or both.

Conversely, the recognition of ADHD may be better if services for epilepsy are involved; or the tolerance of parents for disruptive behaviour may be either lowered or increased by the knowledge that there is a brain disorder. Epilepsy may also evoke a pathogenic environment: family relationships are not in themselves thought to create ADHD, but they can modulate its impact and therefore its presentation to services; and the presence of high levels of critical expressed emotion by parents can worsen the course of children with ADHD, making it more likely that they will develop antisocial symptoms, and therefore that they will remain in touch with services.

The therapeutic interventions for ADHD in children with epilepsy may therefore include increasing the anticonvulsant dosage (to achieve better control of seizures, e.g. at night-time); the reduction of anticonvulsant medication (to avoid toxicity to which high blood levels and low folate levels may be a clue); the use of stimulants (which are not contraindicated in epilepsy, contrary to the teachings of many textbooks); the counselling of parents and others concerning the nature of the child's problems, or more focused measures (such as expressed emotion reduction) to modify the impact of relationship adversity upon the child; the introduction of specific behaviour therapy; or the treatment (with drugs or other methods) of the disorders such as catatonia that have masqueraded as ADHD in the first place.

The general lesson to be remembered, for epilepsy as for other brain disorders, is that the brain disorder is not an alternative to ADHD. ADHD is not a neurological diagnosis but a description of behaviour. It may still be present whatever neurological condition is also present, and in general its treatment follows the same principles as would be the case in children with otherwise normal brains.

REFERENCES

APA (1994) *Diagnostic and Statistical Manual of Mental Disorders, 4th edn (DSM-IV)*. Washington, DC: American Psychiatric Association.

Banaschewski T, Coghill D, Santosh P, Zuddas A, Asherson P, Buitelaar J,Danckaerts M, Dopfner M, Faraone SV, Rothenberger A, Sergeant J, Steinhausen HC, Sonuga-Barke EJ, Taylor E (2006) Long-acting medications for the hyperkinetic disorders: A systematic review and European treatment guideline. *Eur Child Adolesc Psychiatry*. [Epub ahead of print.]

Carter CM, Urbanowicz M, Hemsley R (1993) Effects of a few food diet in attention deficit disorder. *Arch Dis Child* 69: 564–568.

Conners CK (1997) *Conners' Rating Scales: Revised Technical Manual*. New York: Multi-Health Systems.

Dunn DW, Austin JK, Harezlak J, Ambrosius WT (2003) ADHD and epilepsy in childhood. *Dev Med Child Neurol* 45: 50–54.

Gesch CB, Hammond SM, Hampson SE, Eves A, Crowder MJ (2002) Influence of supplementary vitamins, minerals and essential fatty acids on the antisocial behaviour of young adult prisoners. Randomised, placebo-controlled trial. *Br J Psychiatry* 181: 22–28.

Goodman R (1997) The Strengths and Difficulties Questionnaire. *J Child Psychol Psychiatry* **38**: 581–586.

Hazell PL, Stuart JE (2003) A randomized controlled trial of clonidine added to psychostimulant medication for hyperactive and aggressive children. *J Am Acad Child Adolesc Psychiatry* **42**: 886–894.

MTA Cooperative Group (1999a) A 14-month randomized clinical trial of treatment strategies for attention-deficit/hyperactivity disorder. *Arch Gen Psychiatry* **56**: 1073–1086.

MTA Cooperative Group (1999b) Moderators and mediators of treatment response for children with attention-deficit/hyperactivity disorder: the Multimodal Treatment Study of Children with Attention-Deficit/Hyperactivity Disorder. *Arch Gen Psychiatry* **56**: 1088–1096.

Richardson AJ, Montgomery P (2005) The Oxford–Durham study: a randomized, controlled trial of dietary supplementation with fatty acids in children with developmental coordination disorder. *Pediatrics* **115**: 1360–1366.

Santosh PJ, Taylor E, Swanson J, Wigal T, Chuang S, Davies M, Greenhill L, Newcorn J, Arnold LE, Jensen P, Vitiello B, Elliott G, Hinshaw S, Hechtman L, Abikoff H, Pelham W, Hoza B, Molina B, Wells K, Epstein J, Posner M (2006) Refining the diagnoses of inattention and overactivity syndromes: A reanalysis of the Multimodal Treatment Study of attention deficit hyperactivity disorder (ADHD) based on ICD-10 criteria for hyperkinetic disorder. *Clin Neurosci Res* (in press).

Swanson JM, Kraemer HC, Hinshaw SP, Arnold LE, Conners CK, Abikoff HB, Clevenger W, Davies M, Elliott GR, Greenhill LL, Hechtman L, Hoza B, Jensen PS, March JS, Newcorn JH, Owens EB, Pelham WE, Schiller E, Severe JB, Simpson S, Vitiello B, Wells K, Wigal T, Wu M (2001) Clinical relevance of the primary findings of the MTA: success rates based on severity of ADHD and ODD symptoms at the end of treatment. *J Am Acad Child Adolesc Psychiatry* **40**: 168–179.

Taylor EA, Schachar R, Thorley G, Wieselberg HM, Everitt B, Rutter M (1987) Which boys respond to stimulant medication? A controlled trial of methylphenidate in boys with disruptive behaviour. *Psychol Med* **17**: 121–143.

Taylor E, Sergeant J, Doepfner M, Gunning B, Overmeyer S, Mobius HJ, Eisert HG (1998) Clinical guidelines for hyperkinetic disorder. European Society for Child and Adolescent Psychiatry. *Eur Child Adolesc Psychiatry* **7**: 184–200.

Taylor E, Dopfner M, Sergeant J, Asherson P, Banaschewski T, Buitelaar J, Coghill D, Danckaerts M, Rothenberger A, Sonuga-Barke E, Steinhausen HC, Zuddas A (2004) European clinical guidelines for hyperkinetic disorder—first upgrade. *Eur Child Adolesc Psychiatry* **13** Suppl 1: 17–30.

WHO (1993) *The ICD-10 Classification of Mental and Behavioural Disorders: Diagnostic Criteria for Research.* Geneva: World Health Organization.

APPENDIX 11.1
GUIDANCE FOR PRIMARY CARE IN ADHD*

Attention-Deficit / Hyperactivity Disorder

Attention-deficit/hyperactivity disorder (ADHD) (most popular term for hyperkinetic disorder – F90)* (Clinical Term: Attention deficit disorder Eu97)

*ADHD is a term taken from DSM-IV. In its US definition it is a much broader category.

Presenting complaints

Most commonly presents in childhood as a result of complaints by parents or teachers about problems in behaviour and for learning.

Diagnostic features

All of the following:

- Six of nine features of inattention: careless with detail; fail to sustain attention; appears not to listen; does not finish instructed tasks; poor self-organization; avoids tasks requiring sustained mental effort; loses things; easily distracted; seems forgetful
- Three of five features of hyperactivity: fidgets; leaves seat when should be seated; runs/climbs excessively and inappropriately; noisy in play; persistent motor activity unmodified by social context.
- One of four features of impulsivity: blurts out answers before question completed; fails to wait turn or queue; interrupts others' conversation or games; talks excessively for social context.
- Pattern of behaviour pervasive across at least two types of situation; information about school behaviour is therefore very valuable.
- Onset no later than age 7.
- Causing significant distress or impaired functioning.
- Not better explained by another psychiatric disorder.

Excitability, impatience and defiant angry outbursts are common, but as these have many other causes, they do not establish the diagnosis by themselves.

Differential diagnosis and co-existing conditions

- Normal boisterousness or dreaminess
- Conduct or oppositional disorders – F91
- Learning disability (mental retardation) – F70
- Disinhibited attachment disorder
- Depressive – F32#, especially in adolescent boys
- Emotional disorders with onset specific to childhood – F93
- Hearing impairment and epileptic seizures should be asked about.

Comorbidity is common:

- developmental disorders (of reading, motor coordination, speech and language)
- antisocial behaviour
- illicit substance use
- emotional and mood disorders
- tic disorders and Tourette syndrome
- autistic spectrum disorder.

*Reproduced from the *WHO Guide to Mental and Neurological Health in Primary Care* (as downloaded from the WHO Collaborating Centre at http://www.mentalneurologicalprimarycare.org/downloads/primary_care/Attention-deficicit_disorder.pdf [sic]; references omitted). Code numbers refer to ICD-10 classifications.

Essential information for patient and family

- It is essentially a syndrome with various causes, predominantly genetic but including low birthweight, serious early neglect, and fetal alcohol exposure.
- It is not directly a result of upbringing, but a child's behaviour may make it difficult for parents to be positive and supportive.
- Manifestations at school may differ from the picture at home.
- Recognizing comorbidity can avoid some of the arguments that may otherwise arise about diagnosis.

General management and advice to patient and family

- Treat as a chronic disorder.
- If you suspect a child has the condition, refer.
- Maintain consistency and structure: routines, stated expectations of behaviour, family rules. Allowing the child to race around in an ungoverned way in an attempt to diminish hyperactivity will not work. In contrast structured exercise might be helpful, particularly in improving sleep.
- Ensure the child has adequate sleep.
- Establish constructive communication with school to:
  – ensure teachers are informed
  – detect special educational needs
  – monitor progress (particularly if child is on medication).
- Keep confrontations to a minimum.
- Make a positive effort to have enjoyable interactions with child: play and praise.
- Positive interactions should outweigh negative interactions. This should be the basis for any disciplinary intervention; for example the 1–2–3 rule:
  1. Instruct the child to do something or desist
  2. Threat that if not complied with, the child will go to time out
  3. Time out – child placed out of communicative contact for one minute per year of age.
  Set realistic expectations, short-term goals, and praise success.
- Some children will become more excitable and active with certain foods. These vary from child to child, and parents will usually have identified them. Colouring and preservative exclusion can often be helpful, but radical exclusion diets should only be used under supervision from a paediatric dietician.
- There have been anecdotal reports of helpful change with some dietary additives, for example fish oils, evening primrose oil, zinc, with no evidence of harmful effects; some can be prescribed.

Medication

- Medication should always be considered in severe cases; this should follow a specialist assessment.
- Stimulant medication (methylphenidate, dexamphetamine) is the most effective means of controlling core symptoms. It should be initiated only at specialist secondary care level (the paediatrician or child and adolescent psychiatrist). Primary care has an important role in supporting treatment and families. Shared care protocols vary but primary care tasks typically include the following:
  – repeat prescriptions
  – checking height and weight and entering these on a growth chart
  – adjusting doses within narrow limits
  – reporting and managing adverse effects
  – encouraging child's positive view of treatment (not as coercion).
- Specialists are responsible for clear monitoring, supervision and dosage recommendation.
- Stimulant drugs are controlled and need to be prescribed in the doctor's writing using words and figures to describe dosage and numbers of tablets to be prescribed. They do not, however, lead to dependence in children for whom they are prescribed.
- Extended-release preparations are often preferred to avoid the necessity of drugs being given at school.
- Second-line drugs include imipramine, bupropion, atomoxetine, risperidone and melatonin. At the time of writing these are not necessarily licensed but may still be appropriate under specialist supervision.

Referral

ADHD should be considered in any child with hyperactive behaviour or inattentiveness reported by teachers. The diagnosis can be difficult in young children and where there is comorbidity. Many localities have a specialist ADHD clinic; otherwise there may be a choice between a paediatric clinic and Child and Adolescent Mental Health Services.

Resources for patients and families

ADDISS (The Attention Deficit Disorder Information and Support Service)
Tel: 020 8906 9068; website: http://www.addiss.co.uk
Advice, support, local self-help groups, conferences and literature.

CHADD (Children and Adults with ADHD)
Website: http://www.chadd.org
This is an American support group and a good source of information for parents.

The Mental Health Foundation produces the information booklet *All About ADHD*.
Publications, The Mental Health Foundation, 7th Floor, 83 Victoria Street, London SW1H 0HW
Tel: 020 7802 0304; website: http://www.mentalhealth.org.uk

Leaflets are available from the Royal College of Psychiatrists
Website: http://www.rcpsych.ac.uk

12
ADHD IN PRESCHOOL CHILDREN

Margaret Thompson and Edmund Sonuga-Barke

ADHD can present in young children, and is often associated with long-term educational failure, social exclusion, delinquency and substance abuse (Swanson et al. 1998), as demonstrated in both community (Richman et al. 1982; Sonuga-Barke et al. 1994, 1997; Taylor et al. 1996) and clinical samples (Barkley et al. 1990, Mannuzza et al. 1990, Robins 1991, Farrington 1995, DuPaul et al. 2001).

There is good clinical evidence of a syndrome in school-aged children, but what is the evidence of the disorder in preschool children?

In a study of 131 preschool children with ADHD and 131 without ADHD (Kadesjö et al. 2001) the main discriminating features were found to be overactivity, distractability and inattention. Interestingly, on interview the parents with more psychosocial problems themselves outlined more problems with their children with ADHD, than did the parents with fewer psychosocial problems, who underestimated the problems present in their children.

A factor analysis of the Behaviour Check List (Richman 1977) performed on a community sample (birth cohort) of 1047 3-year-olds indicated that factors for overactivity and inattention were present (Sonuga-Barke et al. 1997) and that these factors distinguished children with hyperactivity from children who had symptoms of conduct disorder. Moreover, children with conduct disorder were more likely to have mothers who were single, and were more likely to be more socially disadvantaged. By 8 years, children who had been hyperactive at 3 were more likely to have behaviour problems.

The ADHD diagnosis is still most commonly made when children reach middle childhood (around 8 years). Recently, however, there has been a noticeable increase in the number of preschool children receiving the diagnosis and subsequently being treated with psycho-stimulants, especially in the USA (Zito et al. 2000). This change in clinical practice has led to a lively debate about the nature and significance of preschool hyperactivity (i.e. preschool children's overactive, impulsive and inattentive behaviour). This issue has been pursued from the point of view of two different, but not mutually exclusive, frameworks. There has been debate as to whether ADHD in any age-group constitutes a disorder, whether it is a temperamental trait or a categorical disorder. The later situation will contribute to the importance of deciding at what point the presenting symptoms will constitute a condition.

It is important to differentiate between abnormal and normal, age-appropriate behaviour, and parent expectations (Egeland et al. 1990). In young children the presentation of a psychiatric problem will depend on the views of professionals and parents as to what normal expectations of behaviour should be, and, just as importantly, on whether the child's behaviour impinges on their carer to cause distress, or on the rest of the child's environment

– for example, whether the leaders of a play group can tolerate a child's difficult behaviour. The clinician will seek to assess whether hyperactive behaviour is indeed detrimental to the child's emotional and physical well-being in the present or for the future.

The presenting symptoms of overactivity, distractability and inattention need to be seen in the context of a developmental framework. Campbell (1995) suggests that a disorder should be deemed to be present if there is a pattern or constellation of symptoms, if it has at least short-term stability, if it is pervasive, and if it is relatively severe with a loss of normal functioning. There should therefore be interference with the child's ability to negotiate developmental challenges. Campbell also reminds us of the importance of developmental windows for the development of language, self-regulation and moral realism, and suggests that the child might be disadvantaged if other processes prevent them from reaching appropriate developmental milestones.

In thinking about indicators of risk–disorder pathways it is important to recognize that preschool hyperactivity rarely presents on its own (e.g. Lavigne et al. 1996) but is usually accompanied by symptoms of oppositional disorder (Campbell et al. 1994, Speltz et al. 1999, Keenan and Wakschlag 2000, DuPaul et al. 2001). Indeed, many studies suggest that defiance, tantrums, and aggression are the most frequent reasons for referral in young children and the most common diagnosis in preschool children is oppositional defiant disorder (Eyberg et al. 1995, Lavigne et al. 1998, Keenan and Wakschlag 2000).

Interestingly this combination of problems is predicted by severity of initial problems, which in turn predicts problem persistence (Moffitt 1993, Pierce et al. 1999, Speltz et al. 1999, Campbell 2002). In this way, severity of preschool hyperactivity and comorbid conduct problems appear to combine to represent an important indicator of continuity between early signs of risk and later disorder. Although the association between these two components is well established, much more research is required to tease apart the nature of their causal relation. Existing data suggest that while preschool hyperactivity may represent a second order risk for the onset of antisocial and oppositional behaviour, there are likely to be other cases where either the situation is reversed or the two problems emerge simultaneously during development.

However, longitudinal studies following children from the preschool period to school entry and beyond suggest that preschool hyperactivity is stable in only a proportion of cases (Lavigne et al. 1998, Mathiesen and Sanson 2000). In high-risk and clinically referred samples (i.e. those whose behaviour warrants a diagnosis of ADHD), persistence of problems is somewhat greater, but most children identified as having a disorder in preschool have improved considerably by school entry (Campbell et al. 1994, Lavigne et al. 1998, Marakovitz and Campbell 1998).

If early intervention is to be possible, it would therefore be very useful to be able to predict which children who display preclinical patterns of early hyperactivity go on to develop ADHD or other disorders. Indicators of this trajectory into disorder might take the form of putative risk factors, differences in early behaviour and cognitive functioning or the environment in which they live. Our ability to estimate risk on the basis of our current understanding of genetic and environmental causal factors is limited, so it may be more fruitful to attempt to address this question by studying observable indicators of risk–disorder.

What makes it more likely for children with early hyperactivity to continue to have problems?

We know that children need consistent, predictable parenting which sends out positive messages to the child that what s/he is doing is appropriate and acceptable to his/her parents. Children also need to learn strategies for solving problems. Parents need to use 'scaffolding techniques' appropriately, that is to guide their child by teaching them enough for them to be able to progress to the next stage without being too intrusive and undermining. This will allow their child to have problem-solving techniques for future use. They need to practice these techniques constantly and use 'teachable moments' to reinforce these messages. Teaching should be fun and be positive. Children need to be able to explore language and develop vocabulary in order to communicate and to understand emotions – to develop 'an emotional literacy'. By developing these skills they will learn to control their emotions and their behaviour – learn to self-regulate. Should parenting be hostile, coercive, intrusive and non-respectful to the child, the child will struggle to gain self-control and will not be so able to explore and experiment with language and emotion (Patterson et al. 1989, Morrell and Murray 2003). Individual differences also play a part. Children who also have developmental delay in language, physical control or learning will find it more difficult to control their hyperactivity and inattention. Abnormalities of neuropsychological function lead directly to disorganized behaviour and reluctance to delay (see Chapter 1).

Preschool children who present with problems with hyperactivity and dysregulation (temper tantrums, aggression) may have parents who by their positive parenting can contain their child's behaviour and also help him/her to learn positive ways of gaining self-control and attain school readiness. Should the school also have a positive approach to the problems of these children then the ADHD will be contained and oppositional defiant disorder will not develop. However, if the parents cannot contain the child, and the school does not have a positive targeted programme, then the child's problems may further develop and become set.

Medication

Psychostimulants are the preferred treatment for this disorder in older children, and there is evidence for efficacy of psychostimulants on school performance, social skills and inter-action, and behavioural symptoms (Spencer et al. 2000) and on mother–child relationships (Barkley 1988).

There has been an increase in the USA during the last five years of the use of psycho-stimulants (mainly methylphenidate) in preschoolers, even in children as young as 2 years, with an increase from 1.1 to 3.5 per 1000 in 2-year-olds (Zito et al. 2000).

There is concern about side-effects in this age-group (Firestone et al. 1998), particularly with respect to the developing dopamine systems and neurodevelopment, which has been emphasized by MRI and animal research. There is lack of evidence for long-term effectiveness (Bennett et al. 1999) and ethical objections to altering children's behaviour and intellectual style (Perring 1997).

There have been few trials in preschool children. Spencer et al. (2000) found only eight such trials (out of 200 reviewed); moreover, not all the children in these trials were preschoolers, and most trials contained children with learning difficulties. Two studies had been on children with developmental difficulties; the response rate was 80–90% in children with no developmental difficulties, 71–73% in those with developmental problems with changes in attention and symptoms of hyperactivity. Barkley (1988) found positive changes in mother–child relationships. More side-effects seemed to be found than in trials with older children.

If medicine is to be used (see Chapter 11), then the starting dosage should be low and the drug should be titrated slowly. Careful monitoring should take place to look for side-effects, including weight and height falling through the percentiles.

Psychosocial intervention (PSI)

The MTA trial in school-aged children suggested that an intensive PSI was less effective than algorithm-based psychostimulant intervention on hyperactive symptoms, though when these children were followed up beyond 14 months the effect size for those on medication was nearer that for the PSI group in the medium term.

When presented in combination with psychostimulants, PSI produced only a small increase in effect size but the amount of medication needed was less (MTA 1999a,b). However, considering the theoretical discussion above about pathways to disorder and also the developmental argument against using medication in young children, PSI might usefully be introduced before patterns of behaviour set in. Pelham et al. (1998) have reviewed parenting packages for preschoolers with ADHD.

We have developed a parenting package for parents of preschool children, the New Forest Parenting Package (NFPP). Targeted at ADHD symptoms, the NFPP is an 8-week package delivered for 60–75 minutes in the patient's home. Each week we tackle a different strand, but repeat as we go along to re-enforce the messages. This has proved effective in a randomized control trial, with an effect size of 0.87 with 53% achieving scores within normal ranges, which is as good as using medication only would be, with fewer side-effects. The effect was maintained at 15 weeks following the end of the package (Sonuga-Barke et al. 2001).

Before starting a parenting package it is important to engage the family. It is also important, as in all assessments, to take a good history to outline the features of the child (a description of the behaviour, include any birth issues and developmental delay). An assessment of the mother's and father's personalities is important – are they depressed, and have they themselves got ADHD, as this will impinge on their ability to take on parenting advice which demands organization and consistency (Sonuga-Barke et al. 2002). It is also important to establish the parents' motivation to make changes in their parenting, and it is relevant to check it is the right time for the family, for example that there is no new baby due, the relationship between the parents is positive, and there is no holiday or move planned.

It is often the mother with whom you will do the work, but it is helpful if she can have a partner or friend or other relative with her for the first appointment in order to support her and reinforce the ideas. For some sessions it is good to have the child there so that the therapist can 'model' ideas with the child.

197

THE NEW FOREST PARENTING PACKAGE

There are five strands to the package:

1. *Psycho-education*

   Time spent explaining a simple outline of the theoretical underpinning to ADHD, including the part genetics plays, is important. This leads on to a discussion about the symptoms of ADHD, so that the parent can understand why the child behaves the way s/he does. The therapist should then discuss the need for a more targeted and focused approach to parenting such children.

2. *The mother–child relationship*

   The mother–child relationship is important as this is the 'vehicle' to contain the changes in the parenting.

   We discuss how to recruit attention, encourage eye contact, use short sentences and keep commands simple.

   We discuss how to keep calm, using a psychological technique known as the 'perspex shield'. Just as riot police use shields to protect themselves, so we suggest that mothers learn to use a cue such as rubbing their ears to bring down a 'perspex shield' in their mind, behind which they will not be able to feel the emotions raised by their children's difficult behaviour.

   We talk to mothers about the importance of praising their children as much as possible. We discuss the importance of language and how by using language they can extend play.

   We explain about the importance of criterion-based learning within the proximal zone of the child. We explain about the importance of scaffolding and building up children's skills. Within the package we will give examples and encourage the importance of 'teachable moments'.

3. *Play*

   We explain about the importance of play and using 'alpha commands', i.e. positive comments at all times without qualification.

   We re-emphasize the importance of using language to extend play.

   We explain that hyperactive children find it hard to wait and will get bored easily. It is important to prepare for play. The advice is to use toys and games that can be played quickly – e.g. play dough, Lego® or card games – in order to teach the child how to learn to lose, but to give them a chance to play again quickly. Ludo is a good example (with only one token each). Long games are not helpful: the child gets bored. We suggest that parents play games that they enjoy and do not suggest games that take time when they (the parents) are tired.

4. *Behaviour strategies*

   This is a strand throughout the whole 8 weeks. Time out from positive reinforcement is not tackled until later on in the package. We suggest that time out should be adjusted for the particular child. The technique of 'talk down' is explained: this is a method for allowing the child to calm down with the parents' help.

   We use reward charts, encouraging the child if possible to make one with the mother.

   Mothers are taught to use appropriate sanctions and limit-setting.

5. *Increasing attention*

We work on helping the child to learn to wait for things they want. We teach the parents to help the child cue into events using a count-down technique, e.g. "10 minutes to meal time". It helps to use timing cues like egg timers or kitchen clocks. Some games will improve attention and coping with turn taking, e.g. card games such as 'pairs' or 'snap'. Other games help improve auditory memory, e.g. 'Simon Says', 'I went to market and I bought . .'.

CASE STUDIES

1. After a normal birth, and development at milestones, Martin has been consistently 'on the go' ever since he started walking. He will climb a great deal, but rarely injures himself. He can be kept to task if someone is with him; but if left alone he gets cross, and starts rushing around or doing naughty things like drawing on the walls. He can be very cross if does not get his own way.

Following a careful assessment at age 3 years, the mother was offered a parenting package. She worked hard with the therapist and Martin did well. When it was time to start school the school was prepared for him and so far he has made good progress.

2. Johnny is 4 years old. He was born at 40 weeks, following a long labour and forceps delivery. Initial Apgar score was 6 (low). Developmental milestones have been normal, except that he was slow to speak. He has been excessively on-the-go since he started walking. He climbs everything available, puts himself into danger, and is a frequent attender at the hospital's accident and emergency department. He flits from toy to toy with poor attention and is distracted easily. The playgroup finds him difficult too; he is aggressive and oppositional, and has major temper tantrums.

His mother was offered a parenting package, and it seemed to improve the situation. Nevertheless, when Johnny started school, he found it difficult to sit still, to organize his work, to work in groups, and to take turns. His language was still not at the level of his peers, and he often found it difficult to understand what the teacher asked of him. Support and ideas were offered to the school. It seemed, however, that Johnny's problems would persist, fit the category of ADHD, and include executive function disorder and problems with inhibition. It is likely that he will need to be placed on medication if the strategies at school do not settle him enough. Continued monitoring is a requirement.

REFERENCES

Barkley RA (1988) The effects of methylphenidate on the interactions of preschool ADHD children with their mothers. *J Am Acad Child Adolesc Psychiatry* **27**: 336–341.

Barkley RA, Fischer M, Edelbrock CS, Smallish L (1990) The adolescent outcome of hyperactive children diagnosed by the research criteria: 1 and 8 year prospective follow-up study. *J Am Acad Child Adolesc Psychiatry* **29**: 546–557.

Bennett FC, Brown RT, Craver J, Anderson D (1999) Stimulant medication for the child with attention-deficit/hyperactivity disorder. *Pediatr Clin North Am* **46**: 929–944.

Campbell SB (1995) Behaviour problems in preschool children: a review of recent research. *J Child Psychol Psychiatry* **36**: 113–149.

Campbell SB (2002) *Behavior Problems In Preschool Children: Clinical And Developmental Issues. 2nd edn.* New York: Guilford Press.

Campbell SB, Pierce EW, March CL, Ewing LJ, Szumowski EK (1994) Hard-to-manage preschool boys: symptomatic behavior across contexts and time. *Child Dev* **65**: 836–851.

Dupaul G, McGoey K, Eckert T, Vanbrackle J (2001) Preschool children with attention-deficit/hyperactivity disorder: impairments in behavioral, social, and school functioning. *J Am Acad Child Adolesc Psychiatry* **40**: 508–515.

Egeland B, Kalkoske M, Gottesman N, Erickson MF (1990) Pre-school behaviour problems: stability and factors accounting for change. *J Child Psychol Psychiatry* **31**: 891–909.

Eyberg SM, Boggs SR, Algina J (1995) Parent-child interaction therapy - a psychosocial model for the treatment of young children with conduct problem behaviors and their families. *Psychopharmacol Bull* **31**: 83–91.

Farrington DP (1995) The Twelfth Jack Tizard Memorial Lecture: The development of offending and antisocial behaviour from childhood: key findings from the Cambridge Study in Delinquent Development. *J Child Psychol Psychiatry* **36**: 929–964.

Firestone P, Musten LM, Pisterman S, Mercer J, Bennett S (1998) Short-term side effects of stimulant medication are increased in preschool children with attention-deficit/hyperactivity disorder: A double-blind placebo-controlled study. *J Child Adolesc Psychopharmacol* **8**: 13–25.

Kadesjö C, Kadesjö B, Hagglof B, Gillberg C (2001) ADHD in Swedish 3- to 7-year-old children. *J Am Acad Child Adolesc Psychiatry* **40**: 1021–1028.

Keenan K, Wakschlag LS (2000) More than the terrible twos: the nature and severity of behavior problems in clinic-referred preschool children. *J Abnorm Child Psychol* **28**: 33–46.

Lavigne JV, Gibbons RD, Christoffel KK, Arend R, Rosenbaum D, Binns H, Dawson N, Sobel H, Isaacs C (1996) Prevalence rates and correlates of psychiatric disorders among preschool children. *J Am Acad Child Adolesc Psychiatry* **35**: 204–214.

Lavigne JV, Arend R, Rosenbaum D, Binns HJ, Christoffel KK, Gibbons RD (1998) Psychiatric disorders with onset in the preschool years: I. Stability of diagnoses. *J Am Acad Child Adolesc Psychiatry* **37**: 1246–1254.

Mannuzza S, Klein RG, Konig PH, Giampino TL (1990) Childhood predictors of psychiatric status in young adulthood of hyperactive boys: a study controlling for chance associations. In: Robins L, Rutter M, eds. *Straight and Devious Pathways from Childhood to Adulthood.* Cambridge: Cambridge University Press, pp. 279–299.

Marakovitz SE, Campbell SB (1998) Inattention, impulsivity and hyperactivity from preschool to school age: performance of hard-to-manage boys on laboratory measures. *J Child Psychol Psychiatry* **39**: 841–851.

Mathiesen KS, Sanson A (2000) Dimensions of early childhood behavior problems: Stability and predictors of change from 18 to 30 months. *J Abnorm Child Psychol* **28**: 15–31.

Moffitt TE (1993) The neuropsychology of conduct disorder. *Dev Psychopathol* **5**: 135–151.

Morrell J, Murray L (2003) Parenting and the development of conduct disorder and hyperactive symptoms in childhood: a prospective longitudinal study from 2 months to 8 years. *J Child Psychol Psychiatry* **44**: 489–508.

MTA (1999a) A 14-month randomized clinical trial of treatment strategies for attention deficit/hyperactivity disorder. The MTA Cooperative Group. Multimodal Treatment Study of Children with ADHD. *Arch Gen Psychiatry* **56**: 1073–1086.

MTA (1999b) Moderators and mediators of treatment response for children with attention-deficit/hyperactivity disorder: The Multimodal Treatment Study of children with Attention-Deficit/Hyperactivity Disorder. *Arch Gen Psychiatry* **56**: 1088–1096.

Patterson GR, Debaryshe BD, Ramsey E (1989) A developmental perspective on antisocial behavior. *Am Psychol* **44**: 329–335.

Pelham WE, Wheeler T, Chronis A (1998) Empirically supported psychosocial treatments for attention deficit hyperactivity disorder. *J Clin Child Psychol* **27**: 190–205.

Perring C (1997) Medicating children: the case for Ritalin. *Bioethics* **11**: 228–240.

Pierce EW, Ewing LJ, Campbell SB (1999) Diagnostic status and symptomatic behavior of hard-to-manage preschool children in middle childhood and early adolescence. *J Clin Child Psychol* **28**: 44–57.

Richman, N. (1977) Is a behaviour check list for preschool children useful? In: Graham PJ, ed. *Epidemiological Approaches to Child Psychiatry.* London: Academic Press, pp. 125–136.

Richman N, Stevenson J, Graham P (1982) *Preschool to School: a Behaviour Study.* London: Academic Press.

Robins L (1991) Conduct disorders. *J Child Psychol Psychiatry* **32**: 193–212.

Sonuga-Barke EJS, Lamparelli M, Stevenson J, Thompson M, Hendy A (1994) Behaviour problems and pre-school intellectual attainment: the associations of hyperactivity and conduct problems. *J Child.Psychol Psychiatry* **35**: 949–960.

Sonuga-Barke E, Thompson MJJ, Stevenson J, Vinney D (1997) Patterns of behaviour problems among pre-school children. *Psychol Med* **27**: 909–918.

Sonuga-Barke EJ, Daley D, Thompson MJJ, Laver-Bradbury C, Weeks A (2001) Parent based therapies for attention deficit/hyperactivity disorder: a randomized controlled trial with a community sample. *J Am Acad Child Adolesc Psychiatry* **40**: 402–408.

Sonuga-Barke E, Daley D, Thompson M (2002) Does maternal AD/HD reduce the effectiveness of parent training for pre-school children's AD/HD? *J Am Acad Adolesc Psychiatry* **41**: 696–702.

Speltz M, McClellan, DeKlyen M, Jones K (1999) Preschool boys with oppositional defiant disorder: clinical presentation and diagnostic change. *J Am Acad Child Adolesc Psychiatry* **38**: 838–845.

Spencer T, Biederman J, Wilens T (2000) Pharmacotherapy of attention deficit hyperactivity disorder. *Child Adolesc Psychiatr Clin N Am* **9**: 77–97.

Swanson JM, Sergeant JA, Taylor E, Sonuga-Barke EJS, Jensen PS, Cantwell DP (1998) Attention-deficit hyperactivity disorder and hyperkinetic disorder. *Lancet*: **351**: 429–433.

Taylor E, Chadwick O, Heptinstall E, Danckaerts M (1996) Hyperactivity and conduct problems as risk factors for adolescent development. *J Am Acad Child Adolesc Psychiatry* **35**: 1213–1226.

Zito JM, Safer Dj, DosReis S, Gardner JF, Boles M, Lynch F (2000) Trends in the prescribing of psychotropic medications to preschoolers. *JAMA* **283**: 1025–1030.

13
HYPERACTIVITY DISORDERS IN CHILDREN WITH MENTAL RETARDATION

Emily Simonoff

Although cognitive impairment is recognized as a frequent feature of hyperactivity disorders, significant intellectual disability and its relationship to hyperactivity has had surprisingly little consideration. The need to consider hyperactivity disorders that occur in the context of mental retardation arises for a number of reasons. While the causes of hyperactivity disorders with and without associated mental retardation overlap, there are risk factors for hyperactivity that are uncommon in the general population but play an important role in those with mental retardation. The types of comorbid disorders tend to vary according to cognitive level. The major hyperactivity-specific assessment measures have been designed for and standardized among typically developing children and there remains much uncertainty about the best assessment methods in those with mental retardation. Finally, while there is very much less research regarding treatment of hyperactivity disorders in mental retardation, the limited evidence suggests somewhat differing results.

Throughout this chapter, the term 'mental retardation' is used to refer to the state where individuals have an intelligence quotient, or equivalent measure of cognitive ability, of less than 70. The favoured terminology varies across countries, culture and time. In due course, most terms have taken on a pejorative connotation, presumably reflecting the attitudes of society to those who are less intellectually able. However, mental retardation remains the term in use in the *International Statistical Classification of Diseases and Related Health Problems* (ICD-10; WHO 1992) and the *Diagnostic and Statistical Manual of Mental Disorders* (DSM-IV; APA 1994), and this provides clarity for most clinicians, regardless of any social connotations. The subclassification used in both the ICD-10 and DSM-IV into mild (IQ 50–69), moderate (IQ 35–49), severe (IQ 20–34) and profound mental retardation (IQ <20) also provides an index in relation to the extent of disability, although of course at the more impaired end, measurement of mental retardation relies more heavily on functional ability and accounts from informants than formal cognitive testing. The definition of mental retardation used by the American Association on Mental Retardation (2002) also stipulates the presence of impairment in adaptive behaviour (Table 13.1). This fits in with usual clinical practice, where a diagnosis is given only when secondary impairment is present. However, there are limitations with this requirement. Most particularly, the prerequisite of functional impairment makes it impossible to examine how adaptive behaviour relates to lower cognitive ability. Such a classification will mask the group of individuals

TABLE 13.1
Classification of mental retardation

ICD-10 (WHO 1992)	American Association on Mental Retardation (2002)
General: Arrested or incomplete development of the mind, characterized by impairment of skills that contribute to the overall level of intelligence	*General:* Mental retardation is a disability characterized by significant limitations both in intellectual functioning and adaptive behaviour, originating before age 18

Subclassification	Heading	Definition	Requirement
Mild	F70	IQ 50–69	1. Significant limitations in intellectual functioning
Moderate	F71	IQ 35–49	2. Significant limitations in adaptive behaviour as
Severe	F72	IQ 20–34	expressed in conceptual, social and practical
Profound	F73	IQ <20	adaptive skills
Other	F78		3. Onset before age 18
Unspecified	F79		

Subheadings relating to behavioural impairment
.0   No or minimal behavioural impairment
.1   Significant behavioural impairment
      requiring attention or treatment
.8   Other behavioural impairment
.9   Without mention of behavioural impairment

with low cognitive ability who are functioning well, and will exaggerate the relationship between mental retardation and psychiatric disorder. Furthermore, the distinction between impact on adaptive functioning due to low cognitive ability and that due to psychopathology in the context of low cognitive ability is infrequently made but needs to be explored. For research purposes, it is therefore useful to keep separate the domains of cognitive ability and impairment in adaptive behaviour.

Throughout this chapter, the term 'hyperactivity disorders' refers to a diagnosis, whether under the American DSM or European ICD classification. 'Hyperactivity' refers to the dimension of symptoms. Most of the research on hyperactivity in mental retardation has taken place in the USA and has made use of patient groups classified under different definitions of ADHD. Almost nothing is known about the impact of different classification systems on the research findings.

Definition and classification
There is an ongoing debate as to whether the same sets of diagnoses and diagnostic criteria should be applied to individuals with mental retardation as to those of average intellectual ability. Those favouring a different system point to the qualitative differences in symptomatology. Many psychiatric disorders include, if not require, the presence of mental phenomena that are cognitively complex both in their experience and their communication to others. For example, in those with severe mental retardation features of depression such as the feelings of hopelessness and helplessness may not be possible to elicit (Clarke and Gomez 1999, Matson et al. 1999). The concern is not just one of impaired communication in expressing such mental experiences, but also that the experience requires an intellectual

level that people with more severe retardation may not achieve. As a consequence, behavioural equivalents of mental symptoms have been suggested (Meins 1995). In a similar vein, the attribution of aggressive or destructive behaviour as antisocial assumes the perpetrator can anticipate and understand the consequences of their behaviour. Where this is not the case, many would argue the behaviour is importantly different from that seen in cognitively average people, even if the consequences and distress to others is similar. Much of this thinking has been incorporated in the *Diagnostic Criteria for Learning Disability* (DC-LD; Royal College of Psychiatrists 2001), where alternative diagnostic criteria for a number of psychiatric disorders have been proposed for individuals with severe and profound mental retardation.

Others have argued for aetiology-based diagnostic systems, pointing out that atypically developing individuals may show patterns of emotional and behavioural symptoms that do not fit neatly into classification systems designed for typically developing individuals. Those with behavioural phenotypes show consistent patterns of emotional and behavioural disturbance that often do not relate directly to the available diagnostic categories. For example, the pattern of overeating, self-injurious behaviour and explosive outbursts seen in Prader–Willi syndrome is a combination idiosyncratic to the syndrome that is not seen in typically developing individuals.

There are also arguments to maintain the same diagnostic system for those with significant mental retardation. Differing classification systems make comparisons between those with and without mental retardation difficult to interpret. Different classification systems for those with mental retardation require validation of each diagnosis in the usual ways. While many of the potential abuses of classification systems have been addressed in the ICD and DSM, they may occur anew in a system specific to those with mental retardation. Defining behavioural equivalents, for example to depressed mood, could lead to problems similar to the concept of 'masked depression' in children, where a range of behaviours were conceptualized incorrectly as depressive equivalents. Any move to alter the currently available systems requires independent validation that takes account of functional impairment, prognosis and treatment, all of which may also require different measures from those used in people of average intellect.

Diagnosis of hyperactivity disorders in mental retardation

The general concern about diagnostic classification in mental retardation is applicable to hyperactivity disorders. The diagnostic criteria for hyperactivity disorders rely primarily upon observations of behaviour, whether reported by parents and teachers, or directly assessed by clinicians, rather than inference of mentalizing states. There are several difficulties in applying diagnostic criteria. First, individual symptoms may be problematic to interpret. Within the DSM system, where a symptom count approach is taken, individual items may be difficult to evaluate or not applicable. Items such as "often has difficulty organizing tasks and activities" may tap into cognitive deficits that are a component of intellectual disability, as well as of ADHD. In evaluating symptoms such as "difficulty following through on instructions", examples in which the child's comprehension of instructions is certain may be difficult to obtain. The item "often loses things necessary for tasks or activities" cannot be assessed if it is inappropriate to give the child responsibility for keeping their property. Second, there may be problems specific to mental retardation in the accounts of hyperactivity symptoms volunteered by parents and teachers. For example, levels of motor activity and sustained attention change extensively with age in the typically developing child. For the most part, parents, teachers and clinicians appear to take account of this adequately in their ratings of children. There is some suggestion that, as a general rule, teachers' ratings may be more accurate, possibly because of their more extensive experience of children at a particular developmental level (Simonoff et al. 1998). However, there have been virtually no empirical studies of the ways in which those rating behaviour in children with mental retardation take account of their developmental level. In theory, there are two competing processes. On the one hand, failure to account adequately for a child's developmental level may lead those rating the child to have inappropriately high expectations, and to report more abnormality. Personal experience suggests that, while parents and teachers are usually very accurate in estimating the mental age at which a child is functioning, their communication with and expectations of the child may be somewhat greater than is appropriate for his/her mental age. Alternatively, parents, teachers and clinicians may be affected by *diagnostic overshadowing* (Reiss and Szyszko 1983). This term was coined to describe the process where psychiatric symptoms are less likely to be identified as indicative of mental disorder when the individual also has mental retardation. Thus, restless, inattentive behaviour may be viewed as a behavioural component of mental retardation, rather than a separate problem.

Third, no systematic approach has been formally elucidated to account for mental retardation when diagnosing hyperactivity disorders. Amongst most clinicians, the convention is to take account of developmental level in judging the degree of overactivity, inattentiveness and impulsivity. This approach is endorsed by the DSM. Thus, a 10-year-old functioning at the developmental level of a typical 4-year-old would be judged in relation to what would be usual for a 4-year-old. This process is not exact as there are no available age norms for these areas of behaviour. Where there is a significant difference between verbal and nonverbal abilities, it is unclear which to use. One suggestion is to take into account the nature of the task in which the child is engaged, so that when doing manual tasks, nonverbal ability would be the gauge, and when examining predominantly verbal tasks, such as following oral instructions or watching television, verbal ability would be the yardstick.

There are no specific alterations to the two classification systems (DSM-IV and ICD-10) for ADHD and hyperkinetic disorder in people with mental retardation bar the stipulation that the behaviour should be out of keeping with the child's developmental level. No specific guidelines are given, and none of the research interviews either operationalize a methodology for doing so or have developed standardizations and validation. Abnormalities in developmentally appropriate attention and impulse control can be more difficult to evaluate than overactivity, and many of the individual items in the DSM criteria may not be directly applicable to individuals with severe or profound mental retardation. It is likely that greater reliance is therefore placed on overactivity.

Both the ICD and DSM exclude the diagnosis of ADHD/hyperkinetic disorder when schizophrenia and other psychotic disorders or a pervasive developmental disorder (PDD) is present. The classification systems deal somewhat differently with anxiety and mood disorders: ICD-10 precludes the diagnosis of hyperkinetic disorder in the presence of either of these, while DSM-IV requires consideration as to whether either an anxiety or mood disorder would better explain the clinical features. The theoretical basis for diagnostic exclusions is weak, as comorbidity is common in child psychiatric disorders (Caron and Rutter 1991). In some instances, it may be clinically helpful in assessing complex cases to determine a primary diagnosis and establish treatment priorities. However, there are also instances in which applying the exclusion when another disorder is present will lead to a failure to treat associated hyperactivity. The PDD exclusion arises frequently in children with mental retardation. With the increasing rate of PDD diagnoses (Fombonne 1999), at least in part due to increased recognition of more subtle social communication abnormalities, the diagnosis of a PDD is common among children with mental retardation (Gillberg and Wing 1999) and produces a substantial number in whom a hyperactivity disorder is not considered if the exclusion is followed. Clinicians recognize a group of children with autism and other PDDs in whom overactivity and general inattentiveness are distinct features causing independent impairment. Within the ICD classification, some may be appropriately accounted for by the PDD diagnosis *overactive disorder associated with mental retardation and stereotyped movements*. However, this classification is limited to those of IQ <50, and emphasizes the stereotyped behaviours rather than problems with social reciprocity and communication. It is unclear whether this has greater utility than the joint diagnoses of a PDD and hyperkinetic disorder.

Aetiology

Aetiological factors for hyperactivity in mental retardation can be conceptualized according to whether they are risk factors that play an equivalent role at all levels of cognitive ability or are relatively specific for individuals with mental retardation. Within the cognitively average population, genetic factors play a major causal role in both hyperactivity symptoms and disorders (Thapar et al. 1999). Behaviour genetic (twin and adoption) studies indicate that these genetic factors are largely multiple genes, each accounting for a small proportion of the overall risk but in combination being responsible for about 60–80% of individual variability. Some of these susceptibility genes have been identified, e.g. the dopamine D4 receptor and the dopamine transporter, but they account for only a small proportion of the overall genetic risk, thus indicating that other susceptibility genes are yet to be identified.

There are no behaviour or molecular genetic studies of hyperactivity focusing on individuals with mental retardation. Epidemiological studies suggest that hyperactivity is increased among those with mental retardation. This could occur for several reasons. First, risk factors for hyperactivity in the general population may also increase the chance of cognitive impairment and mental retardation. Second, there may be a causal relationship between mental retardation and hyperactivity. Kuntsi et al. (2004) showed that the observed correlation between symptoms of hyperactivity and cognitive ability, in a general population sample of twins, was largely due to genetic effects. However, the alternative causal model was not tested and therefore cannot be excluded.

Twin studies also suggest there are shared genetic risk factors between hyperactivity and specific cognitive problems, such as spelling disability (Stevenson et al. 1993). These statistical methods do not identify the genes involved in shared genetic risk. It is not known whether the genes that influence the risk of hyperactivity and cognitive variation in the general population also play a role in those with mental retardation because these studies did not include subjects with mental retardation. However, support for the role of genes influencing both hyperactivity and cognition comes from the findings of several genome-wide scans of ADHD. The first (Fisher et al. 2002) identified two regions of possible linkage, 2g24 and 16p13, that overlap with regions reported in genome scans of autism (International Molecular Genetic Study of Autism Consortium 2001). An extension of work from this group (Ogdie et al. 2003) subsequently reported that four of six regions of possible interest overlap with regions of interest reported for either autism – 16p13 (Philippe et al. 1999), 17p11 (International Molecular Genetic Study of Autism Consortium 2001), and 5p13 (Liu et al. 2001) – or dyslexia – 6p21 (Fisher et al. 1999, Grigorenko et al. 2000). A third genome scan (Bakker et al. 2003) reported 10 regions of interest, of which one (chromosome 15q15) overlaps with that reported for autism in a number of studies (Audi et al. 1998, Philippe et al. 1999, Risch et al. 1999, Shao et al. 2002) and also dyslexia Grigorenko et al. 1997). The findings of regions of shared interest between ADHD and dyslexia were confirmed by Loo et al. (2004), who, using the same sample as Fisher et al. (2002), reported that areas of possible linkage on 17p and 2p overlap with regions reported for reading retardation. Genome scans highlight regions of potential interest, rather than identifying individual susceptibility genes. It is possible that the overlapping regions of linkage occur because they contain separate susceptibility genes for hyperactivity and other disorders. Nevertheless, these intriguing findings raise the possibility of a shared genetic vulnerability for a range of neurodevelopmental disorders.

There are also a number of recognized genetic disorders in which both mental retardation and hyperactivity are prominent features, often to the extent of being part of a behavioural phenotype. Those genetic disorders where hyperactivity is a common feature are listed in Table 13.2. The genetic mechanisms underlying these disorders are varied and include a single gene defect (e.g. neurofibromatosis, Sotos syndrome), an expanding trinucleotide repeat (e.g. fragile X syndrome), and submicroscopic deletions (Smith–Magenis and Williams syndromes). These disorders account for only a minority of cases of hyperactivity and mental retardation. They are, however, important to recognize because of the potential genetic implications for other family members and the knowledge of associated physical and behavioural problems and prognosis for the affected individuals.

Although family-wide environmental factors associated with both hyperactivity and mental retardation cannot be excluded, the psychosocial disadvantage reported in mild mental retardation (Broman et al. 1987) is not generally seen in studies of hyperactivity disorders (Taylor et al. 1991). Severe environmental deprivation can lead to both low IQ and a range of psychiatric disorders with features of hyperactivity and autism (Rutter et al. 1999). It is interesting to note that cognitive function tends to recover first, at least when deprivation terminates fairly early in childhood (O'Connor et al. 2000). With respect to individual-specific environmental risk, certain risk factors – prenatal, e.g. exposure to alcohol (Aronson et al. 1997, Aronson and Hagberg 1998); perinatal, e.g. preterm birth with hypoxia (Mervis et al. 1995, Hille et al. 2001, Anderson et al. 2003); and postnatal, e.g. encephalitis, lead

TABLE 13.2
Medical disorders commonly presenting with mental retardation and hyperactivity as frequent features*

Disorder	Abnormality
Neurofibromatosis	Single gene mutation (autosomal dominant) with variable expression, chromosome 2p, high rate of spontaneous mutations
Sex chromosome anomalies: XXY and XYY	
Angelman syndrome	Abnormality of *UBE3A* gene, occurring in imprinted region of chromosome 15q: single gene mutation, deletion of paternal copy of gene, maternal uniparental disomy (two copies of maternal gene)
Fragile X syndrome	Expanded trinucleotide repeat in *FMR1* gene on X chromosome
Noonan syndrome	Single gene mutation, chromosome 12q24
Smith–Magennis syndrome	Submicroscopic deletion, chromosome 17p11
Sotos syndrome	Single gene mutation
Velo-cardio-facial syndrome	Submicroscopic deletion ion chromosome 22q
Williams syndrome	Sibmicroscopic deletion, chromosome 7q11, affecting elastin gene

*Although hyperactivity has been described as a clinical feature, in the majority of cases there has been no systematic research to determine the proportion of cases in which diagnostic criteria are met.

toxicity (Raab et al. 1985, Thompson et al. 1989 – increase the chance of both cognitive impairment and hyperactivity. Traumatic brain injury (Max et al. 1998), especially when severe, may cause a secondary hyperactivity disorder, although the features are often somewhat different, with greater social disinhibition and more specific memory problems.

Clinical features

PREVALENCE AND RISK FACTORS

Hyperactivity disorders are one of the most common reasons for children with mental retardation to present to mental health services, with one study reporting ADHD in 42% of clinic presentations (Hardan and Sahl 1997). In contrast to research among children of average cognitive ability, there are very few epidemiological studies indicating the prevalence of hyperactivity disorders in children with mental retardation. Dekker and Koot (2003a) used the Diagnostic Interview Schedule for Children (DISC) to assess a large sample of Dutch school-age children attending special schools for the "educable" (IQ 60–80) and "trainable" (IQ<60). Overall, the rate of DSM-IV ADHD was 14.8%, decreasing to 6.8% when an additional impairment criterion was included. Emerson (2003) conducted a secondary analysis of the British Household Survey of children aged 5–15 years. Intellectual disability was defined according to parental reports either of a history of severe early language delay or of attendance at a school for learning disability, and the absence of contradictory information from teachers. ICD-10 hyperkinetic disorder was diagnosed by the Development and Well-being Assessment (DAWBA; Goodman et al. 2000). The rate of hyperkinetic disorder amongst those with intellectual disability was 8.9%, a 10-fold increase over the rate of 0.9% in the rest of the population.

In their Norwegian study, Stromme and Diseth (2000) ascertained children with mental retardation through registers and teacher/clinician nominations, and used semi-structured interviews based on ICD-10 criteria and observation to identify psychiatric disorders. Hyperkinetic disorder was diagnosed in 16% of the sample. Gillberg et al. (1986) studied a sample of Swedish school children with moderate and severe mental retardation in whom semi-structured parental interviews and observation were completed. No cases of hyperkinetic disorder were reported among the 73 with severe mental retardation, in contrast to a rate of 11% in the 91 with mild mental retardation.

While each study has limitations, these vary across the different reports and there is a consistent finding of rates of hyperactivity disorders of between 8% and 16%. Studies ascertaining children though attendance in special schools (e.g. Gillberg et al. 1986, Stromme and Diseth 2000, Dekker and Koot 2003a) not surprisingly report higher rates than the British Household Survey, which commenced with a general population sample. These studies using registers and special schools are likely to have subjects with greater impairment in adaptive functioning and overall lower IQ. The absence of hyperkinetic disorder in the severely retarded sample reported by Gillberg et al. (1986) differs from the results of (Dekker and Koot 2003a), who found no effect of the child's educational level. However, the latter sample were relatively able, were not formally assessed for autism, and were noted to include few children with severe physical disorder or sensory disability.

There is also an inconsistency between the same two studies with respect to sex differences in prevalence. The Dekker and Koot study found no sex differences, while Gillberg et al. reported that males were 3.5 times more likely to be affected. The failure in the Dekker and Koot study to find a sex bias highlights the possibility that the effect of mental retardation may override other, sex-based risk factors that operate in the general population.

These findings also raise questions about whether the severity of mental retardation is a further risk factor for hyperactivity. Within general population studies, there is evidence for a gradient between IQ and probability of hyperactivity (Kuntsi et al. 2004). Dekker and Koot reported that level of education, a proxy for degree of mental retardation, did not affect the rate of diagnosed ADHD, while Gillberg et al. reported no cases of hyperkinesis among the more severely retarded. In the latter instance, it may be that the high rate of autism in those with severe mental retardation played an important role in reducing diagnoses of hyperkinesis. As this was not included in the formal diagnostic assessment in the Dutch study, it may have had less effect. In support of the Gillberg et al. findings are those of Einfeld and Tonge (1996). These authors conducted an epidemiological study of psychiatric symptoms in children with mental retardation in New South Wales, Australia, whose degree of retardation varied from mild to profound, using the Developmental Behaviour Checklist (DBC; Einfeld and Tonge 1996). The Disruptive scale of the DBC, which includes items on hyperactivity, showed a linear decrease in scores as level of retardation became more severe. The fact that hyperactivity disorders are more difficult to diagnose with certainty in the more severely mentally retarded may play a role in this funding. In contrast, Chadwick et al. (2000) examined behavioural problems, including overactivity, among children attending schools for severe mental retardation. Ratings using the Disability Adjustment

Schedule (Holmes et al. 2002) and both the parent and teacher forms of the Aberrant Behavior Checklist (Aman 1986) showed that children functioning at a lower mental age were significantly more overactive. There is, then, no consistency in the findings with regard to risk of hyperactivity and severity of mental retardation.

FAMILY RISK FACTORS

Remarkably little is known about the role of family factors and hyperactivity in mental retardation, a topic so fully studied in the general population. Dekker and Koot (2003b) examined the role of family factors in predicting psychiatric disorder among their Dutch sample with mental retardation. History of psychiatric disorder in a parent, family dysfunction and low parental educational level all predicted a disruptive disorder. ADHD was not differentiated from antisocial behaviour in these analyses, and it is uncertain how specific these risk factors are for hyperactivity, particularly given the different family risk factors for antisocial behaviour and hyperactivity among children of average cognitive ability (Taylor et al. 1986). Although there may be strong biological risk factors for hyperactivity in the context of mental retardation, other factors could augment this risk. Hessl et al. (2001) reported that the quality of the home environment and parental psychopathology increased the risk of behaviour problems in children with fragile X syndrome. It appears that children with mental retardation are likely to be vulnerable to similar environmental risk factors as typically developing children, although whether their sensitivity to such risk factors is similar, greater or smaller, is unknown.

COGNITIVE DEFICITS

Early work on cognitive processes in people with mental retardation has attempted to identify specific deficits compared to chronological or mental age peers. Much of the work, undertaken in the 1960s and 1970s, can be criticized for considering mental retardation as a unitary condition, and failing to take account of the role that the aetiology of mental retardation may have in influencing cognitive processes. It is now clear that cognitive profiles, as well as behaviour, can vary substantially according to aetiology. For example, individuals with Down syndrome show problems with short-term memory and inhibition that are greater than what would be expected by their overall ability (Pennington et al. 2003), while those with Williams syndrome have a particular skill in lexical decoding (Laing et al. 2001). Furthermore, some conditions associated with mental retardation, including Down syndrome and fragile X, show a decline over time in developmental trajectory, so that IQ decreases with age.

Relatively little systematic work has been done to determine whether the differences in cognitive tasks between children of average intellectual ability with and without hyperactivity are similar to those in children with mental retardation. Crosby (1972) found that on simple vigilance tasks, such as continuous performance tests, children with mental retardation performed equivalently to mental-age-matched controls, although Tomporowski (1990) reported that differences between individuals with learning disability and average-intellect controls were greater on more complex tasks. Yet other studies suggest that the ability to remain focused on a task may be as good or better in those with mental retardation, but there is reduced task efficiency and flexibility (Krakow and Kopp 1983, Loveland 1987).

Findings with regard to selective attention have varied in whether individuals with mental retardation show poorer performance than controls. It may be that selective attention in individuals with mental retardation is more dependent on task difficulty (Sen and Clarke 1968, Turnure 1970) and the type of distraction used (Belmont and Ellis 1968), and this could be responsible for the variation in results. Where the distractor is more similar to the task, making discrimination more difficult, individuals with mental retardation are more likely to show a poorer performance than chronological age controls (Pearson et al. 1997). There is evidence that at least some people with mental retardation may have impaired working memory (Mackie and Mackay 1982, Pennington et al. 2003), and this may affect their performance on tasks of attention that are either more complex and/or involve longer latencies between stimulus and response. This may interfere with performance on more complex attentional tasks.

Melnyk and Das (1992) divided children with mental retardation into 'poor' and 'good' attenders. On an auditory sustained attention task, there were no significant group differences, although the poor attenders showed a trend toward decline in performance. Pearson et al. (1996) compared children with mild and severe mental retardation with and without a diagnosis of ADHD on a range of attentional measures. Although the group with ADHD showed more errors of omission and commission on a continuous performance test, the decline over time in performance, typically seen in children of average intellectual ability with ADHD, was not present.

In examining selective visual attention, Melnyk and Das (1992) found a significantly worse performance in their 'poor attenders' group, and Pearson et al. (1991) also reported poorer selective visual attention in their ADHD group, as indexed by a slower response time and greater error rate, especially when the distractor was salient to the task.

The limited work on impulsivity in children with mental retardation suggests that the rates may be greatest in those with an organic basis for their intellectual disability (Rotundo and Johnson 1981, Dykens et al. 1989).

Pearson et al. (1997) suggest that some of these differences between hyperactive children with and without mental retardation could be due to underlying cognitive patterns that differentiate children with and without mental retardation, regardless of hyperactivity. Thus the 'cognitive inertia' that has been described in mental retardation could blunt the decline in performance in sustained attention tasks. The range of assessments applicable to children with mental retardation needs extension to provide tasks that measure the functions shown to discriminate ADHD in children of average intelligence.

COMORBIDITIES

Like children in the general population, those with mental retardation and one psychiatric disorder are at increased risk of a further psychiatric disorder. Dekker and Koot (2003a) reported that 14% of their Dutch sample had two or more DSM-IV disorders (36% of those with one disorder had at least one further disorder). Those with ADHD were most likely to have a disruptive comorbid disorder. The type of comorbidity may vary according to cognitive level. In mild mental retardation, comorbidity may be similar to that seen in the general population, with oppositional and conduct disorders being most common. As the degree of retardation increases, autistic disorders appear to become more common.

Hyperactivity is a persisting problem with a range of secondary impairments and psychosocial consequences among children and adolescents with mental retardation. In a 1–5 year follow-up of children with ADHD and mental retardation, Handen et al. (1997) noted that all areas of psychiatric symptoms measured, except conduct problems, improved over the follow-up period. However, two-thirds still showed high (>98th centile) hyperactivity scores on the Conners scales, and two-thirds were on stimulant medication for hyperactivity. Inpatient psychiatric admission was common (11/51). Another 3–5 year follow-up study confirmed the presence of persistent levels of hyperactivity. Irritability and stereotyped behaviours were also ongoing problems (Aman et al. 2002a). Five of the 25 children followed up had been admitted to hospital for accidental injury during the intervening period. Both studies reported high rates of school suspension and problems with the law. Given that the oldest children in both studies were in early adolescence, these problems could be expected to increase subsequently.

Assessment

In a child presenting with mental retardation and a possible hyperactivity disorder, the aims of assessment are as follows.
1. Note symptoms and behaviours that are of most concern to parents, other adults and the child.
2. Assess the symptoms of hyperactivity in the context of the child's developmental level and across situations to determine whether symptoms of overactivity, inattention and impulsivity are present.
3. If hyperactivity is present, consider the differential diagnosis for these symptoms; this includes considering the role of medical disorders and medication the child may be taking.
4. Evaluate areas of possible comorbidity.
5. Establish level of adaptive functioning and identify possible psychosocial impairment.
6. Identify the treatment and management strategies currently and previously employed by carers and teachers, and their effectiveness.
7. Evaluate the current need for treatment, feasibility of alternative treatment options, and parent and child attitudes to alternatives.

History taking should begin by identifying activities in which the child regularly participates that will provide examples of activity level, attention and impulsivity. The aim is to gain a clear account of the child's typical behaviour when engaged in tasks within his/her capability but where performance will be altered by symptoms of hyperactivity. It is essential to establish that the demands of activities are within the child's cognitive ability. Where a child's cognitive level is uncertain, supporting evidence should be elicited to demonstrate the child's ability to complete the task successfully. Even accounts of the child's behaviour watching television need to be considered in relation to the child's understanding of the language and complexity of the programmes being viewed.

Family norms and expectations should be enquired about, and accounts of behaviour contextualized in relation to these. For example, it is unhelpful to ask about a child's ability to sit still at mealtimes when the family does not sit together to eat; in such instances alternatives should be sought. Exemplar activities that parents regularly monitor should be sought in preference to others that they do not observe. For this reason, computer games as well as activities undertaken out of parents' view are not good examples. It is not uncommon for parents to report that children can occupy themselves for substantial periods of time with computer games and videos in their bedroom, while the child demonstrates overactivity and inattention in a range of other activities.

Having identified a range of activities, a careful account of the child's behaviour should be recorded. The quality of the child's behaviour and the length of time s/he attends to the activity should be quantified. Some parents may find it difficult to be specific about timing, and it may be helpful to compare the child's time spent on a task with the parent's ability to carry out daily tasks at the same time, as a way of gaining approximate timings. Finally, it is important to determine whether the account given by the parent reflects the child's behaviour in other settings, both in school and leisure activities. Where behavioural differences occur, reasons for the variation should be sought. Situational demands, structure, aspects of the environment and response from others can all influence behaviour. Age at onset can be particularly difficult to establish in children with mental retardation. If the child has attended a special school from an early age, symptoms of hyperactivity may have been dealt with by extra classroom support and not mentioned to parents. Therefore, it may be useful to focus on whether there have been qualitative changes in the child's behaviour. Fluctuations and sudden onset should be excluded, as these may indicate an underlying medical disorder; epilepsy in particular should be considered. In children with frequent seizures, peri-ictal behaviour should be excluded in the evaluation of hyperactivity.

RATING SCALES

Behavioural ratings provide a helpful addition to the clinical assessment. A rating scale that covers a range of symptom domains alerts the clinician to additional concerns that may not be mentioned as part of the presenting problems. They also provide a useful standardized metric against which the clinician can compare his/her evaluation. Rating scales are also a medium for obtaining information from a range of sources that cannot be directly questioned during the history taking, including teachers and other carers.

The scales available for rating psychopathology in the general population of children and adolescents are often applicable to those with mild mental retardation, especially those attending mainstream schools. These include broad measures such as the Child Behavior Checklist (CBC; Achenbach and Edelbrock 1985) and the Strengths and Difficulties Questionnaire (SDQ; Goodman 1997) as well as specific measures of hyperactivity such as the Conners (Conners 1989) and DuPaul Rating Scales (DuPaul et al. 1998). Measures employed in the general population have good standardization with cut-offs that robustly screen for disorder. However, these standardizations are not specific for those with mental retardation and may be misleading. When considering the use of such measures in children with more severe retardation, the appropriateness of the questions must also be evaluated. For example, asking about homework or tasks requiring close attention to detail may not apply. Inappropriate questions may lead those completing the questionnaire to doubt whether the clinician appreciates the child's difficulties. As a rule of thumb, the use of questionnaires aimed at the general population should probably be limited to children who are functioning in a mainstream school environment with only moderate amounts of additional support.

There are several general measures of psychopathology aimed specifically at populations with mental retardation (Aman 1991), of which the most carefully standardized and widely used are the Aberrant Behavior Checklist (ABC; Aman and Singh 1985) and the Developmental Behaviour Checklist [DBC; Einfeld and Tonge 2002). Both are suitable for use in children with moderate to profound mental retardation and both cover a wide range of behaviours. The ABC is considerably shorter (58 items) than the DBC (96 items). The ABC can be completed by any adult with knowledge of the child; the DBC has parallel parent/carer and teacher versions. While both have items on hyperactivity, neither questionnaire was originally designed to include a hyperactivity scale. The ABC identifies a 16-item factor called *hyperactivity/noncompliance*; in the DBC, a 6-item factor was derived from secondary analyses. Neither scale has been standardized against diagnosis to establish cut-offs for screening.

In gaining viewpoints from different informants, it is helpful to use the same rating scale to allow comparison of differences in type and degree of symptoms. Such differences need to be understood prior to completing the diagnostic assessment and initiating a treatment programme. In children with mental retardation, unrealistic academic expectations in school is a common reason for school-specific hyperactivity. Alternatively, problems with attention and activity in school may be masked when children have a high level of one-to-one support. Differences in ratings but not actual behaviour may occur when expectations of behaviour vary, when behavioural symptoms are attributed to other causes and when the degree of monitoring of behaviour differs. Because activity and attention levels alter with developmental age, those rating the behaviour need to consider the child in relation to others. For parents this may be measured against the development of their other children, while a teacher in a special school may compare the child to other pupils. Misinterpretation of questions is another common pitfall of rating scales, and the areas that cause difficulty may be somewhat different in mental retardation. Stereotypies, tics, mannerisms and overactivity may be confused. Inattention is often blamed when lack of understanding may be the reason for "not listening" or "not completing instructions".

OBSERVATION
Observation forms an essential part of the diagnostic assessment and most particularly when there are discrepancies between informants. The clinical assessment should always provide opportunities to observe the child. This should focus on the child's behaviour while carrying out tasks that require sustained attention, and others that demonstrate the ability

to plan, to structure and to inhibit his/her responses. Cognitive assessment provides an opportunity for such observation, although the one-to-one, highly structured nature of the situation and the short duration of any single subtest (particularly among those with mental retardation who complete fewer items) should be borne in mind. It is desirable also to observe the child in a less structured play situation that provides appropriate materials for the child's developmental age, as behaviour may differ from that seen during a highly structured activity.

When discrepancies remain between the findings in the clinic and those reported by informants, it is important to conduct a direct observation at school or home to reconcile these differences. Standardized procedures for classroom observation have been shown to be reliable (Abikoff et al. 1977) and to discriminate between children with mental retardation with and without ADHD (Fee et al. 1994). Although time-consuming, this is invariably a useful investment in clarifying the diagnosis and developing a shared view of the child with parents and teachers. For example, a teacher who has viewed the behaviour of a hyperactive child as non-compliant may resist giving medication to the child, may treat the child more negatively, and may have inappropriate expectations until a consensus view is reached. Similarly, if failure to focus on schoolwork is incorrectly perceived as hyperactivity when it is due to autism, treatments that could aggravate autism may be initiated. A school observation also provides the opportunity to educate staff about hyperactivity and other mental disorders.

COGNITIVE ASSESSMENT

It is essential to have a reasonably accurate assessment of the child's developmental level and degree of mental retardation. Ideally this is provided by a cognitive assessment that includes a full-scale IQ. This may not always be available and therefore clinicians should have in reserve a range of alternative assessments. Measures of receptive vocabulary such as the Peabody (Dunn and Dunn 2001) and British Picture Vocabulary Scales (Dunn et al. 1997) are useful because they require limited cooperation from children, are straightforward to interpret, and provide age equivalents down to a mental age of 2½ years. There is a range of nonverbal tests that can be used down to a mental age of 2–3 years of age but many are more complex and require greater experience. Of the more straightforward measures, the Raven's Coloured Progressive Matrices (Raven 1998) is designed for use with typically developing children under 6 years of age. While many clinicians have relied on the Vineland Adaptive Behavior Scales (Sparrow et al. 1994), this is based on parental account and it may be useful to consider assessments that involve the child more directly, such as the Mullen Scales of Early Development (Mullen 1997).

In reviewing the results of cognitive assessments undertaken, it is important to be alert to 'floor effects'. These are particularly likely to occur when the child is assessed by an examiner less experienced with mental retardation. Where scale scores are at the floor of the test, examination of the raw scores is important, as these will reveal whether the child was able to achieve any correct answers. When raw scores are very low, it may be useful to reassess the child with a battery designed for children of lower mental age, to ensure that sufficient items are correctly completed to allow a mental age estimation.

An increasing number of neuropsychological tests are available to assess cognitive processes that may be deficient in hyperactivity disorders. At the time of writing, the Children's Memory Scales (Cohen 1997) is one of the few that has been standardized to provide predicted scores based on full-scale IQ. There is a need to investigate the range of cognitive processes that might be involved in hyperactivity disorders in mental retardation and not to assume that the difficulties will be the same as those seen in average-ability children with hyperactivity.

PHYSICAL EXAMINATION AND INVESTIGATIONS
Physical examination serves three main purposes in the assessment of children with mental retardation and a possible hyperactivity disorder. A good medical and family history should precede the physical examination. The examination should look for physical signs of medical disorders that may cause or be confused with hyperactivity. Thyroid disease may cause a clinical picture similar to hyperactivity, although this is rare. A neurological examination should always be conducted but with special attention when the history suggests head injury or a brain tumour. Hearing and vision should be formally assessed if there is any question of a sensory deficit. Observation should make note of any tics, stereotypies, other abnormal movements or alteration in consciousness.

Where the cause of mental retardation is unknown, the examination should also look for stigmata of disorders causing mental retardation. Identifying the cause of mental retardation may be helpful to families in coming to terms with their child's disability. It may also refine prognosis and have indications for follow-up. In addition, the cause may have genetic implications for other family members. The examination should include an assessment for neurocutaneous stigmata and dysmorphic features. If not previously investigated, blood should be taken for cytogenetic and fragile X testing, especially in those with IQ <50 or where significant dysmorphic features are present. Should a syndrome be suspected, a clinical genetic opinion should be obtained before taking blood as tests for specific disorders may require fresh samples.

The examination should determine whether any physical disorders are present that might affect the use of stimulant or other psychotropic medication. These considerations are much the same as for children with average intellectual ability. Most commonly, abnormalities on cardiovascular examination may require a specialist opinion if stimulant medication is to be considered. Children with epilepsy should have a baseline electroencephalogram (EEG) prior to initiating medication, although the deleterious effect of stimulant medication on seizures has not been demonstrated and there is even a suggestion that stimulants may improve the EEG (Gucuyener et al. 2003).

DIFFERENTIAL DIAGNOSIS AND COMORBIDITY (TABLE 13.3)
The differential diagnosis of a hyperactivity disorder is the same in children with and without mental retardation, but the alternatives change in their likelihood, particularly as mental retardation becomes more severe. It is not uncommon for children to present for assessment of hyperactivity when the extent of their mental retardation (or associated specific speech and language disorder) is not fully appreciated. When this is accounted for,

TABLE 13.3
Differential diagnosis of hyperactivity disorders
in mental retardation

1. Mental retardation only

2. Other psychiatric disorders
    Oppositional and conduct disorder
    Tic disorder
    Autism
    Anxiety
    Major depressive disorder
    Bipolar disorder
    Post-traumatic stress disorder

3. Medical disorders
    Epilepsy
    Motor disorders including Huntington's and
        Sydenham's chorea
    Progressive (dementing) disorder
    Head injury
    Brain tumour
    Hearing or vision deficit
    Hypothyroidism
    Lead toxicity

activity and attention levels may be deemed developmentally appropriate. Alternatively, in cases where hyperactive behaviour is largely confined to the school setting, the child's inability to access the curriculum may account for off-task behaviour. It is wise to be particularly cautious about diagnosing hyperactivity in young children with either global or specific developmental delay as their hyperactivity symptoms may improve significantly with age and educational support. Improvement in communication may be particularly associated with a decrease in hyperactivity symptoms.

In differential diagnosis a question to be asked is whether another disorder accounts for the entirety of the clinical picture and is therefore the sole diagnosis. While parsimony should be practised in identifying psychiatric disorders, this should be balanced against the need to provide treatments that will reduce functional impairment. Discretion is important in determining the treatment approach as hyperactivity disorders are among the more treatable psychiatric conditions in children with mental retardation. Oppositional and conduct disorders are the most common comorbidities and are also important differential diagnoses in children with disruptive behaviour and mild mental retardation. Parents frequently complain that children won't listen, don't do as asked and are destructive. The distinguishing characteristic of a hyperactivity disorder is that these behaviours persist even when the child is motivated to comply. As discussed earlier, it is also important to determine that the child understands what is being asked of him/her and has the cognitive capacity to respond appropriately. It may be useful to elucidate the role of impulsivity in any aggressive behaviour as this may be a target for treatment of hyperactivity. In severe mental retardation, aggressive and destructive behaviour remain common but are usually easy to distinguish by their episodic nature.

Autism and pervasive developmental disorders (PDDs) are much more common in children with mental retardation and are therefore important differential diagnoses. Language and social development should always be covered in the assessment of individuals with mental retardation. Parents and teachers of children with autism/PDD often complain about their poor attention and the activities that attract their interest are frequently unusual or restricted. The differentiation is whether children can attend well to activities that interest them. The two disorders may be comorbid, and where hyperactivity symptoms are severe, autism/PDD may be difficult to detect, even with appropriate questioning. Successful treatment of hyperactivity may clarify the comorbidity. When social withdrawal becomes more pronounced with medication for hyperactivity, it is important to consider whether this might be a side-effect of treatment.

Tic disorders also need consideration both as comorbid and alternative diagnoses. Children with motor and vocal tics may be described by parents and teachers as overactive and disruptive. Some of this may be misconstrual of tics; other aspects may be secondary behaviours that children develop to disguise the tics, and yet others the attentional problems so commonly seen in tic disorders. A careful history followed by adequate observation of the child should expose the motor behaviours, although it is not always easy to distinguish tics from stereotypies.

Anxiety and also severe depression may present with impaired concentration and motor restlessness. In children of average intellect, the distinction is usually straightforward on mental state examination but may be more difficult in children with little or no speech. Recent onset or an association with environmental change or loss, may provide clues as does the full constellation of symptoms and signs. For depression, greater reliance must be placed on the presence of vegetative features and the loss of interest in previously enjoyed activities. People with mental retardation who develop depression may show a decrease in their level of adaptive functioning as well as social withdrawal. The importance of bipolar disorder in childhood is currently much discussed without a consensus having yet been determined, and even less is known about bipolar disorder in childhood mental retardation. However, the symptom overlap of motor restlessness and impaired concentration requires that it is considered. Conventionally, the earlier onset of hyperactivity and the absence of congruence between mood alteration and other behaviours would provide important elements of the differential diagnosis. While some are questioning the minimum diagnostic requirements for bipolar and cyclothymic disorders, hyperactivity disorders remain the better described and validated. At present they should be adopted in preference to bipolar disorder unless there is clear evidence favouring the latter.

It should be remembered that children with mental retardation are more vulnerable to physical and sexual abuse, and these experiences may be particularly difficult for children with limited verbal skills to communicate to their parents or the clinicians. Poor concentration is a frequent feature of post-traumatic stress disorder, and motor restlessness is a very nonspecific symptom seen in children with mental retardation. The recent/late onset and its relation to particular events and the comparison of behaviour before and after the event will help to clarify the picture.

Undiagnosed or inadequately controlled absence or complex partial seizures may appear as inattention. The episodic nature, along with pre-ictal motor features, should provide clues. To masquerade as attentional problems seizure activity will be sufficiently frequent to detect with EEG monitoring. In children with severe or intractable seizures, it may be difficult to disentangle inattention from peri- and post-ictal phenomena; here the aim is to identify relatively seizure-free periods (which in complex epilepsy may first require continuous monitoring to identify the range of seizure type and their manifestations) and to assess behaviour during that time. Other neurological processes can cause the picture of hyperactivity and learning disability. These include acquired brain injury, brain tumours and dementing disorders. In all cases, the history of change should prompt a thorough examination. It is well recognized that children with hyperactivity are at increased risk of accidents that may lead to head injury (Chadwick et al. 1981, Filley et al. 1987), highlighting that children may have both ADHD and a history of head injury.

Treatment

PSYCHOEDUCATION AND SOCIAL CARE

The backbone of intervention is psychoeducation for parents, carers and teachers. This may include education about mental retardation as well as hyperactivity. With regard to mental retardation, it is useful to determine at what level parents and others believe the child is functioning with regard to mental age equivalents. These views can vary widely, with many parents giving accurate estimates of the child's level of development but others underestimating the degree of delay that is present. Parents and other adults may find it particularly difficult to estimate a child's developmental level when there are large discrepancies across cognitive domains. Adults may be particularly inaccurate when a child's attainments, such as reading and spelling, are well above those predicted by ability. This may require considerable time for explanation. Even when parental estimates are accurate, the expectations of and behaviour towards the child may inadvertently be more appropriate for a higher-functioning child. For example, a parent may accurately identify their child's developmental level as typical for a 3-year-old, but the complexity of the parent's communication with the child may be suitable for a mental age of 6 years. It is also important to explore parental expectations with regard to longer-term development. Some parents, whilst acknowledging the current level of functioning, may continue to hope their child will 'grow out of it'. Others may not have considered future education and care implications for the longer-term disability. Such planning is particularly important when a child with mental retardation has another impairing disorder, such as hyperactivity.

A similar process should be conducted with regard to hyperactivity. At present, it seems likely that parents whose children have mental retardation are less likely to consider a hyperactivity disorder than parents with children of average ability. In some cases, parents and other adults may be very clear in their descriptions of the child's symptoms, and the primary task is to relate those symptoms to diagnosis. In others, more explanation is needed about the inconsistency between the child's overall cognitive functioning and levels of overactivity and attention. Wherever possible, it is useful to involve other carers and teachers in the process of psychoeducation. Where this cannot be done personally, provision of written materials is useful. Unfortunately, there is little commercially published material on hyperactivity focused on those with mental retardation.

The process of psychoeducation should take account of the child's environment – home, school and leisure activities. Considerations of safety in the home and play environment is of great importance, and there is often a need for very high levels of supervision. The most important school issues may depend on whether the child attends a mainstream or special school and the amount of individual support s/he is receiving. The key elements are to ensure that the general curriculum is appropriate for the child's intellectual ability, that the mode of presentation is in line with the child's attention span, and that a programme of contingent reinforcement is in place for achievement. Respite care with trained adults is often of benefit to both children and parents, and other structured activities should be planned for school holidays. Respite carers need information and training with respect to mental retardation and hyperactivity to provide safe and appropriate care.

BEHAVIOURAL INTERVENTION

Behavioural treatment is an important approach in hyperactivity disorders but has received very little evaluation among children with mental retardation. One study evaluated the effects of contingent reinforcement over and above those of methylphenidate in three children with mild mental retardation (Johnson et al. 1994). Two of the three children showed further improvement with intervention during an academic task over that observed in the medication-only condition, when contingent reinforcement focused on accuracy of work. The results are limited by the small sample, the narrowness of the observational assessment, and the short-term nature of the follow-up. Furthermore, the results cannot be directly translated to such an intervention in more severe retardation.

In general, children with mental retardation are responsive to the effects of programmes of reinforcement, provided the incentives, their schedule of delivery and the goals are appropriate. The approach should be suitable for the child's developmental age. In children of average cognitive ability, behavioural intervention was at least as helpful as stimulant medication for children with comorbid psychiatric disorders such as anxiety and in helping with secondary impairments such as peer relationships (Owens et al. 2003). This may also be the case in children with mental retardation, where the main effects of a behavioural approach may be to enhance compliant and appropriate behaviour, rather than to eradicate hyperactivity. Behavioural approaches may also be sufficient for the mildest hyperactivity disorders. Some degree of behavioural intervention should always be considered where the behavioural management by parents, teachers and carers is thought to be suboptimal. The aims should be not only to manage hyperactive behaviour but also to ensure that an appropriate regime of expectations and reinforcement is in place.

MEDICATION

Of the medication currently used to treat hyperactivity disorders, methylphenidate has received the most attention in children with mental retardation. Overall, the studies show that behavioural improvement is significantly more likely on stimulants than placebo, but suggest that the response rate is less than that seen in children of average ability. Aman et al. (2003) aggregated the findings of three studies from their group using crossover designs to compare methylphenidate in a single morning dose of 0.4mg/kg versus placebo. Treatment response based on behavioural ratings, whether measured by percentage improvement or effect size, was substantially less than that reported in studies of children of average intellect. These revealed that 44% showed symptom reduction compared to a placebo rate of 30% or more, and only 25% had 50% or greater improvement. These results provided effect sizes of 0.57 for teachers and 0.39 for parents, compared to ones of 0.7–0.8 in many studies of typically developing children and 0.9 in the NIMH Multimodal Treatment Study (MTA 1999).

Dosage may be critical in level of response; two studies have used varying dose and shown this affects response rate. Handen et al. (1992) evaluated behavioural response to placebo and methylphenidate at doses of 0.3 and 0.6 mg/kg in children with mild to moderate mental retardation. While there was some variability according to the measure, 9 out of 14 children showed a response of 1 standard deviation improvement over placebo on the Conners Hyperactivity Index. (Pearson et al. 2003) compared low (0.15 mg/kg), medium (0.3 mg/kg) and high (0.6 mg/kg) doses of methylphenidate with placebo using a crossover design in 24 children with mild mental retardation. Behavioural ratings showed significant symptomatic reduction that was greatest on high dose, in some cases significantly greater than on medium dose. However, parents also reported significant increases in appetite loss and insomnia on the high dose.

The combined findings highlight a number of themes and raise additional questions. Parents were less likely than teachers to report benefits of stimulant medication. None of the trials used three times daily dosing, and it is not known whether this would be beneficial for children with mental retardation. There appear to be the same expected trade-offs between better symptom control and higher rates of adverse effects as dose is increased. It is unclear whether the therapeutic window is smaller for children with mental retardation, or whether the benefits of medication are more limited. However, the findings across studies suggest that low doses may not be the best for all children with mental retardation and hyperactivity. None of the studies have used the method of individual dose titration, but the findings support the idea that this may be the best option. Also, none of the studies maintained children on medication long enough to determine its medium- or longer-term benefits, or the course of adverse effects. Only the studies by Aman and colleagues (Aman et al. 1991, 1993, 2002b) include children with severe mental retardation and his results suggest that those with more severe intellectual disability are less likely to respond to medication (Aman et al. 2003). This finding needs further exploration in a larger study with individual titration to balance behavioural response and adverse effects. A secondary analysis by Handen et al. (1994) indicated that those with more deviant hyperactivity scores were more likely to improve, a finding also seen in studies of children of average intellect. The long-standing clinical view that children with autistic symptoms and disorders may fare poorly on stimulant medication needs systematic evaluation, particularly in light of the increasing awareness of features of autism, which means that a higher proportion of children with mental retardation and hyperactivity are recognized as having autistic features.

In current clinical practice, methylphenidate is therefore the pharmacological treatment of first choice. Although the research findings suggest that higher doses may be best for some children, titration should commence with a low dose, and increases should be performed cautiously. Monitoring should be frequent, as this group of children are more likely to experience adverse effects. Although there has been concern about using methylphenidate in children with epilepsy, the available evidence suggests it is safe to do so (Gross-Tsur et al. 1997, Gucuyener et al. 2003). Although the product license for methylphenidate includes as a contradindication an individual history of tics or a family history of Tourette syndrome, there is evidence that it can be used in children with comorbid tic disorders, without exacerbation of the latter (Gadow et al. 1999).

Should there be grounds for avoiding methylphenidate, or should methylphenidate be ineffective or not tolerated, the choices are those available for hyperactive children of average ability (Pliszka et al. 2000a,b), but there is no systematic evidence base determining their efficacy in children with mental retardation. Despite the lack of evidence, the first approach to alternative medication should employ drugs that are aimed at the treatment of hyperactivity, unless comorbidity is a prominent and impairing feature. There are now several studies showing that low-dose risperidone may be effective for severely disruptive and/or aggressive behaviour in children with mental retardation, with or without autism. These studies indicate a significant decrease in irritability, disruptive behaviour and aggression on daily doses usually of 1–2 mg, and few short-term side-effects (Buitelaar et al. 2001, Van Bellinghen and De Troch 2001, Aman et al. 2002b, Turgay et al. 2002). A role has been suggested for risperidone 'augmentation' in children with hyperactivity disorders and comorbid disorders (Bramble and Cosgrove 2002). To date, the work is descriptive rather than systematic and does not specifically address the reduction in hyperactivity symptoms as opposed to its common comorbidities. Therefore, augmentation should only be considered when impairing symptoms persist and first-line treatment has been optimized. Clarity of the aims of augmentation treatment with baseline and follow-up measures is especially important. Polypharmacy increases the possibility not only of adverse effects but also of drug interactions, and clinical monitoring should therefore be increased.

Research priorities
Programmatic research is required to understand, identify and treat effectively hyperactivity disorders in the context of mental retardation. The establishment of adequate sensitivity and specificity against diagnosis for screening measures is needed. Clinical assessment tools for children with mental retardation also need to be developed, as does a battery of neuropsychological measures that can identify the cognitive profiles that differentiate children with mental retardation who also have hyperactivity. Properly designed trials need to determine the efficacy of both behavioural and pharmacological interventions. A better understanding of the role of comorbidities and underlying genetic disorders in guiding intervention is required.

Given the enduring nature of both disorders, all aspects of this research should be a priority.

REFERENCES

Abikoff H, Gittelman-Klein R, Klen DF (1977) Validation of a classroom observation code for hyperactive children. *J Consult Clin Psychol* **45**: 772–783.

Achenbach TM, Edelbrock C (1985) *Manual for the Child Behavior Checklist and the Revised Child Behavior Profile.* Burlington, VT: University of Vermont.

Aman M (1986) *Aberrant Behavior Checklist – Community.* New York: Slosson Educational Publications.

Aman MG (1991) *Assessing Psychopathology and Behavior Problems in Persons with Mental Retardation: A Review of Available Instruments.* Rockville, MD: Department of Health & Human Services.

Aman MG, Marks RE, Turbott SH, Wilsher CP, Merry SN (1991) Clinical effects of methylphenidate and thioridazine in intellectually subaverage children. *J Am Acad Child Adolesc Psychiatry* **30**: 246–256.

Aman MG, Kern RA, McGhee DE, Arnold LE (1993) Fenfluramine and methylphenidate in children with mental retardation and ADHD: Clinical and side effects. *J Am Acad Child Adolesc Psychiatry* **32**: 851–859.

Aman MG, Armstrong S, Buican B, Sillick T (2002a) Four-year follow-up of children with low intelligence and ADHD: a replication. *Res Dev Disabil* **23**: 119–134.

Aman MG, De Smedt G, Derivan A, Lyons B, Findling RL; Risperidone Disruptive Behavior Study Group (2002b) Double-blind, placebo-controlled study of risperidone for the treatment of disruptive behaviors in children with subaverage intelligence. *Am J Psychiatry* **159**: 1337–1346.

Aman MG, Buican B, Arnold LE (2003) Methylphenidate treatment in children with borderline IQ and mental retardation: analysis of three aggregated studies. *J Child Adolesc Psychopharmacol* **13**: 29–40.

Aman MG, Singh NN (1985) The Aberrant Behavior Checklist: A behavior rating scale for the assessment of treatment effects. *Am J Ment Defic* **89**: 485–491.

American Association on Mental Retardation (2002) Definition of mental retardation. http://www.aamr.org/Policies/faq_mental_retardation.shtml

Anderson P, Doyle LW; Victorian Infant Collaborative Study Group (2003) Neurobehavioural outcomes of school-age children born extremely low birth weight or very preterm in the 1990s. *JAMA* **289**: 3264–3272.

APA (1994) *Diagnostic and Statistical Manual of Mental Disorders, 4th edn (DSM-IV).* Washington DC: American Psychiatric Association.

Aronson M, Hagberg B (1998) Neuropsychological disorders in children exposed to alcohol during pregnancy: a follow-up study of 24 children to alcoholic mothers in Göteborg, Sweden. *Alcohol Clin Exp Res* **22**: 321–324.

Aronson M, Hagberg B, Gillberg C (1997) Attention deficits and autistic spectrum problems in children exposed to alcohol during gestation: a follow-up study. *Dev Med Child Neurol* **39**: 583–587.

Audi L, Mantzoros CS, Vidal-Puig A, Vargas D, Gussinye M, Carrascosa A (1998) Leptin in relation to resumption of menses in woman with anorexia nervosa. *Mol Psychiatry* **3**: 544–547.

Bakker SC, van der Meulen EM, Buitelaar JK, Sandkuijl LA, Pauls DL, Monsuur AJ, van't Slot R, Minderaa RB, Gunning WB, Pearson PL, Sinke RJ (2003). A whole-genome scan in 164 Dutch sib pairs with attention-deficit/hyperactivity disorder: suggestive evidence for linkage on chromosomes 7p and 15q. *Am J Hum Genet* **72**: 1251–1260.

Belmont JM, Ellis NR (1968) Effects of extraneous stimulation upon discrimination learning in normals and retardates. *Am J Ment Defic* **72**: 525–532.

Bramble DJ, Cosgrove PVF (2002) Parental assessments of the efficacy of risperidone in attention deficit hyperactivity disorder. *Clin Child Psychol Psychiatry* **7**: 225–233.

Broman S, Nichols PL, Shaughnessy P, Kennedy W (1987) *Retardation in Young Children: A Developmental Study of Cognitive Deficit.* Hillsdale, NJ: Lawrence Erlbaum.

Buitelaar JK, van der Gaag RJ, Cohen-Kettenis P, Melman CT (2001) A randomized controlled trial of risperidone in the treatment of aggression in hospitalized adolescents with subaverage cognitive abilities. *J Clin Psychiatry* **62**: 239–248.

Caron C, Rutter M (1991) Comorbidity in child psychopathology: concepts, issues and research strategies. *J Child Psychol Psychiatry* **32**: 1063–1081.

Chadwick O, Rutter M, Brown G, Shaffer D, Traub M (1981) A prospective study of children with head injuries: II. Cognitive sequelae. *Psychol Med* **11**: 49–61.

Chadwick O, Piroth N, Walker J, Bernard S, Taylor E (2000) Factors affecting the risk of behaviour problems in children with severe intellectual disability. *J Intellect Disabil Res* **44**: 108–123.

Clarke DJ, Gomez GA (1999) Utility of modified DCR-10 criteria in the diagnosis of depression associated with intellectual disability. *J Intellect Disabil Res* **43**: 413–420.

Cohen MJ (1997) *Children's Memory Scale.* London: Psychological Corporation.

Conners CK (1989) *Conners' Rating Scales Manual.* New York: Multi-Health Systems.

Crosby KG (1972) Attention and distractibility in mentally retarded and intellectually average children. *Am J Ment Defic* **77**: 46–53.

Dekker MC, Koot HM (2003a) DSM-IV disorders in children with borderline to moderate intellectual disability. I: Prevalence and impact. *J Am Acad Child Adolesc Psychiatry* **42**: 915–922.

Dekker MC, Koot HM (2003b) DSM-IV disorders in children with borderline to moderate intellectual disability. II: Child and family predictors. *J Am Acad Child Adolesc Psychiatry* **42**: 923–931.

DuPaul GJ, Power TJ, Anastopoulos AD, Reid R (1998) *ADHD Rating Scale—IV: Checklists, Norms, and Clinical Interpretation.* New York: Guilford Press.

Dunn LM, Dunn LM (2001) *The Peabody Picture Vocabulary Test, 3rd edn.* Circle Pines, NM: American Guidance Services.

Dunn LM, Dunn LM, Whetton C, Burley J (1997) *The British Picture Vocabulary Scales, 2nd edn.* Windsor: NFER-Nelson.

Dykens EM, Hodapp RM, Leckman JF (1989) Adaptive and maladaptive functioning of institutionalized and noninstitutionalized fragile X males. *J Am Acad Child Adolesc Psychiatry* **28**: 427–430.

Einfeld SL, Tonge BJ (1996) Population prevalence of psychopathology in children and adolescents with intellectual disability: II. Epidemiological findings. *J Intellect Disabil Res* **40**: 99–109.

Einfeld SL, Tonge BJ (2002) *Manual for the Developmental Behaviour Checklist, 2nd edn.* Sidney: University of New South Wales and Monash University.

Emerson E (2003) Prevalence of psychiatric disorders in children and adolescents with and without intellectual disabilities. *J Intellect Disabil Res* **47**: 51–58.

Fee VE, Matson JL, Benavidez DA (1994) Attention deficit–hyperactivity disorder among mentally retarded children. *Res Dev Disabil* **15**: 67–79.

Filley CM, Cranberg LD, Alexander MP, Hart EJ (1987) Neurobehavioral outcome after closed head injury in childhood and adolescence. *Arch Neurol* **44**: 194–198.

Fisher SE, Francks C, McCracken JT, McGough JJ, Marlow AJ, MacPhie IL, Newbury DF, Crawford LR, Palmer CG, Woodward JA, Del'Homme M, Cantwell DP, Nelson SF, Monaco AP, Smalley SL (2002) A genomewide scan for loci involved in attention-deficit/hyperactivity disorder. *Am J Hum Genet* **70**: 1183–1196.

Fisher SE, Marlow AJ, Lamb J, Maestrini E, Williams DF, Richardson AJ, Weeks DE, Stein JF, Monaco AP (1999) A quantitative-trait locus on chromosome 6p influences different aspects of developmental dyslexia. *Am J Hum Genet* **64**: 146–156.

Fombonne E (1999) The epidemiology of autism: a review. *Psychol Med* **29**: 1–18.

Gadow K, Sverd J, Sprafkin J, Nolan E, Grossman S (1999) Long-term methylphenidate therapy in children with comorbid attention-deficit hyperactivity disorder and chronic multiple tic disorder. *Arch Gen Psychiatry* **56**: 330–336.

Gillberg C, Wing L (1999) Autism: not an extremely rare disorder. *Acta Psychiatr Scand* **99**: 399–406.

Gillberg C, Persson M, Grufman M, Themner U (1986) Psychiatric disorders in mildly and severely mentally retarded urban children and adolescents: epidemiological aspects. *Br J Psychiatry* **149**: 68–74.

Goodman R (1997) The Strengths and Difficulties Questionnaire: A research note. *J Child Psychol Psychiatry* **38**: 581–586.

Goodman R, Ford T, Richards H, Gatward R, Meltzer H (2000) The Development and Well-Being Assessment: description and initial validation of an integrated assessment of child and adolescent psychopathology. *J Child Psychol Psychiatry* **41**: 645–655.

Grigorenko EL, Wood FB, Meyer MS, Hart LA, Speed WC, Shuster A, Pauls DL (1997) Susceptibility loci for distinct components of developmental dyslexia on chromosomes 6 and 15. *Am J Hum Genet* **60**: 27–39.

Grigorenko EL, Wood FB, Meyer MS, Pauls DL (2000) Chromosome 6p influences on different dyslexia-related cognitive processes: further confirmation. *Am J Hum Genet* **66**: 715–723.

Gross-Tsur V, Manor O, Van Der Meere J, Joseph A, Shalev RS (1997) Epilepsy and attention deficit hyperactivity disorder: is methylphenidate safe and effective? *J Pediatr* **130**: 670–674.

Gucuyener K, Erdemoglu AK, Senol S, Serdaroglu A, Soysal S, Kockar AI (2003) Use of methylphenidate for attention-deficit hyperactivity disorder in patients with epilepsy or electroencephalographic abnormalities. *J Child Neurol* **18**: 109–112.

Handen BL, Breaux AM, Janosky J, McAuliffe S, Feldman H, Gosling A (1992) Effects and noneffects of methylphenidate in children with mental retardation and ADHD. *J Am Acad Child Adolesc Psychiatry* **31**: 455–461.

Handen B, Janosky J, McAuliffe S, Breaux AM, Feldman H (1994) Prediction of response to methylphenidate among children with ADHD and mental retardation. *J Child Adolesc Psychiatry* **33**: 1185–1193.

224

Handen BL, Janosky J, McAuliffe S (1997) Long-term follow-up of children with mental retardation/borderline intellectual functioning and ADHD. *J Abnorm Child Psychol* 25: 287–295.

Hardan A, Sahl R (1997) Psychopathology in children and adolescents with developmental disorders. *Res Dev Disabil* 18: 369–382.

Hessl D, Dyer-Friedman J, Glaser B, Wisbeck J, Barajas RG, Taylor A, Reiss AL (2001) The influence of environmental and genetic factors on behavior problems and autistic symptoms in boys and girls with fragile X syndrome. *Pediatrics* 108: E88.

Hille ET, den Ouden AL, Saigal S, Wolke D, Lambert M, Whitaker A, Pinto-Martin JA, Hoult L, Meyer R, Feldman JF, Verloove-Vanhorick SP, Paneth N (2001) Behavioural problems in children who weigh 1000 g or less at birth in four countries. *Lancet* 357: 1641–1643.

Holmes J, Hever T, Hewitt L, Ball C, Taylor E, Rubia K, Thapar A (2002) A pilot twin study of psychological measures of attention deficit hyperactivity disorder. *Behav Genet* 32: 389–395.

International Molecular Genetic Study of Autism Consortium (2001) A genomewide screen for autism: Strong evidence for linkage to chromosome 2q, 7q and 16p. *Am J Hum Genet* 69: 570–581.

Johnson CR, Handen BL, Lubetsky MJ, Sacco KA (1994) Efficacy of methylphenidate and behavioral intervention on classroom behavior in children with ADHD and mental retardation. *Behav Modif* 18: 470–487.

Krakow JB, Kopp CB (1983) The effects of developmental delay on sustained attention in young children. *Child Dev* 54: 1143–1155.

Kuntsi J, Eley TC, Taylor A, Hughes C, Asherson P, Caspi A, Moffitt TE (2004) Co-occurrence of ADHD and low IQ has genetic origins. *Am J Med Genet B Neuropsychiatr Genet* 124: 41–47.

Laing E, Hulme C, Grant J, Karmiloff-Smith A (2001) Learning to read in Williams syndrome: looking beneath the surface of atypical reading development. *J Child Psychol Psychiatry* 42: 729–739.

Liu J, Nyholt DR, Magnussen P, Parano E, Pavone P, Geschwind D, Lord C, Iversen P, Hoh J, Ott J, Gilliam TC; Autism Genetic Resource Exchange Consortium (2001) A genomewide screen for autism susceptibility loci. *Am J Hum Genet* 69: 327–340.

Loo SK, Fisher SE, Francks C, Ogdie MN, MacPhie IL, Yang M, McCracken JT, McGough JJ, Nelson SF, Monaco AP, Smalley SL (2004) Genome-wide scan of reading ability in affected sibling pairs with attention-deficit/hyperactivity disorder: unique and shared genetic effects. *Mol Psychiatry* 9: 485–493.

Loveland KA (1987) Behavior of young children with Down syndrome before the mirror: Exploration. *Child Dev* 58: 768–778.

Mackie R, Mackay CK (1982) Attention vs. retention in discrimination learning of low-MA retarded adults and MA-matched nonretarded children. *Am J Ment Defic* 86: 543–547.

Matson JL, Rush KS, Hamilton M, Anderson SJ, Bamburg JW, Baglio CS, Williams D, Kirkpatrick-Sanchez S (1999) Characteristics of depression as assessed by the Diagnostic Assessment for the Severely Handicapped—II (DASH-II). *Res Dev Disabil* 20: 305–313.

Max JE, Arndt S, Castillo CS, Bokura H, Robin DA, Lindgren SD, Smith WL, Sato Y, Mattheis PJ (1998) Attention-deficit hyperactivity symptomatology after traumatic brain injury: a prospective study. *J Am Acad Child Adolesc Psychiatry* 37: 841–847.

Meins W (1995) Symptoms of major depression in mentally retarded adults. *J Intellect Disabil Res* 39: 41–45.

Melnyk L, Das J (1992) Measurement of attention deficit: Correspondence between rating scales and tests of sustained and selective attention. *Am J Ment Retard* 96: 599–606.

Mervis CA, Decoufle P, Murphy CC, Yeargin Allsopp M (1995) Low birthweight and the risk for mental retardation later in childhood. *Paediatr Perinat Epidemiol* 9: 455–468.

MTA (1999) A 14-month randomized clinical trial of treatment strategies for attention-deficit hyperactivity disorder. The MTA Cooperative Group. Multimodal Treatment Study of Children with ADHD. *Arch Gen Psychiatry* 56: 1073–1086.

Mullen EM (1997) *Mullen Scales of Early Learning*. Los Angeles: Western Psychological Services.

O'Connor TG, Rutter M, Beckett C, Keaveney L, Kreppner JM (2000) The effects of global severe privation on cognitive competence: extension and longitudinal follow-up. English and Romanian Adoptees Study Team. *Child Dev* 71: 376–390.

Ogdie MN, Macphie IL, Minassian SL, Yang M, Fisher SE, Francks C, Cantor RM, McCracken JT, McGough JJ, Nelson SF, Monaco AP, Smalley SL (2003) A genomewide scan for attention-deficit/hyperactivity disorder in an extended sample: suggestive linkage on 17p11. *Am J Hum Genet* 72: 1268–1279.

Owens EB, Hinshaw SP, Kraemer HC, Arnold LE, Abikoff HB, Cantwell DP, Conners CK, Elliott G, Greenhill LL, Hechtman L, Hoza B, Jensen PS, March JS, Newcorn JH, Pelham WE, Severe JB, Swanson JM, Vitiello

B, Wells KC, Wigal T (2003) Which treatment for whom for ADHD? Moderators of treatment response in the MTA. *J Consult Clin Psychol* **71**: 540–552.

Pearson DA, Pumariega AJ, Seilheimer DK (1991) The development of psychiatric symptomatology in patients with cystic fibrosis. *J Am Acad Child Adolesc Psychiatry* **30**: 290–297.

Pearson DA, Yaffee LS, Loveland KA, Lewis KR (1996) Comparison of sustained and selective attention in children who have mental retardation with and without attention deficit hyperactivity disorder. *Am J Ment Retard* **100**: 592–602.

Pearson DA, Norton AM, Farwell EC (1997) Attention-deficit/hyperactivity disorder in mental retardation: Nature of attention deficits. In: Burack JA, Enns JT, eds. *Attention, Development, and Psychopathology.* New York: Guilford Press, pp. 205–221.

Pearson DA, Santos CW, Roache JD, Casat CD, Loveland KA, Lachar D, Lane DM, Faria LP, Cleveland LA (2003) Treatment effects of methylphenidate on behavioral adjustment in children with mental retardation and ADHD. *J Am Acad Child Adolesc Psychiatry* **42**: 209–216.

Pennington BF, Moon J, Edgin J, Stedron J, Nadel L (2003) The neuropsychology of Down syndrome: evidence for hippocampal dysfunction. *Child Dev* **74**: 75–93.

Philippe A, Martinez M, Guilloud-Bataille M, Gillberg C, Rastam M, Sponheim E, Coleman M, Zappella M, Aschauer H, Van Maldergem L, Penet C, Feingold J, Brice A, Leboyer M (1999) Genome-wide scan for autism susceptibility genes. Paris Autism Research International Sibpair Study. *Hum Mol Genet* **8**: 805–812.

Pliszka SR, Greenhill LL, Crismon ML, Sedillo A, Carlson C, Conners CK, McCracken JT, Swanson JM, Hughes CW, Llana ME, Lopez M, Toprac MG (2000a) The Texas Children's Medication Algorithm Project: Report of the Texas Consensus Conference Panel on Medication Treatment of Childhood Attention-Deficit/Hyperactivity Disorder. Part I. Attention-Deficit/Hyperactivity Disorder. *J Am Acad Child Adolesc Psychiatry* **39**: 908–919.

Pliszka SR, Greenhill LL, Crismon ML, Sedillo A, Carlson C, Conners CK, McCracken JT, Swanson JM, Hughes CW, Llana ME, Lopez M, Toprac MG (2000b) The Texas Children's Medication Algorithm Project: Report of the Texas Consensus Conference Panel on Medication Treatment of Childhood Attention-Deficit/Hyperactivity Disorder. Part II: Tactics. *Am Acad Child Adolesc Psychiatry* **39**: 920–927.

Raab GM, Fulton M, Laxen DPH, Thomson GOB (1985) The Edinburgh Lead Study: aspects of design and progress. *Statistician* **34**: 45–57.

Raven JC (1998) *Raven's Progressive Matrices.* Windsor: NFER-Nelson.

Reiss S, Szyszko J (1983) Diagnostic overshadowing and professional experience with mentally retarded persons. *Am J Ment Defic* **87**: 396–402.

Risch N, Spiker D, Lotspeich L, Nouri N, Hinds D, Hallmayer J, Kalaydjieva L, McCague P, Dimiceli S, Pitts T, Nguyen L, Yang J, Harper C, Thorpe D, Vermeer S, Young H, Hebert J, Lin A, Ferguson J, Chiotti C, Wiese-Slater S, Rogers T, Salmon B, Nicholas P, Petersen PB, Pingree C, McMahon W, Wong DL, Cavalli-Sforza LL, Kraemer HC, Myers RM (1999) A genomic screen of autism: evidence for a multi-locus etiology. *Am J Hum Genet* **65**: 493–507.

Rotundo N, Johnson EG (1981) Verbal control of motor behaviour in mentally retarded children: A re-examination of Luria's theory. *J Ment Defic Res* **25**: 281–290.

Royal College of Psychiatrists (2001) *Diagnostic Criteria for Psychiatric Disorders for Use with Adults with Learning Disabilities and Mental Retardation.* London: Gaskell.

Rutter M, Andersen-Wood L, Beckett C, Bredenkamp D, Castle J, Groothues C, Kreppner J, Keaveney L, Lord C, O'Connor TG (1999) Quasi-autistic patterns following severe early global privation. English and Romanian Adoptees (ERA) Study Team. *J Child Psychol Psychiatry* **40**: 537–549.

Sen A, Clarke AM (1988) The effects of distraction during and after learning a serial recall task. *Am J Ment Defic* **73**: 46–49.

Shao Y, Wolpert CM, Raiford KL, Menold MM, Donnelly SL, Ravan SA, Bass MP, McClain C, von Wendt L, Vance JM, Abramson RH, Wright HH, Ashley-Koch A, Gilbert JR, DeLong RG, Cuccaro ML, Pericak-Vance MA (2002) Genomic screen and follow-up analysis for autistic disorder. *Am J Med Genet* **114**: 99–105.

Simonoff E, Pickles A, Hervas A, Rutter M, Silberg JL, Eaves LJ (1998) Genetic influences on childhood hyperactivity: Contrast effects imply parental rating bias, not sibling interaction. *Psychol Med* **28**: 825–837.

Sparrow S, Balla D, Cichetti D (1984) *Vineland Adaptive Behavior Scales.* Circle Pines, MN: American Guidance Services.

Stevenson J, Pennington BF, Gilger JW, DeFries JC, Gillis JJ (1993) Hyperactivity and spelling disability: testing for a shared genetic aetiology. *J Child Psychol Psychiatry* **34**: 1137–1152.

226

Stromme P, Diseth TH (2000) Prevalence of psychiatric diagnoses in children with mental retardation: data from a population-based study. *Dev Med Child Neurol* **42**: 266–270.

Taylor E, Schachar R, Thorley G, Wiselberg M (1986) Conduct disorder and hyperactivity: I. Separation of hyperactivity and antisocial conduct in British child psychiatric patients. *Br J Psychiatry* **149**: 760–777.

Taylor E, Sandberg S, Thorley G, Giles S (1991) *The Epidemiology of Childhood Hyperactivity*. Oxford: Oxford University Press.

Thapar A, Holmes J, Poulton K, Harrington R (1999) Genetic basis of attention deficit and hyperactivity. *Br J Psychiatry* **174**: 105–111.

Thomson GO, Raab GM, Hepburn WS, Hunter R, Fulton M, Laxen DP (1989) Blood-lead levels and children's behaviour—results from the Edinburgh Lead Study. *J Child Psychol Psychiatry* **30**: 515–528.

Tomporowski PD (1990) Sustained attention in mentally retarded persons. In: Fraser WI, ed. *Key Issues in Mental Retardation Research*. New York: Routledge, pp. 249–306.

Turgay A, Binder C, Snyder R, Fisman S (2002) Long-term safety and efficacy of risperidone for the treatment of disruptive behavior disorders in children with subaverage IQs. *Pediatrics* **110**: e34.

Turnure J, Zigler E (1964) Outer-directedness in the problem solving of normal and retarded children. *J Abnor Soc Psychol* **69**: 427–436.

Van Bellinghen M, De Troch C (2001) Risperidone in the treatment of behavioral disturbances in children and adolescents with borderline intellectual functioning: a double-blind, placebo-controlled pilot trial. *J Child Adolesc Psychopharmacol* **11**: 5–13.

WHO (1992) *International Statistical Classification of Diseases and Related Health Problems, 10th edn (ICD-10)*. Geneva: World Health Organization.

14
THE CLINICAL ASSESSMENT AND TREATMENT OF ADHD IN ADULTS

Philip J Asherson and JJ Sandra Kooij

Most child and adolescent mental health services recognize the existence of, and need for treatment in ADHD. Many specialist multidisciplinary ADHD clinics have been developed in recent years, and many paediatricians have included the treatment of ADHD as an important part of their clinical activity. A good deal of the justification for this increase in therapeutic activity has been the demonstration that ADHD is indeed a predictor of adult mental health problems. General adult psychiatry, however, has not followed suit in identifying and treating substantial numbers of affected people. It is likely nonetheless that an increasing load in adult psychiatry will develop. An increasing number of young people will come into adult life while still receiving stimulant medication or other treatment for ADHD, and adult psychiatrists are likely to be consulted. An increasing number of adults are likely to recognize themselves as having been disabled by ADHD and therefore seek assistance. In many cases, individuals with adult ADHD who require specific treatment for the condition will have been treated unsuccessfully for disorders with overlapping symptom profiles such as anxiety, depression, bipolar disorder or antisocial personality disorder. Courts increasingly wish to know whether adults who appear to have ADHD will benefit from treatment for misdemeanours that are either the result of impulsiveness (e.g. hitting out, getting into fights) or inattentiveness leading to neglect (e.g. inadequate child care, car accidents).

Review of prospective follow-up studies suggests that childhood ADHD often persists into adult life, not always as a categorical diagnosis, but often as a contribution to poor social adjustment and personality problems. Clinical correlates reported with adult ADHD include impairments on tests of attention and impulsiveness, and high levels of comorbidity with concurrent depressive disorder, anxiety disorder, antisocial personality disorder and alcohol and drug use disorders (Biederman et al. 1993; Mannuzza et al. 1993; Taylor et al. 1996; Kooij et al. 2001a, 2004). Many investigators interpret the pattern of behaviours associated with ADHD as a heightened need for stimulation and reinforcement, which may therefore be related to novelty seeking or sensation seeking tendencies (Downey et al. 1997).

The ADHD criteria were not written with adults in mind, so it is likely that some adults, who do not meet current operational criteria for the diagnostic category, will be impaired by ADHD-related symptoms. Importantly, double-blind placebo-control trials inform us that the same stimulant drugs effective in children are also an effective means of reducing ADHD symptoms in adulthood (Wender et al. 1985, Wilens et al. 1995, Kooij et al. 2004,

Spencer et al. 2005). The missing piece of hard evidence is whether the reduction of symptoms in this way also promotes better social adjustment. Clinical experience, however, shows improvement in relationships, social functioning, adjustment to working conditions, abstinence from drugs and alcohol, and better driving performance. Drug treatment for ADHD should therefore be a part of the therapeutic resources available within general adult psychiatry.

Awareness of the condition can lead to fruitful clinical interventions. Training of general psychiatrists in the clinical evaluation and management of ADHD is therefore a high priority. Although it has been suggested that ADHD is a self-limiting condition that rarely requires treatment in adult life, there is no good evidence for this assertion. Longitudinal studies that have followed children with a diagnosis of ADHD into young adulthood find that around two-thirds have persistent symptoms of ADHD associated with significant clinical impairments (Faraone et al. 2006). Epidemiological studies suggest a prevalence between 2% and 5% for ADHD in adults (Weiss et al. 1985, Murphy and Barkley 1996c, Kessler et al. 2005a, Kooij et al. 2005). Furthermore, child and adolescent psychiatrists see many patients with ADHD who have continued difficulties as they grow older and are aware of the need for continued treatment during the transition from child to adult services. They are also aware of the high level of clinically significant ADHD symptoms among many parents of their child patients (Murphy and Barkley 1996b); data on familial risks suggest a rate of ADHD among parents of ADHD probands of around 20% (Faraone et al. 2000).

Experience of psychiatrists working with adult ADHD is consistent with this view. At the inaugural meeting of the European Network for Adult ADHD in September 2003, which 28 clinicians from 12 European countries attended, it was striking that a common perspective on the best way to diagnose and treat adult ADHD was held by group members (see also: www.adult-adhd.net). The impression was that direct clinical experience across diverse European countries was very similar, suggesting that adult ADHD is a robust and stable concept with clear clinical implications. Nevertheless, little systematic research has been carried out on the long-term consequences and response to treatment in this group of patients.

Definition of ADHD in adults

There are no separate criteria for ADHD in adults. The DSM-IV criteria defined by the American Psychiatric Association (APA 1994) are the most widely used and include the three subtypes of ADHD: inattentive, hyperactive/impulsive, and combined. Many clinicians consider that inattention is the key feature of ADHD, and is it notable that most children who receive an ADHD diagnosis in UK clinics have either the combined type (CT) or inattentive (I) subtypes, but rarely the hyperactive/impulsive (H/I) subtype. This is in keeping with experience from adult ADHD clinics, but contrasts with non-clinical adult populations where surveys find a high rate of the H/I subtype (Kessler et al. 2005a, Kooij et al. 2005). The reasons for this difference between clinical and epidemiological samples are not well understood but suggest that adults with the H/I subtype may be less impaired. More research is required into the development of ADHD across the lifespan.

The World Health Organization (ICD-10) criteria for hyperkinetic disorder (WHO 1992) define a subgroup of the DSM-IV category of ADHD and represent a more restricted application of the diagnostic criteria. Most clinicians, however, prefer to follow the broader DSM-IV guidelines as this fits better with clinical practice and current research. All groups attending the European Network for Adult ADHD use the DSM-IV definition. Under both sets of criteria, there are no special definitions for ADHD in adults. The same set of 18 core symptoms and behaviours are listed under both DSM-IV and ICD-10, 9 symptoms describing inattentive behaviours and 9 describing hyperactive and impulsive behaviours. Current DSM-IV criteria use the same fixed threshold for the number of symptoms required to make the diagnosis in both children and adults, namely 6 out of the 9 inattentive behaviours for the I subtype, 6 out of the 9 hyperactive/impulsive behaviours for the H/I subtype, or both for the CT diagnosis. According to DSM-IV definitions of ADHD the diagnosis can be 'in partial remission' in adolescents and adults who no longer meet the full criteria. It is important to recognize that many adults who fulfilled operational criteria for ADHD as children no longer have a sufficient number of current ADHD symptoms to reach full current criteria for ADHD, even though persistence of some symptoms continues to cause substantial clinical impairments. The strict usage of the diagnostic criteria will therefore lead to under-representation of the problem. Epidemiological data support the validity of applying a lower threshold in adults (e.g. 4 or 5 out of 9 criteria), as this lower threshold correlates significantly with impairment (Buitelaar 2002, Kooij et al. 2005). The DSM-IV description "in partial remission" does not seem to do justice to the significant impairments seen in adults no longer meeting the full DSM criteria but still suffering from the effects of ongoing ADHD symptoms in adult life; adults seem to outgrow the (child) criteria rather than the disorder. One solution is to use the same thresholds for retrospective diagnosis of ADHD in childhood, but developmentally referenced (lower) thresholds in adults.

A related issue is the formulation of ADHD symptoms in the DSM-IV. The DSM-IV criteria were designed to be evaluated following parent and teacher reports, as opposed to the more common use of self-report in adults. The emphasis has been less on psychopathology than on descriptions of observed behaviours. As a consequence the descriptions in DSM-IV are not always easy to apply to adults. In adults, attention problems tend to be particularly disabling as organizational demands increase, impulsivity changes quality and has very different consequences, and the aimless hyperactivity of childhood may become more purposeful (e.g. sporting activities, work that allows for restless behaviour) or may present as feelings of inner restlessness. Adults are also more able to adapt and compensate for problems with attention, hyperactivity and impulsivity. Clinical and research experience supports the idea that definitions of ADHD should be adapted for different developmental stages and for self-report.

Comorbidity and differential diagnosis
ADHD is frequently accompanied by comorbid disorders, especially anxiety, mood, substance use and personality disorders. Comorbidity is the rule in clinical series, with up to 75% having at least one other comorbid disorder, and 33% having two or more other disorders (Biederman et al. 1993; Murphy and Barkley 1996a; Kooij et al. 2001a, 2004). However, as indicated above, it is important to distinguish between comorbid disorders and symptoms related to ADHD that overlap with other common psychiatric disorders. For this

reason, assessment of adult ADHD needs to be thorough. Differential diagnostic considerations are an important part of the diagnostic process, and have consequences for treatment as well as the order of treatment. More information about differential diagnosis and comorbidity can be found below.

Age of onset

The DSM-IV age of onset criterion ("some symptoms should be met before the age of 7 years") may sometimes be difficult to evaluate retrospectively. Nevertheless, establishing the early age of onset of some symptoms is critical to establishing the diagnosis, and sufficient retrospective data should be gathered to be confident about early childhood onset.

The current age criterion, however, may be too restricted for clinical practice since some symptoms that begin before the age of 7 years do not give rise to significant impairments until much later. This is especially true for inattention, which may go unnoticed in early childhood but becomes more evident during the increasing demands of secondary school education and early adolescence. Another consideration is that individuals providing a self-report of their own childhood behaviours are rarely able to give an accurate account before the age of 10–12 years. Moreover, follow-up studies among children with age of onset before and after the age of 7 years showed no differences in severity of symptoms, treatment outcome or prognosis (Applegate et al. 1997, Barkley and Biederman 1997). For these reasons it has been suggested that a broader criterion of symptoms being met before the age of 12 years be used when the diagnosis is being evaluated for the first time in adulthood, especially where other characteristic features of the disorder are present.

Gender issues and differences in ADHD subtypes

Special attention should be paid to the diagnosis in women. As males have dominated child clinic samples of ADHD, female manifestations and sex differences have been relatively neglected in the clinical and research literature. Studies of the level of ADHD symptoms in general population samples find that girls as a group have less ADHD symptoms than boys, when evaluated using ADHD rating scales. However, it is also likely that girls are less frequently referred since they are less likely to have comorbid oppositional and conduct disorder problems and a bit more likely to have inattentive rather than more overt hyper-active/impulsive symptoms; however, just as in boys the majority of girls have the combined subtype. A third reason might be that the disorder in girls is less well known among general practitioners, leading to a negative referral bias. As a consequence, in adulthood women with ADHD are under-identified and therefore less likely to receive treatment. It is important to note that the higher prevalence of anxiety and depressive disorders in women can conceal underlying ADHD and influence diagnosis and treatment.

Women presenting for evaluation of ADHD for the first time in adulthood are more likely to be in the over-30 age-group, whereas men most often present in their twenties. In contrast to studies of ADHD in children, both clinical and epidemiological studies find that the male–female ratio for adult ADHD is approximately equal (Murphy and Barkley 1996a, Pineda et al. 1999, Rowland et al. 2002, Kooij et al. 2005). The male preponderance seen in child ADHD clinics is no longer seen, with almost as many females as males seeking help for adult ADHD. The reasons for this change in gender distribution are not well understood and deserver further investigation.

The assessment process

Diagnosis should be based on a careful and systematic assessment of the developmental psychiatric history, not just on the current mental state examination and adult psychiatric history. The lifetime history of ADHD symptoms and behaviours is chronic and persistent from early childhood, in contrast with many other psychiatric conditions diagnosed in adults, which generally have a later onset and a more episodic course. The specific symptoms of ADHD when recognized for the first time in an adult will therefore appear to be behavioural traits, rather than symptoms, in the sense that there is no change from a premorbid state. For example, affective disorders such as anxiety, depression and manic depression are all viewed as a definite change in the mental state from the premorbid state, but clearly this is not the case for a disorder that starts in early childhood. For this reason it is easy to see that in some cases ADHD will be mistaken for a personality disorder, particularly if there are associated emotional and behavioural problems.

A major issue faced by clinicians is to decide at what level of severity the behaviours and symptoms of ADHD become significant. This is an area that requires more research to be precise and at this time no specific guidelines exist for calling each of the 18 items, especially in the adult age group. In the absence of precise definitions for each symptom, the principle that needs to be adopted is that each should be maladaptive and inconsistent with developmental age. Some of the symptoms should be pervasive, occurring in two or more settings (typically home, work/college, social situations) and be associated with significant impairments in social, academic or occupational function. ADHD symptoms should not be better explained by another disorder, and this can be evaluated by establishing whether they occur exclusively during the course of conditions such as mood disorders, anxiety disorders, schizophrenia and personality disorders.

As described above, establishing the early age of onset is key to the evaluation. It is therefore essential to evaluate a lifetime history of impairment related to the presence of ADHD symptoms in at least two situations such as school, work, home or interpersonal contacts. Although they are neither necessary nor sufficient for diagnosis, associated features like mood lability and temper outburst need to be evaluated, and comorbid psychiatric conditions identified. To get a complete overview of lifetime medical history it is important to enquire about psychiatric symptoms occurring throughout the lifespan and previous treatments for psychiatric and medical conditions.

Establishing an accurate record of early adult and childhood symptoms using retrospective accounts remains controversial, although the task of collecting accurate accounts of past behaviour is in fact central to understanding many psychiatric disorders. This is therefore a process with which all general adult psychiatrists should be familiar. Self-reports for current and retrospective symptoms generally show moderate correlations with observer reports. Judgements will have to be formed on the reliability of the account and whether the patient has good insight into the symptoms and behaviours at each time-point. Diagnosis based on the single use of self-report is not impossible, but clearly provides less certainty than using the combination of self-report and observer reports.

The importance of using information from multiple informants is underscored by follow-up data in adolescents with ADHD. It has been shown that higher persistence rates of ADHD are recorded using parent reports than using self-report, with parent reports being more strongly associated with clinical impairments (Barkley 1997). This reflects a substantial risk of under-diagnosis, rather than the more commonly assumed problem of over-diagnosis, using self-report alone. On the other hand, epidemiological studies have shown that lower levels of the core symptoms of ADHD are often recognized in the absence of significant impairment, suggesting that in a proportion of cases self-report may lead to over-diagnosis. Despite these concerns over the accuracy of self-report for ADHD symptoms, the usual clinical experience is similar to that for other non-psychotic psychiatric conditions; in many cases both the individual with ADHD and the informant agree on the major items. Sometimes it may be difficult for parents or siblings to acknowledge the level of symptoms in the patient, especially when ADHD symptoms run in the family. However, as with psychiatric assessments of other common conditions, informant report is helpful to corroborate the account, provide more detailed objective observations of behaviour, and find out more about the impact of the behaviours on interactions with close relatives, friends and work colleagues.

For the observer reports, partner/spouses seem the most appropriate persons to report on current symptoms, and parents (if available) or other family members for the retrospective recall of childhood symptoms. As short assessments seem to increase the risk for both under- and over-diagnosis, it is important that sufficient care is taken in the assessment of a lifetime history of symptoms and impairment. The use of information from multiple informants usually requires a more extended psychiatric assessment of around 2–3 hours.

Clinical features

DSM-IV Items

Central to the assessment is evaluation of each of the 18 core symptoms of ADHD. These are listed in Appendix 14.1, with descriptions of how each of the symptoms may present in adulthood. As described above it is important to confirm the presence of sufficient symptoms in childhood (6 out of 9 items for each symptom domain) and persistence of some or all of the symptoms causing continued impairment into adult life. For current ratings, 4 or 5 out of 9 may be considered sufficient, although individuals not meeting the full DSM-IV criteria as adults are usually described as being in 'partial remission'. However, this is a semantic argument and does not reflect the main aim of the clinical assessment, which is to identify whether ADHD symptoms causing significant functional impairments have persisted into adulthood and therefore require treatment.

Mood Symptoms

In addition to the DSM-IV symptom checklist, there are other important symptoms that commonly occur in adults with ADHD. Problems with mood lability, emotional over-reactivity and temper outburst are seen in up to 90% of patients (Kooij et al. 2001a) and in some cases are the main presenting complaint. These often appear to be part of the ADHD syndrome when they have an early age of onset, occur across the lifespan in association with the main ADHD symptoms, and do not fluctuate (are non-episodic). Clinical experience shows that these symptoms often respond to stimulant medication in the same time-course as the main ADHD symptoms, and should therefore be regarded as part of the ADHD condition and not always as a separate mood disorder. Careful evaluation will need to be made of any affective symptoms that occur, to differentiate these from more typical onset of anxiety or mood disorders (see below).

THOUGHT PROCESSES

A common account from individuals with ADHD is of having a "distractible mind" or a mind that is "in a fog". Individuals report the experience of ceaseless mental activity and thoughts that are constantly on the go, or that their mind is constantly full of thoughts. Thoughts are often described as uncontrolled in the sense that multiple thoughts occur at the same time, one overlapping the other and distracting each other. Thoughts are sometimes described as flitting from one thing to another or jumping around between topics. When extreme, such thought processes may be confused with the speeding of thoughts and flight of ideas observed in bipolar disorder. However, individuals with ADHD do not describe their thoughts as clear or focused, they do not have typical flight of ideas, and the thought content is not grandiose. They do not perceive their thoughts as running faster than usual, rather that they are uncontrolled, constant and unfocused. As with the other features of ADHD such descriptions of thought processes are not periodic but begin early in life and are persistent and non-fluctuating. They are often described as exhausting, not allowing the individual to relax or have a quiet mind and may give rise to initial insomnia. Another feature of this symptom is the sensitivity to stimulant medication since this is often one of the first symptoms to respond to the immediate effects.

Ceaseless or uncontrolled mental activity may also mimic anxious worrying or rarely obsessional thoughts. Individuals with ADHD often have a number of difficulties in their day-to-day life such as problems at work or in their social contacts, and these concerns often form the content of their thoughts. The combination of realistic worries, low self-esteem and ceaseless thought process can appear remarkably similar to more common anxiety states. The main differences are the age of onset, the persistence over time, the lack of association to particular triggers, the absence of somatic symptoms of anxiety, and immediate response to stimulant medication.

Diagnostic instruments

There are several screening instruments and diagnostic interviews available to use during the assessment process. The most widely used screening instruments for current symptoms are based on the DSM-IV criteria and include the Barkley adult ADHD rating scale (Barkley and Murphy 1998) and the Conners Adult ADHD rating scale (Conners et al. 1998). The ADHD rating scale consists of the 18 DSM-IV criteria for self-report use and is often used for screening as well as treatment response (Spencer et al. 1995; DuPaul et al. 1998; Kooij et al. 2004, 2005). A recent development by Kessler and colleagues (2005b) in conjunction with the World Health Organization is the Adult ADHD Self-Report Scale (ASRS-v1.1) that reworded the 18-item checklist for ADHD to make the questions more appropriate for adults. A subset of 6 items from the ASRS was subsequently found to be sensitive to the diagnosis and can be used as an initial short set of screening items. The Brown ADD Scale (BADDS) is frequently used in US clinics and consists of a broader range of inattention symptoms and organizational difficulties, including several items related to emotional regulation (Brown 1996). The BADDS does not investigate hyperactive/impulsive behaviour, which limits its use for evaluation of H/I and combined subtypes. For the retrospective diagnosis of ADHD in childhood a commonly used screening instrument is the Wender–Utah Rating Scale (WURS; Ward et al. 1993), although the Barkley and Conner scales also include checklists that are used retrospectively to obtain information on childhood symptoms. These and other rating scales can be found online at http://www.neurotransmitter.net/adhdscales.html.

To guide the assessment process diagnostic interviews are available that systematically enquire about the major symptoms and related behaviours, comorbid syndromes and clinical outcome. These include the BADDS Diagnostic Form (Brown 1996), the Conners Adult ADHD Diagnostic Interview for DSM-IV (Epstein et al. 1999), the structured Diagnostic Interview Schedule DIS-L (part of the DIS-IV) (Robins et al. 1981) and the Dutch semi-structured interview for adult ADHD (SGIK) (Kooij 2002).

As for most other psychiatric disorders, there are no direct biological tests with sufficient sensitivity and specificity. Structural imaging, functional imaging and direct measurement of striatal dopamine transporter density using SPECT (single photon emission computed tomography) have all shown group differences between ADHD probands and controls. The most commonly used neuropsychological tests likewise show deficits at the group level. On an individual level, patients may be sufficiently aroused by the novelty of the setting to perform well, but many individuals will show deficits on tests of attention, executive function, timing tasks and response inhibition. The observation that individuals with ADHD perform better when sufficiently rewarded or stimulated by a task is reflected in the common complaint that "I get bored far more quickly than other people". An extensive research literature demonstrates that individuals with ADHD do not generally have core deficits of attention or response inhibition (in the sense that individuals have different IQ levels), but rather show variability of responses more characteristic of altered regulatory control of cognitive processes. High stimulus rates and tasks performed under rewarding conditions are associated with improvements in performance to the extent that differences between cases and normal controls may disappear entirely during the test situation. For that reason, neurocognitive testing still plays no major role in the diagnostic assessment of adult ADHD.

Treatment
IMPACT OF DIAGNOSIS AND TREATMENT
As ADHD is a developmental disorder persisting across the lifespan, the impact of the disorder on adults can be considerable. Many adults with ADHD report a life full of problems and frustrations that stemmed directly from attention deficits, impulsive and overactive behaviour and mood lability. Others often perceive behaviours related to ADHD as the result of being *lazy*, *stupid*, or just *difficult*. Individuals with ADHD often say they have always known that they were different from other people their own age, but never knew what was

wrong. As a result, the diagnosis of ADHD is often received with considerable relief since it provides an explanation for lifetime problems and the potential for effective treatment where significant symptoms persist. This initial relief is sometimes followed by feelings of anger; "Why didn't I receive this diagnosis earlier on?", "I could have finished my education", or "Maybe my relationship/marriage wouldn't have failed". Diagnosis alone often has a great impact, as finally an overview and understanding of lifetime patterns of behavioral problems is achieved. Many individuals need time to accept the diagnosis and its consequences. Finally, if treatment is successful, new opportunities arise, and many patients need to learn new skills to cope with them.

ADHD symptoms can be treated effectively in adults as well as in children. Numerous studies have shown the beneficial effects of stimulant medication on the core symptoms of ADHD. The number of drug trials in adults is far less than that for childhood ADHD, but these consistently demonstrate similar response rates. Due to the demands and responsibilities of adult life and the ability of many adults to develop strategies to cope with ADHD symptoms, a range of targeted psychosocial and psychological treatments are likely to be beneficial; however, there have been few attempts to quantify the benefits of such interventions. Treatment offers hope of a better life by reducing the level of ADHD symptoms that give rise to psychosocial impairments and enabling individuals to overcome dysfunctional patterns of behaviour. Areas of improvement include:
• Levels of distress from ADHD symptoms
• Psychological functioning and self-confidence
• Family/relational functioning
• Interpersonal (broader than family) functioning
• Professional/academic functioning
• Driving performance
• Risk of alcohol and substance abuse (including smoking).

OPTIMAL TREATMENT ALGORITHM
Treatment always starts with careful diagnostic assessment of ADHD, accompanying symptoms and behaviours and comorbid disorders. Comorbidity is common, with most individuals with adult ADHD having one or more associated psychiatric disorders. However, care must be taken to differentiate associated symptoms of ADHD such as mood lability, irritability and low self-esteem from distinct (comorbid) psychiatric disorders. Differential diagnostic considerations are an important part of the diagnostic process and have consequences for treatment and the order of treatment. As for most other psychiatric conditions, treatment should take a multimodal approach including psycho-education, pharmacotherapy and psychotherapeutic interventions such as coaching, cognitive behavioural therapy and counselling.

PSYCHO-EDUCATION
Psycho-education should describe the major features of ADHD to patients and family, provide an understanding of how ADHD symptoms have affected their lives, and describe the most appropriate forms of treatment. Advice on the prevalence of ADHD (around

2–5%) and the increased risk to first-degree relatives (around 15–20%) should be discussed. It is useful to point out that ADHD represents the extreme of a set of characteristics that are distributed throughout the general population, and are quantitatively rather than qualitatively different from normality; thus other family members may be more likely to show some of the characteristics but will not necessarily show the same psychosocial impairments. Some discussion of the role of heritability, biological brain processes and environmental risk factors involved in ADHD may be helpful.

Ideally, psycho-education should be offered at the end of the diagnostic assessment to all persons involved: patients, their spouses/partners and other close family members. The reason for this extensive psycho-education is that after so many years of problems and disturbed relationships, every person involved should share the same information on diagnosis and treatment. Often this process offers new insights into the shared history of the patient and the difficulties across the years. Every family member gets the opportunity to ask questions and to get a better understanding of the causes of past and present difficulties. Relationship problems often decline after this sharing of information.

PHARMACOTHERAPY FOR ADULT ADHD

Stimulants (methylphenidate or dexamphetamine) are the first choice treatments for ADHD in both children and adults. The evidence base for the effectiveness and relative safety of these medications in children is considerable (Taylor et al. 2004), and there is now an increasing amount of data concerning efficacy in adults (Spencer et al. 1995, 2005; Conners et al. 2002; Kooij et al. 2004). Meta-analysis suggests that the short-term effectiveness of stimulants in adult life shows similar effect sizes to that seen in child and adolescent samples (Faraone et al. 2004), providing assurance for clinicians that the diagnosis and treatment of ADHD can be applied with validity in adulthood.

The effects of stimulants on the core ADHD symptoms are different from many other treatments in psychiatry being more similar to the immediate effects of anti-anxiety or sedative short-acting benzodiazepines. The therapeutic effects begin within 30 minutes of a starting dose and continue (depending on dose and individual pharmacokinetic profiles) for around 2–4 hours for methylphenidate and a little longer for dexamphetamine. It is therefore necessary to take a dose every 2–4 hours throughout the day to obtain a sustained effect. Nearly all patients benefit from the use of a timer to help remember to take the medication on time. Compliance problems are the main limitation to the effectiveness of methylphenidate in adult patients. To increase the ease of taking methylphenidate, improve compliance and smooth out the effects of short-acting medications, long-acting preparations are now marketed; these need to be taken only once per day. This is particularly useful for adults with ADHD who suffer from lifetime complaints such as forgetfulness and disorganization (Banaschewski et al. 2006).

The one area where different parameters may operate compared to the treatment of children, is dosage level. Titration to an effective dose is important (Faraone et al. 2004). Spencer et al. (2005) found that daily doses up to 1.0 mg/kg/day and a three times daily dose regime could be required to ensure adequate coverage for adults. The most common dose range used in European adult ADHD clinics for immediate-release methylphenidate is 10–20 mg taken 3–5 times daily, with both higher and lower dosing required in individual cases. The use of extended-release stimulants has been less extensively investigated in the adult ADHD population but the similar effect sizes for immediate-release methylphenidate suggest that the guidelines for their use in older children and adolescents should be followed for adults. As with immediate-release preparations, titration to a clinically effective dose is required. One large trial of *Concerta XL* (Biederman et al. 2006) involved a randomized, 6-week, placebo-controlled, parallel design study in 103 adult patients with DSM-IV ADHD. Dosage could be titrated up to 1.3 mg/kg/day; the average daily dose used in this study was 72 mg, and the maximum was 108 mg.

For an adult with a long working day and responsibilities in the evening, or where marked behavioural symptoms such as irritability and impulsivity appear once the effects of medication wear off, the use of once-daily extended-release methlyphenidate may need to be supplemented with immediate-release medication. Careful consideration of the timing of reappearance of symptoms and the pharmacokinetic profile of each drug should be considered in deciding whether to opt for a supplement of immediate-release stimulant medication or a change to atomoxetine (see below).

A recent alternative that may be considered the second line of treatment, *atomoxetine* is a specific noradrenergic reuptake inhibitor (SNRI). This new medication is currently licensed in the USA for the treatment of ADHD in both children and adults. It has recently been licensed for children with ADHD in several European countries, as well as for continued use in adulthood but only when the medication was started in childhood. This is the first major alternative to conventional stimulant drugs that act primarily by inhibiting reuptake of dopamine and the direct release of dopamine.

Similar treatment effect sizes to those seen in children have been shown in drug trials of atomoxetine (Michelson et al. 2003, Simpson and Plosker 2004, Adler et al. 2005). The potential advantages include reduced potential for drug misuse, extended action throughout the day, and a different profile of side-effects and hazards. The usual dose for adults is 80–100 mg taken once per day.

Third choices are antidepressants, particularly those that have noradrenergic effects such as desipramine (Wilens et al. 1996). Hyperactive and impulsive behaviours in both children and adults with ADHD have also been shown to diminish using tricyclic antidepressants, although they leave inattention symptoms untreated.

Other choices comprise medications like guanfacine, modafinil and bupropion that have recently been studied and proven effective in adult ADHD (Taylor and Russo 2001, Turner et al. 2004, Wilens et al. 2005). Some of these are available in Europe, but none is currently registered for ADHD. Clonidine, an alpha-2-adrenergic receptor agonist, is effective for hyperactive and impulsive behaviour in children but not for inattention. The side-effects like sedation and hypotension limit its use in adults (Kooij et al. 2001a).

Licensing of ADHD treatments
At the time of writing, drug treatments for adult ADHD are not licensed for use within the adult population in any European country (in contrast, several medications for adult ADHD have been licensed in the USA). This means that current prescriptions are written 'off-label'.

The exception is atomoxetine, which is licensed for use in adults but only when treatment was initiated in childhood or adolescence. Nevertheless, since both stimulants and atomoxetine are effective in adults with ADHD, the recommendation from experts in the management of adult ADHD is for their clinical use, both for individuals who started treatment in childhood/adolescence and for those receiving a first-time diagnosis of ADHD in adulthood.

In most cases, lack of licensing in the adult population has not come about from failed licensing applications, but rather from an historical lack of interest in treating ADHD in adults from both clinicians and drug companies. It is envisaged that this situation will change in the near future since several extended-release preparations are undergoing European trials in adult ADHD samples to demonstrate the safety and efficacy levels required by the licensing agencies. The treatment of adults is likely to remain a specialist interest in the short term, although in the medium term we expect that an increasing number of adult psychiatrists and adult mental health services will incorporate treatment of ADHD into their general practice.

Lifetime treatment
As the full ADHD syndrome does not always appear to persist into adulthood, it has been suggested that the group of adults with ADHD may be a more severe subgroup and perhaps have a higher genetic loading. Medication treatment of ADHD does not cure the disorder as symptoms return immediately following the discontinuation of medication. Therefore, lifetime medication is a possibility in many cases, and this will need to be reviewed at regular intervals. It is suggested that regular follow-up of the need for stimulant medication is performed at least once every few years. If the medication is discontinued, evaluation of the level of symptoms and of psychosocial functioning off medication for a few months should facilitate the decision how to proceed. If symptoms return and lead to impairment in work and/or social relationships, continued prescription of medication is advised. These questions need to be investigated in proper follow-up studies of adults.

Attitude towards stimulants
Although stimulants are the most studied and most effective treatment for ADHD, their use, particularly in adults, remains controversial across most European countries. Hesitancy and uncertainty about using drugs classified as controlled drugs that are not licensed for use in adult ADHD and are related to substances of abuse, is understandable. Interestingly, this hesitancy appears to stem mainly from professionals, rather than individuals with ADHD who are aware of the benefits of successful control of ADHD symptoms. Furthermore, the high level of hesitancy is not shared by child and adolescent mental health services that are aware of the potential benefits and relative safety of stimulants in children (although there was strong initial resistance to the use of stimulants in children when they were first introduced). It is therefore an unusual scenario that a treatment considered suitable for treatment in children is not generally accepted for use in adults, and it creates a particular problem for individuals making the transition from child to adult psychiatric services. Doctors treating adult patients have generally been resistant to the use of stimulants because they are not used to prescribing these medications in adults and because of unsubstantiated

concerns over their abuse potential (see ADHD and substance use disorders below). This is due to the fact that for a long time ADHD has been considered a disorder limited to childhood. There is also the more pragmatic concern that prescriptions for controlled drugs take longer to write out and therefore have a high nuisance value to busy psychiatrists and family practitioners. Continued research into the safety and efficacy of stimulants in adult patients is clearly a high priority, as is professional training.

COACHING

Coaching is a structured, supportive therapy that can be offered individually or in group sessions. The purpose of coaching is to learn new problem-solving skills for identified practical problems. Due to the early onset and persistence of ADHD, patients have often failed to learn to cope with the practical and organizational demands of daily life. Skills such as time management, and the use of tools such as checklists and handheld computers can be trained in a step-by-step programme. The support and recognition of typical ADHD difficulties by group members is an additional and powerful treatment tool during coaching in the group setting. Themes of coaching include acceptance of the disorder, learning to deal with time management, learning to limit activities to 'one goal at a time', organizing home management and finances, and dealing with relationship difficulties.

PSYCHOTHERAPY

There is little research available yet about the efficacy of psychotherapeutic treatments for adult ADHD. Cognitive behaviour therapy has recently been studied in addition to stimulant treatment for residual symptoms, and was found more effective than medication alone (Safren et al. 2005). The ability of individuals to make best use of cognitive approaches may correlate with general cognitive ability, since clinical experience indicates that some bright individuals develop effective strategies to cope with the symptoms of ADHD. However, this usually entails a high cost in the amount of time and effort required to complete many tasks. Other forms of psychotherapy such as counseling or client-based psychotherapies will have an important role in helping some individuals come to terms with and understand better the way that ADHD has influenced their personal and emotional lives. Treatment with stimulants presents great opportunities but is also a time of great change. Considerable anger and regret may form around missed opportunities, and individuals may need considerable support to take best advantage of improvements in their cognitive function.

THE ORDER OF TREATMENT IN CASES OF COMORBIDITY

The order of treatment of ADHD and comorbid disorders always depends on the severity of the different disorders and a clinical judgement on which disorder is driving the current level of behavioural impairments or mental state changes. It is therefore important to provide a diagnostic formulation based upon consideration of the possible differential diagnoses. A critical aspect of the formulation is to draw the distinction between symptoms that commonly co-occur with ADHD and major psychiatric disorders that require targeted treatments.

ADHD and mood symptoms

A volatile and irritable mood is frequently seen in adult ADHD and is not usually the consequence of comorbid depression or bipolar disorder. In this case treatment should be targeted at ADHD. On the other hand this symptom clearly overlaps with that seen in major affective disorders, and care must be taken to ensure that mood lability does not occur solely within the context of such disorders. This is determined by attending to the time-course of the symptoms (i.e. early onset, chronic trait-like course, frequency of mood swings 4–5 times a day, no recent deterioration or severe exacerbation in ADHD) and the detailed psychopathology (i.e. extreme mood swings, low or high moods sustained for longer periods, and association with other features of major affective disorder in depressive disorders).

Individuals with ADHD may present with major depression. In this case treatment of depression would become the priority because of the severe and immediate risks of untreated depression. Moreover, persistence of major depression will interfere with the interpretation of the efficacy of treatment for ADHD. The severity of ADHD symptoms and the need for stimulant medication can be considered once improvement has been seen for the depression. Data on the combined use of antidepressants and stimulants are lacking, although clinical experience suggests that the combination of antidepressants with stimulants is effective and safe.

The frequency of comorbid bipolar disorder with ADHD is currently subject to discussion and research due to the symptom overlap (irritability, volatility, overactive thought processes, restlessness, overactive behaviour, impulsive behaviour), especially in the case of juvenile-onset bipolar disorder. However, the distinction is a little easier to make in adults, and the overlap with bipolar I (manic–depressive) disorder is rarely a diagnostic dilemma. ADHD compared to bipolar disorder usually has a much earlier age of onset and a chronic persistent course. Mood swings are less extreme and more frequent (around 4–5 times a day), are interspersed by short periods of normal mood, and there are no extended periods of very low or high moods. Episodic grandiosity and sexual disinhibition are not features of ADHD. Thoughts may be ceaseless and unfocused (a distracted mind) but are not speeded up, do not show flight of ideas, and are not experienced as unusually clear or special. Adults with ADHD generally feel exhausted by their symptoms and complain of difficulty sleeping. Finally, adults with ADHD may have a family history of ADHD and other developmental disorders but rarely of bipolar disorder or schizophrenia. In cases of comorbid bipolar disorder with ADHD, (differential) diagnosis may be difficult.

ADHD and anxiety symptoms

Individuals with ADHD commonly report high levels of anxiety on rating scales. However, a more detailed enquiry about the psychopathology shows that in some cases the ADHD syndrome mimics apparent anxiety symptoms, and the primary treatment should therefore target ADHD. For example, individuals with ADHD frequently have difficulty coping with social situations (especially social groups) because they are unable to focus on conversations and tend to 'tune out'. They may as a consequence worry about how they will cope in such situations (i.e. an understandable concern) and as a result avoid group interactions. A similar scenario can occur with simple tasks such as shopping because of their experience of forgetting things and high levels of disorganization and frustration. The difficulties coping with simple everyday tasks that most of us take for granted are a source of considerable concern, and are often accompanied by avoidance of stressful tasks and poor self-esteem. In combination with ceaseless mental activity, these legitimate concerns and responses take on the appearance of a mild to moderate anxiety state, although lacking the systemic manifestations of anxiety disorders. Some patients try to cope with disorganization by getting overly rigid and perfectionist, in order to have some control over the chaos. This behaviour can mimic obsessive–compulsive disorder, but does not have the function to avert fear. It serves to control complete chaos. As with the major affective disorders, the key to understanding the comorbid symptoms is to focus on the precise phenomenology and consider whether they have a similar onset and time course to the ADHD symptoms or the extent to which they appear to be explained by and are the consequence of core ADHD symptoms.

Of course it is also the case that many individuals with ADHD will develop more typical anxiety states, and it will then be important to consider whether primary treatment should be targeted at the anxiety disorder. A judgement will need to be made on the severity of the anxiety and the strength of the current relationship between the anxiety and the ADHD symptoms. Three main courses of action can be then be considered: (1) medication for anxiety (e.g. SSRI) followed by medication for ADHD (e.g. stimulant medication); (2) medication for ADHD followed by medication for anxiety; or (3) stimulant medication for ADHD followed by cognitive–behavioural treatment for anxiety.

Untreated anxiety symptoms can deteriorate using stimulant medication due to the slight increase of pulse rate that accompanies stimulant treatment. In such cases first pharmacotherapeutic treatment of the anxiety disorder (especially panic disorder) is advised. Although it is possible to introduce two medications at the same time, it is usually advisable to introduce them one at a time. If the anxiety symptoms are severe and warrant immediate treatment then follow the first option, but consider introducing stimulant medication early on if ADHD symptoms are considerable since they may contribute to maintenance of the anxiety state. Finally, psychological interventions are far more likely to succeed once some control has been gained over the core ADHD symptoms using stimulants.

ADHD and substance use disorders
ADHD is a risk factor for substance use disorders through three potential mechanisms: (1) increased levels of reward seeking (risk taking) behaviours; (2) increased levels of conduct disorder and antisocial behaviours that are themselves associated with substance abuse; and (3) self-medication for ADHD symptoms. It should be remembered that children with ADHD often show a very poor academic performance compared to their ability, and have difficulties in developing healthy social interactions and a tendency to act in an impulsive way that may lead them to keep company with other individuals showing poor social integration. Family background and other environmental risks are another set of factors to take into consideration. The reason for the increased level of substance use disorders among individuals with ADHD is therefore necessarily complex.

In most cases severe substance use disorders should be treated first because of the known risks and impairments associated with such behaviour. Ongoing substance abuse will interfere with evaluation of ADHD treatment response, interactions will emerge, and side-effects can be intensified. Therefore all substance use should be minimized before the start of medication for ADHD.

However, it is important to recognize the role that persistent ADHD symptoms play in maintaining substance abuse. For example, street amphetamine, cocaine and ecstasy may be used to calm the mental and physical restlessness associated with ADHD. The same is true for alcohol. Cannabis is often used to relax and to fall asleep. An interesting related phenomenon that illustrates the immediate reward-seeking behaviours of some individuals with ADHD (related to the increased risk of substance abuse) is the high rate of gambling.

For these reasons it has been argued that it is important to use stimulant medication to decrease the level of ADHD symptoms in comorbid adult ADHD and substance use disorders. Case reports support the view that treatment of ADHD with stimulants may diminish the need for substance use in adults. A recent study and meta-analysis of previous studies confirms reports that treatment of ADHD with stimulants does indeed reduce the risk of substance abuse in adolescents (Wilens et al. 2003). The concerns of some professionals that use of stimulants in ADHD may lead to drug abuse (a gateway hypothesis) are not supported by available evidence.

ADHD and personality disorders
The relationship of ADHD to personality disorders is complex and to some extent semantic, although there is no doubt that ADHD is a risk factor for the development of conduct disorder and maladaptive social behaviours. Confusion, however, stems from the early onset and persistence of ADHD symptoms that therefore appear to be traits or personality characteristics rather than symptoms, the difference in definition being that symptoms represent a change from a *normal* premorbid state, such as the onset of adult depression or psychosis, while traits are considered to be enduring characteristics. Current psychiatric training tends to focus on this distinction and provides conceptualizations that do not fit well with the diagnosis of ADHD. First, because of the trait-like quality of ADHD phenomena, significant psychopathology often goes unnoticed (not recognized as a symptom) or is regarded as a personality trait that is not amenable to pharmacotherapy and is relatively resistant to psychological interventions. Second, because ADHD phenomena are frequently associated with persistent disruptive and oppositional behaviours, it is again assumed that this represents an ingrained and therapeutically resistant set of behaviours. Further confusion stems from the definitions of cluster B personality disorders, like antisocial and borderline personality disorder, that include symptoms of impulsivity, anger outbursts and mood swings which are also common features of ADHD.

The issue for diagnosis and treatment is to recognize when there is evidence for ADHD; that is whether the operational criteria were fulfilled in early childhood, and whether sufficient ADHD symptoms have persisted and continue to bring about significant (clinical) impairments. While the diagnostic focus should be on the main symptoms that define inattention, overactivity and impulsivity, it is also important to remember that irritable behaviour and mood swings are common components of the ADHD syndrome. Care must be taken to distinguish uncontrolled, impulsive, oppositional and antisocial behaviours that arise in the context of a specific ADHD syndrome from those that do not. For this reason it is often useful to make particular enquiries about symptoms that are more specific to ADHD such as short attention span, distractibility, forgetfulness, disorganization, physical restlessness and over-talkativeness, rather than focus on the occurrence of maladjusted and aggressive behaviour (which does not define ADHD).

Where ADHD and personality disorder occur together, treatment of ADHD can effectively diminish problems of inattention, impulsivity, mood swings and associated aggressive behaviour and may lead to more adherence to other treatment programmes, like psychotherapy for personality disorders. Therefore, treatment of ADHD is advised before starting treatment of personality disorders.

It should, however, be recognized that although stimulant medication may treat the specific symptoms of ADHD, overall prognosis may be poor for individuals who cannot engage in behavioural or psychotherapeutic interventions aimed at altering maladaptive patterns of behaviour or are unable to make these changes for themselves. In a few cases compliance with stimulants can be poor, even when informants such as parents and close friends report an improved behavioural response. This is usually because the increased focus and ability to reflect on patterns of behaviour that accompany treatment of ADHD may be difficult to tolerate for individuals with many years of disruptive and antisocial behaviour. It may be easier and more exciting for them to remain in the relative haze and fog of untreated ADHD.

ADHD and psychotic disorders
Psychotic symptoms should be diagnosed and treated using conventional antipsychotic medication. Severe inattention may rarely mimic the thought disorder symptoms seen in some psychoses, such as derailment, tangentiality, circumstantiality and flight of ideas. Careful monitoring of both psychotic symptoms and ADHD symptoms is advised, but it may be very difficult to distinguish residual and negative symptoms of schizophrenia from persistence of ADHD symptoms. In general the use of stimulants (dopamine agonists) is not advised for treatment of ADHD in case of comorbid psychotic symptoms, and in a few cases it is possible that stimulants might trigger a relapse (or first episode) of a psychotic illness. Alternative treatments for ADHD could be considered such as noradrendaline reuptake inhibitors (atomoxetine, reboxetine) or tricyclic anti-depressants. In some cases stimulants have been used alongside traditional antipsychotics and, despite the apparent contradiction in such a regime, have been successful in controlling both conditions; for this reason it is reasonable to keep such a combination where it has already been initiated and appears to be successful.

Concluding remarks
Morbidity and mortality are both increased in ADHD. As stated before, ADHD is frequently accompanied by a number of other psychiatric disorders. Somatic illnesses that have been suggested to be more frequent in ADHD are asthma, allergies, and impairments resulting from accidents (including dog bites, fire-setting injuries and traffic accidents) and lifestyle

(i.e. leading a hard life: smoking, alcohol and drug abuse, and lack of adequate healthcare) (Leibson et al. 2001, Mitchell et al. 2003). Adults with ADHD are at increased risk of having children with the same disorder, so that the risks of disorders and impairment easily multiply in families with ADHD. In terms of the costs to society, for children with ADHD these are estimated to be double those for normal controls, based on substantially more inpatient as well as outpatient hospitalizations and emergency department visits (Leibson et al. 2001, Chan et al. 2002). The costs of treatment and other healthcare costs of patients with ADHD and their family members, and the costs of work loss have been shown to be substantial (Birnbaum et al. 2005). Undiagnosed and untreated ADHD will lead to inefficient health care use and less satisfactory outcomes. It is therefore in everyone's interest that clinicians begin to take the disorder in adults seriously and provide appropriate diagnostic and treatment services.

An important issue is who should be carrying out these assessments. At the present time only very few psychiatrists with expertise in general adult psychiatry have acquired the necessary knowledge, and it remains the case that the majority do not yet recognize the clinical needs of this group. However, the ability to diagnose and treat ADHD does not require skills that are not already widely available, in the sense that professional staff with a good understanding of how to diagnose and treat adults for other common psychiatric disorders already have the clinical skills to make the diagnosis and manage these cases appropriately. General adult psychiatrists, for example, are well versed in the detailed psychopathology and clinical course of anxiety and affective disorders, and are therefore in the best position to make the appropriate differential diagnosis. What is now required is additional training to raise the level of awareness of ADHD as it presents in adults and the best forms of management. Specialist clinics have a key role to play in advising, supporting and training clinicians in this area, and, as with other psychiatric disorders, can assist in the management of clinically more complex cases. The experience of adult psychiatrists who have taken this step has been extremely rewarding due to the availability of effective treatments for this important clinical group.

REFERENCES

Adler LA, Spencer TJ, Milton DR, Moore RJ, Michelson D (2005) Long-term, open-label study of the safety and efficacy of atomoxetine in adults with attention-deficit/hyperactivity disorder: an interim analysis. *J Clin Psychiatry* **66**: 294–299

APA (1994) *Diagnostic and Statistical Manual of Mental Disorders, 4th edn (DSM-IV)*. Washington, DC: American Psychiatric Association.

Applegate B, Lahey BB, Hart EL, Biederman J, Hynd GW, Barkley RA, Ollendick T, Frick PJ, Greenhill L, McBurnett K, Newcorn JH, Kerdyk L, Garfinkel B, Waldman I, Shaffer D (1997) Validity of the age-of-onset criterion for ADHD: a report from the DSM-IV field trials. *J Am Acad Child Adolesc Psychiatry* **36**: 1211–1221.

Banaschewski T, Coghill D, Santosh P, Zuddas A, Asherson P, Buitelaar J, Danckaerts M, Dopfner M, Faraone SV, Rothenberger A, Sergeant J, Steinhausen HC, Sonuga-Barke EJ, Taylor E (2006) Long-acting medications for the hyperkinetic disorders: a systematic review and European treatment guideline. *Eur Child Adolesc Psychiatry* (epub ahead of print).

Barkley RA (1997) *ADHD and the Nature of Self Control*. New York: Guilford Press.

Barkley RA, Biederman J (1997) Toward a broader definition of the age-of-onset criterion for attention-deficit hyperactivity disorder. *J Am Acad Child Adolesc Psychiatry* **36**: 1204–1210.

Barkley RA, Murphy KR (1998) *Attention-Deficit Hyperactivity Disorder. A Clinical Workbook, 2nd edn.* New York: Guilford Press.

Biederman J, Faraone SV, Spencer T, Wilens T, Norman D, Lapey KA, Mick E, Lehman BK, Doyle A (1993) Patterns of psychiatric comorbidity, cognition and psychosocial functioning in adults with attention deficit hyperactivity disorder. *Am J Psychiatry* **150**: 1792–1798.

Biederman, J, Mick, E, Surman, C, Doyle, R, Hammerness, P, Harpold, T, Dunkel, S, Dougherty, M, Aleardi, M, Spencer, T (2006) A randomized, placebo-controlled trial of OROS methylphenidate in adults with attention-deficit/hyperactivity disorder. *Biol Psychiatry* **59**: 829–835.

Birnbaum HG, Kessler RC, Lowe SW, Secnik K, Greenberg PE, Leong SA, Swensen AR (2005) Costs of attention deficit-hyperactivity disorder (ADHD) in the US: excess costs of persons with ADHD and their family members in 2000. *Curr Med Res Opin* **21**: 195–206.

Brown TE (1996) *Attention-Deficit Disorder Scales.* San Antonio: Psychological Corporation.

Buitelaar JK (2002) Epidemiological aspects: what have we learned over the past decade? In: Sandberg S, ed. *Hyperactivity and Attention Disorders of Childhood, 2nd edn.* Cambridge: Cambridge University Press, pp. 30–63.

Chan E, Zhan C, Homer CJ (2002) Health care use and costs for children with attention-deficit/hyperactivity disorder: national estimates from the medical expenditure panel survey. *Arch.Pediatr.Adolesc.Med* **156**: 504–511.

Conners CK (2002) Forty years of methylphenidate treatment in attention-deficit/ hyperactivity disorder. *J Atten Disord* **6** Suppl 1: S17–S30.

Conners CK, Erhardt D, Sparrow E, Conners MA (1998) *CAARS Adult ADHD Rating Scales.* New York: Multi Health Systems.

Downey KK, Stelson FW, Pomerleau OF, Giordani B (1997) Adult attention deficit hyperactivity disorder: psychological test profiles in a clinical population. *J Nerv Ment Dis* **185**: 32–38.

DuPaul GJ, Power TJ, Anastopolous AD, Reid R (1998) *ADHD Rating Scale-IV. Checklists, Norms and Clinical Interpretation.* New York: Guilford Press.

Epstein J, Johnson D, Conners K (1999) *Conners Adult ADHD Diagnostic Interview for DSM-IV (CAADID).* New York: Multi Health Systems.

Faraone SV, Biederman J, Monuteaux MC (2000) Toward guidelines for pedigree selection in genetic studies of attention deficit hyperactivity disorder. *Gen Epidemiol* **18**: 1–16.

Faraone SV, Spencer T, Aleardi M, Pagano C, Biederman J (2004) Meta-analysis of the efficacy of methylphenidate for treating adult attention-deficit/hyperactivity disorder. *J Clin Psychopharmacol* **24**: 24–29.

Faraone SV, Biederman J, Mick E (2006) The age-dependent decline of attention deficit hyperactivity disorder: a meta-analysis of follow-up studies. *Psychol Med* **36**: 159–165.

Kessler RC, Adler L, Ames M, Barkley RA, Birnbaum H, Greenberg P, Johnston JA, Spencer T, Ustun TB (2005a) The prevalence and effects of adult attention deficit/hyperactivity disorder on work performance in a nationally representative sample of workers. *J Occup Environ Med* **47**: 565–572.

Kessler RC, Adler L, Ames M, Demler O, Faraone S, Hiripi E, Howes MJ, Jin R, Seknik K, Spencer T, Ustun TB, Walters EE (2005b) The World Health Organization Adult ADHD Self-Report Scale (ASRS): a short screening scale for use in the general population. *Psychol Med* **35**: 245–256.

Kooij JJ (2002) [*ADHD in Adults. Introduction to Diagnosis and Treatment.*] Lisse: Swets & Zeitlinger (Dutch).

Kooij JJ, Aeckerlin LP, Buitelaar JK (2001a) [Functioning, comorbidity and treatment of 141 adults with attention deficit hyperactivity disorder (ADHD) at a psychiatric outpatients department.] *Ned Tijdschr Geneeskd* **145**: 1498–1501 (Dutch).

Kooij JJ, Middelkoop HA, van Gils K, Buitelaar JK (2001b) The effect of stimulants on nocturnal motor activity and sleep quality in adults with ADHD: an open-label case–control study. *J Clin Psychiatry* **62**: 952–956.

Kooij JJ, Burger H, Boonstra AM, Van der Linden PD, Kalma LE, Buitelaar JK (2004) Efficacy and safety of methylphenidate in 45 adults with attention-deficit/hyperactivity disorder (ADHD). A randomized placebo-controlled double-blind cross-over trial. *Psychol Med* **34**: 973–982.

Kooij JJ, Buitelaar JK, van den Oord EJ, Furer JW, Rijnders CA, Hodiamont PP (2005) Internal and external validity of attention-deficit hyperactivity disorder in a population-based sample of adults. *Psychol Med* **35**: 817–827.

Leibson CL, Katusic SK, Barbaresi WJ, Ransom J, O'Brien PC (2001) Use and costs of medical care for children and adolescents with and without attention-deficit/hyperactivity disorder. *JAMA* **285**: 60–66.

Mannuzza S, Klein RG, Bessler A, Malloy P, LaPadula M (1993) Adult outcome of hyperactive boys. Educational achievement, occupational rank, and psychiatric status. *Arch Gen Psychiatry* **50**: 565–576.

Michelson D, Adler L, Spencer T, Reimherr FW, West SA, Allen AJ, Kelsey D, Wernicke J, Dietrich A, Milton D (2003) Atomoxetine in adults with ADHD: two randomized, placebo-controlled studies. *Biol Psychiatry* **53**: 112–120.

Mitchell RB, Nanez G, Wagner JD, Kelly J (2003) Dog bites of the scalp, face, and neck in children. *Laryngoscope* **113**: 492–495.

Murphy K, Barkley RA (1996a) Attention deficit hyperactivity disorder in adults: comorbidities and adaptive impairments. *Compr Psychiatry* **37**: 393–401.

Murphy KR, Barkley RA (1996b) Parents of children with attention-deficit/hyperactivity disorder: psychological and attentional impairment. *Am J Orthopsychiatry* **66**: 93–102.

Murphy K, Barkley RA (1996c) Prevalence of DSM-IV symptoms of ADHD in adult licensed drivers: implications for clinical diagnosis. *J Atten Disord* **3**: 147–161.

Pineda D, Ardila A, Rosselli M, Arias BE, Henao GC, Gomez LF, Mejia SE, Miranda ML (1999) Prevalence of attention-deficit/hyperactivity disorder symptoms in 4- to 17-year-old children in the general population. *J Abnorm Child Psychol* **27**: 455–462.

Robins LN, Helzer JE, Croughan J, Ratcliff KS (1981) National Institute of Mental Health Diagnostic Interview Schedule. Its history, characteristics, and validity. *Arch Gen Psychiatry* **38**: 381–389.

Rowland AS, Lesesne CA, Abramowitz AJ (2002) The epidemiology of attention-deficit/hyperactivity disorder (ADHD): a public health view. *Ment Retard Dev Disabil Res Rev* **8**: 162–170.

Safren SA, Otto MW, Sprich S, Winett CL, Wilens TE, Biederman J (2005) Cognitive–behavioral therapy for ADHD in medication-treated adults with continued symptoms. *Behav Res Ther* **43**: 831–842.

Simpson D, Plosker GL (2004) Atomoxetine: a review of its use in adults with attention deficit hyperactivity disorder. *Drugs* **64**: 205–222.

Spencer T, Wilens T, Biederman J, Faraone SV, Ablon JS, Lapey K (1995) A double-blind, crossover comparison of methylphenidate and placebo in adults with childhood onset attention deficit hyperactivity disorder. *Arch Gen Psychiatry* **52**: 434–443.

Spencer T, Biederman J, Wilens T, Doyle R, Surman C, Prince J, Mick E, Aleardi M, Herzig K, Faraone S (2005) A large, double-blind, randomized clinical trial of methylphenidate in the treatment of adults with attention-deficit/hyperactivity disorder. *Biol Psychiatry* **57**: 456–463.

Taylor E, Chadwick O, Heptinstall E, Danckaerts M (1996) Hyperactivity and conduct problems as risk factors for adolescent development. *J Am Acad Child Adolesc Psychiatry* **35**: 1213–1226.

Taylor E, Dopfner M, Sergeant J, Asherson P, Banaschewski T, Buitelaar J, Coghill D, Danckaerts M, Rothenberger A, Sonuga-Barke E, Steinhausen HC, Zuddas A (1996) European clinical guidelines for hyperactivity disorder – first upgrade. *Eur Child Adolesc Psychiatry* **13** Suppl 1: 17–30.

Taylor FB, Russo J (2001) Comparing guanfacine and dextroamphetamine for the treatment of adult attention-deficit/hyperactivity disorder. *Clin Psychopharmacol* **21**: 223–228.

Turner DC, Clark L, Dowson J, Robbins TW, Sahakian BJ (2004) Modafinil improves cognition and response inhibition in adult attention-deficit/hyperactivity disorder. *Biol Psychiatry* **55**: 1031–1040.

Ward MF, Wender PH, Reimherr FW (1993) The WURS: A rating scale to aid in the retrospective diagnosis of attention deficit disorder in childhood. *Am J Psychiatry* **150**: 885–890.

Weiss G, Hechtman L, Milroy T, Perlman T (1985) Psychiatric status of hyperactives as adults: A controlled prospective 15-year follow-up of 63 hyperactive children. *J Am Acad Child Psychiatry* **24**: 211–220.

Wender PH, Reimherr FW, Wood D, Ward M (1985) A controlled study of methylphenidate in the treatment of attention deficit disorder, residual type, in adults. *Am J Psychiatry* **142**: 547–552.

Wilens TE, Biederman J, Spencer TJ, Prince J (1995) Pharmacotherapy of adult attention deficit/hyperactivity disorder: a review. *J Clin Psychopharmacol* **15**: 270–279.

Wilens TE, Biederman J, Prince J, Spencer TJ, Faraone SV, Warburton R, Schleifer D, Harding M, Linehan C, Geller D (1996) Six-week, double-blind, placebo-controlled study of desipramine for adult attention deficit hyperactivity disorder. *Am J Psychiatry* **153**: 1147–1153.

Wilens TE, Faraone SV, Biederman J, Gunawardene S (2003) Does stimulant therapy of attention-deficit/hyperactivity disorder beget later substance abuse? A meta-analytic review of the literature. *Pediatrics* **111**: 179–185.

Wilens TE, Haight BR, Horrigan JP, Hudziak JJ, Rosenthal NE, Connor DF, Hampton KD, Richard NE, Modell JG (2005) Bupropion XL in adults with attention-deficit/hyperactivity disorder: a randomized, placebo-controlled study. *Biol Psychiatry* **57**: 793–801.

WHO (1992) *International Statistical Classification of Diseases and Related Health Problems, 10th edn (ICD-10)*. Geneva: World Health Organization.

The aim of this guide is to provide a comprehensive list of the 18 items that are required to make a diagnosis of ADHD according the DSM-IV. These items are the same as those listed in ICD-10; however, ICD-10 insists that every item must be present in more than one environment (e.g. home and school or work). Under DSM-IV some of the symptoms must be present in two or more settings, but there is no requirement that each item must fulfil the criteria of pervasiveness. Symptoms must be maladaptive and inconsistent with developmental level. Overall, there must be clear evidence of clinically significant impairment in social, academic or occupational functioning.

In adults, there should be two parts to the diagnostic interview. The 18 item list is the same for each, but the symptoms are likely to be reflected in different types of behaviours at the different ages:
• Childhood mental state and behaviours (off medication)
• Current mental state and behaviours (off medication)

Age of onset in early childhood: It is critical that a good account is taken of childhood psychopathology. A diagnosis of ADHD can be made only with an onset of some symptoms prior to the age of 7 years. Due to the problems with obtaining reliable retrospective accounts from such an early age, it is usually acceptable to use the less stringent criterion of onset by age 12 when making the diagnosis in adults.

In addition to taking a history from the individual being assessed, it is usual to enquire after childhood symptoms and behaviour from one or both parents. If this is not possible an older sibling may be able to give an accurate account. Problems at school may be established from individual and informant accounts, and verified from school records. It is often useful to interview the informant with the proband to obtain a consensus account of childhood symptoms. In case of disagreement between informants, the most reliable informant(s) should be followed.

Symptoms are not better accounted for by another disorder: They should not occur exclusively during the course of a pervasive developmental disorder (autism or Asperger syndrome), schizophrenia or other psychotic disorders, mood disorders, anxiety disorders, dissociative disorders or a personality disorder.

Some impairment from the symptoms is present in two or more settings: Impairment must be observed at home as well in other settings such as school or work.

Clear evidence of clinically significant impairment in social, academic or occupational function: The criterion of clinically significant impairment is an important one and can affect many different aspects of an individual's life. Guidelines for impairment are given below.

Adult (current) symptoms
Following the assessment interview it should be possible to include or exclude the following 18 DSM-IV items of ADHD. Examples of each item and how they apply to adults is given below. Note that there is overlap between some of the symptoms. Some symptoms may be observed in the mental state, although most will need to be enquired after.

INATTENTION
A1a
Often fails to give close attention to detail: Difficulty remembering where they put things. In work this may lead to costly errors. Tasks that require detail and are tedious (e.g. income tax returns) become very stressful. This may include overly perfectionistic and rigid behaviour, needing too much time for tasks involving details in order to prevent forgetting any of them.

A1b
Often has difficulty sustaining attention: Inability to complete tasks such as tidying a room or mowing the lawn,

without forgetting the objective and starting something else. Inability to persist with boring jobs. Inability to sustain sufficient attention to read a book that is not of special interest, although there is no reading disorder. Inability to keep accounts, write letters or pay bills. Attention, however, often can be sustained during exciting, new or interesting activities like using the internet, chatting, computer games, etc. This does not exclude the criterion when boring activities are not completed.

A1c
Often does not seem to listen when spoken to: Adults receive complaints that they do not listen, that it is difficult to gain their attention. Even where they appear to have heard, they forget what was said and follow instructions or the flow of a conversation. These complaints reflect a sense that they are "not always in the room", "not all there", "not tuned in".

A1d
Fails to follow through on instructions and complete tasks: Adults may observe difficulty in following other people's instructions. Inability to read or follow instructions in a manual for appliances. Failure to keep commitments undertaken (e.g. work around the house).

A1e
Difficulty organizing tasks or activities: Adults note recurrent errors (e.g. lateness, missed appointments, missing critical deadlines). Sometimes a deficit in this area is seen in the amount of delegation to others, e.g. secretary at work or spouse at home.

A1f
Avoids or dislikes sustained mental effort: Putting off tasks such as responding to letters, completing tax returns, organizing old papers, paying bills, establishing a will. One can enquire about specifics then ask why particular tasks were not attended to. These adults often have a tendency for procrastination.

A1g
Often loses things needed for tasks: Misplacing purse, wallet, keys, and assignments from work, where car is parked, tools, and even children!

A1h
Easily distracted by extraneous stimuli: Subjectively experience distractibility and describe ways in which they try to overcome this. This may include listening to white noise, multi-tasking, requiring absolute quiet or creating an emergency to achieve adequate states of arousal to complete tasks; many projects ongoing simultaneously; and trouble with completion of tasks.

A1i
Forgetful in daily activities: May complain of memory problems. They head out to the supermarket with a list of things, but end up coming home having failed to complete their tasks or having purchased something else.

HYPERACTIVITY
A2a
Fidgets with hands or feet: This item may be observed, but it is also useful to ask about this. Fidgeting may include picking their fingers, shaking their knees, tapping their hands or feet and changing position. Fidgeting is most likely to be observed while waiting in the waiting area of the clinic.

A2b
Leaves seat in situations in which remaining seated is usual: Adults may be restless, e.g. frustrated while dining out in restaurants, and unable to sit during conversations, meetings and conferences. This may also manifest as a strong internal feeling of restlessness when waiting.

A2c
Wanders or runs about excessively, or frequent subjective feelings of restlessness: Adults may describe their subjective sense of always needing to be "on the go", or feeling more comfortable with stimulating activities (e.g. skiing) than with more sedentary types of recreation. They may pace during the interview.

A2d

Difficulty engaging in leisure activities quietly: Adults may describe an unwillingness/dislike to ever just stay home or engage in quiet activities. They may complain that they are workaholics, in which case detailed examples should be given.

A2e

Often "on the go" or acts as if driven by a motor: Significant others may have a sense of the exhausting and frenetic pace of these adults. ADHD adults will often appear to expect the same frenetic pace of others. Holidays may be described by others as draining since there is no opportunity for rest.

A2f

Talks excessively: Excessive talking makes dialogue difficult. This may interfere with a spouse's sense of "being heard" or achieving intimacy. This chatter may be experienced as nagging and may interfere with normal social interactions. Clowning, repartee or other means of dominating conversations may mask an inability to engage in give-and-take conversation.

IMPULSIVITY

A2g

Blurts out answers before questions have been completed: This will usually be observed during the interview. This may also be experienced by probands, as a subjective sense of other people talking too slowly and of finding it difficult to wait for them to finish. Tendency to say what comes to mind without considering timing or appropriateness.

A2h

Difficulty waiting in turn: Adults find it difficult to wait for others to finish tasks at their own pace, such as children. They may feel irritated waiting in line at bank machines or in a restaurant. They may be aware of their own intense efforts to force themselves to wait. Some adults compensate for this by carrying something to do at all times.

A2i

Interrupts or intrudes on others: This is most often experienced by adults as social ineptness at social gatherings or even with close friends. An example might be inability to watch others struggle with a task (such as trying to open a door with a key) without jumping in to try for themselves.

Symptoms associated with adult ADHD

Some symptoms are not a requirement for a DSM-IV diagnosis of ADHD but are commonly associated with the disorder and should therefore be looked for:

Procrastination: Seen when assignments are not begun until the day they are due. In adult life procrastination causes potentially serious consequences, such as not paying bills, not completing income tax forms and not answering letters – all of which make life difficult both for the individual and their spouse.

Low tolerance of frustration: This is related to impulsivity and is often described as being on a "short fuse". Relatively minor frustrations cause catastrophic reactions that may manifest as actual loss of temper or by getting in an angry mood. It may occur at home or at work and interferes with relationships in either setting.

Mood lability: Mood lability is very commonly seen (up to 90% of cases). The characteristic mood is highly volatile from one part of the day to the next, changing around 4–5 times a day. Mood changes are not necessarily in response to external events although they may be. The mood is up and down, often for an hour or a few hours. It has been described as like a "roller coaster". Unlike the mood changes seen in unipolar or bipolar affective disorders, the mood swings are not so extreme, do not last for days or weeks at a time, and do not fit into an episodic or cyclical pattern.

Low self-esteem: Diminished self-esteem is very common. It is expected given the life-long problems with rejections and failures that occur more frequently than would be expected given their individual potential. Problems of low self-esteem that start in childhood are often enduring (e.g. following academic failure). Adults often describe feeling "stupid and different" at some time in their life. Even successful individuals feel is if they are a fraud or a nuisance to those around them, and they frequently complain that they are unable to perform at the level that they expect of themselves. Low self-esteem is often pervasive since it started so early in life.

Other common associated symptoms include:
- Underachievement associated with a sense of failure. This may result from academic and social failure at school, frequent changing of jobs due to boredom or understimulation, or being fired for poor performance
- A frequent search for high stimulation
- An intolerance of boredom
- Hyper-focusing: ADHD is not usually the result of a core attention deficit, but distribution (regulation) of attention is problematic
- Trouble going through proper procedures because of boredom and frustration
- Tendency to worry needlessly (worry becomes what attention turns into when it is not focused)
- Sense of insecurity
- Inaccurate self-observation and self-assessment of their impact on others.

Assessment of impairment
Impairment is a requirement for a diagnosis of ADHD. You need to assess whether an individual is impaired relative to his or her own potential, or relative to expected norms. Some very bright individuals are not impaired relative to expected norms, but reveal unequivocal impairment relative to their own potential. It is important to enquire into different areas of life since someone with ADHD may be brilliant at some sorts of work, while feeling totally inadequate because of their inability to be organized or to do work around the house.

Quality of life: Mood lability, a short fuse and constant efforts to correct scatterbrained mistakes are frustrating and demoralizing.

Family life: Even where an adult with ADHD feels fine, interviewing of the patient's spouse/family may reveal significant dysfunction.

Work: While some ADHD individuals find work that is compatible with their symptoms, they may be impaired by not being able to move in new directions where they would otherwise have desired to move. Others may be functioning in attention-demanding professions, but at great emotional cost and without much success. Work may not be commensurate with their intelligence and educational background. This is usually experienced as underachievement.

Love: ADHD is hard on relationships, and some adults with ADHD give up on their capacity for intimacy and lead an isolated existence. They may be unaware of the ways in which their ADHD-caused behaviour patterns have contributed to relationship failures.

Education: Many adults with ADHD are impeded from obtaining an education appropriate to their potential (usually assessed by IQ). A history of academic underachievement or erratic performance represents academic impairment.

Activities of daily life (ADL): Even high-functioning individuals with ADHD may have difficulties with ADL such as shopping, cleaning, dressing or managing money. The deficit is seen not in what the individual can do, but in what s/he actually does – so direct observation or an informant is required to assess this properly.

INDEX

DC-LD (Diagnostic Criteria for Learning Disability), 204
definitions, 21, 53, 95, 115
  hyperactivity, 7, 71
depression, 56, 95
  adults, 241
  as comorbidity, 102
  as differential diagnosis, 101
  learning disability, 203–4, 218
  'masked,' 204
  pharmacotherapy, 123–4, 128, 182, 186, 238
  symptoms, 101
desipramine, 124, 238
Developmental Behavior Checklist, 209, 214
developmental coordination disorder, 82, 188
developmental delay, 90–1, 196, 197
  global, 91, 217
  see also neurodevelopment
developmental disorders, 56
  see also specific disorders
developmental neurobiology (normal), neuroimaging studies, 29, 31
dexamphetamine
  adults, 237
  adverse effects, 119
  efficacy, 173
  information for families, 137–8
  titration, 178–9
Dexedrine, see dexamphetamine
diagnosis, 21, 27, 53–5, 115
  adults, see adults (with ADHD)
  age of child at, 194
  conduct disorder, 9, 55, 95, 96–7
  criteria, 8–9, 9, 75, 229–30
  cultural factors, 11, 54
  differential diagnosis, 94–104, 191, 216–19, 217
    affective disorders vs, 101
    learning disability vs, 95–6, 216–19, 217
    oppositional defiant disorder vs, 96–7
  epilepsy, 92
  hyperkinetic conduct disorder, 9, 94–5
  hyperkinetic disorder, see hyperkinetic disorder (HKD)
  overshadowing, 205
  pathway to, 10–11
  prior to referral, 54–5
    see also referral
  social factors, 11, 54
  validity, 16–17, 18–19, 194
  see also assessment; specific criteria
Diagnostic and Statistical Manual of Mental Disorders (DSM-IV)
  ADHD, 8–9, 9, 53, 183, 229–30
  conduct disorder, 8, 97
  hyperactivity criteria, 9, 9
  learning disability, 202–4

Diagnostic Criteria for Learning Disability (DC-LD), 204
Diagnostic Interview Schedule for Children (DISC), 208
dietary factors, 45
dietary interventions, 16, 22, 172–3, 175
Differential Ability Scales, 79
differential diagnosis, see under diagnosis
diffusion tensor imaging, 36
direct contingency management, 143–4
direct observation, assessment, 71, 76–7, 214–15
Disability Adjustment Schedule, 209–10
DISC (Diagnostic Interview Schedule for Children), 208
distractibility, 2, 3
  see also inattentiveness
dopamine beta hydroxylase (DBH), polymorphism, 42–3
dopamine D_2 receptors, SPECT/PET studies, 35
dopamine D_4 receptor gene (DRD4) polymorphism, 40–1
dopamine D_5 receptor gene (DRD5) polymorphism, 41
dopaminergic neurotransmission
  ADHD aetiology, 6, 17, 88
  animal models of ADHD, 37
  learning disability, 206
  polymorphisms and genetic associations, 40–2
  preschool children, 196
  see also specific components
dopaminergic therapy, periodic limb movement disorder, 163
dopamine transporter (DAT)
  DAT1 polymorphism, 41–2
  functional role, 41
  knockout mice, 37
  SPECT/PET studies, 35
Down syndrome, 210
DRD4 (dopamine D_4 receptor gene) polymorphism, 40–1
DRD5 (dopamine D_5 receptor gene) polymorphism, 41
drug response, neuroimaging studies, 32–3, 34, 35
DSM-IV classification, see Diagnostic and Statistical Manual of Mental Disorders (DSM-IV)
DuPaul Rating Scales, 213
dyslexia, 72, 79, 95, 207
dysomnias, 164
dysphoria, stimulant-related, 121

E
ecstasy, 243
educational impairment, 75–6
electroencephalography, 88
elimination diets, 172–3
EMG, tibialis anterior, 163

255

hyperkinetic disorder criteria, 8, 229–30
learning disability, 202–4, *203*
imipramine, 123–4, 126, 182
  ASD/ADHD, 101
  information for families, 138
  titration, 182–3
impulsiveness, 4–6, 18, 73
  adults, 250
  assessment, 4, 81, 184–5
    ICD-10/DSM-IV criteria, 9, *9*
    PACS Scale, 65–6, 69
  brain lesions, 15
  child neglect association, 16
  learning disability, 211
  subjective experience, 7
inattentiveness, 1–4, 18
  assessment, 73–4, 184–5, 248–9
    cognitive analyses, 2–4, *3*
    ICD-10/DSM-IV criteria, 9, *9*
    PACS Scale, 66–9
    secondary, 95–6
  brain lesions, 15
  child neglect association, 16
information/advice
  for families, 23–6, 112, 192, 193
    pharmacotherapy-related, 134–40
    useful contacts, 24–5
  parenting, 170–1
  primary care, 191–3
  for teachers, 115–17
information processing deficits, 74
  brain lesions associated, 15
inheritance of ADHD, *see* genetic factors
inhibition tasks
  anatomical MRI and, 30–1
  functional MRI and, 32
inhibitory control deficits, 74
insomnia, *see* sleep problems
instructional accommodation, 107–8
intellectual ability, 15–16, 95–6, 105
  assessment, 78–80
  impairment, 187
  learning disability, *see* learning disability
International Molecular Genetic Study of Autism
    Consortium 2001, 207
*International Statistical Classification of Diseases
    and Related Health Problems, see* ICD-10 clas-
    sification
interpersonal relationships, teacher–student, 112
interventions, 21–2, 170–93
  adults, *see* adults (with ADHD)
  attributional training, 111–2
  behavioural management, *see* behavioural therapy
  complementary approaches, 173
  dietary, 16, 22, 172–3, 175
  environmental management, 144–7

goals, 77
initial approaches, 170–2, *171*
learning disabled children, 219–22
monitoring effects, 77–8, 177
parent-based, *see* parents/parenting
pharmacological, *see* pharmacotherapy
preschool children, *see* preschool children
school-based, *see* school-based interventions
interviews, *see* assessment
IQ, *see* intellectual ability
iron deficiency, 16, 88

L

language/speech problems, 81–2
lead exposure, 16, 45
learning disability, 202–27
  aetiology, 206–8, *208*
  aggression, 130, 217
  assessment, 212–19
  autism, 206, 209, 215, 218
  British Household Survey, 208, 209
  classification, 202–4, *203*
  cognitive deficits, 210–1
  as comorbidity, 87, 96, 128, 211–2, 216–9
  definition, 202–4
  as differential diagnosis, 95–6, 216–9, *217*
  family risk factors, 210
  features associated, 186
    depression, 203–4, 218
    restlessness, 96
  hyperkinesis with stereotypies, 104
  hyperkinetic disorder, 205–6, 208–9
  impulsiveness, 211
  intellectual function, 79
  interventions, 219–22
  memory function, 211
  preschool children, 197
  prevalence, 208–10
  research, 222
  risk factors, 208–10
  school failure, 105
  sexual abuse, 218
  tic disorders, 218
linkage analysis, 39

M

macrocephaly, 91
magnesium pemoline, 120, 129
magnetic resonance imaging (MRI)
  anatomical/structural, 29–31
    attention/inhibition tasks and, 30–1
    clinical correlation, 30
    cross-sectional studies, 30
    longitudinal studies, 29–30
    unmedicated children, 29–30
    volumetric techniques, 29

home–school communication, 110
information/education
  parent/child, 112
  teachers, 115–7
self-regulation, 110–1
success, 106–7
whole-school approach, 105
school behaviour, 115–6
  assessment, PACS Scale, 70
  variation, 105–6
seizures, 92, 188, 216, 218–9
  see also epilepsy
selective serotonin reuptake inhibitors (SSRIs), 101
  see also specific drugs
self-attribution, 111–2
self-evaluation, reinforced, 148–9
self-harm, 102
self-regulation, school-based interventions, 110–1
separation anxiety disorder, 98–9
serotonergic neurotransmission
  animal models of ADHD, 38
  functions, 38
  polymorphisms and genetic associations, 42
serotonin receptors, *5HTR 1B* polymorphism, 42
serotonin transporter, *5-HTT/SLC6A*4 genetic polymorphism, 42
sex differences, 72
  adult ADHD, 231–2
  corpus callosum and, 45
  epidemiology, 13–14, 231
  learning disability, 209
  referral and, 54, 231
sexual abuse, learning disabled children, 218
shopping trips, behaviour assessment, 64–5
single parents, 194
single-photon emission computed tomography (SPECT), 34–5, 235
  drug response and, 35
  MRS vs, 33
SLC6A4 gene polymorphism, 42
sleep architecture disturbance, 163–4
sleep hygiene, 166
sleep onset insomnia, 161, 165, 166
sleep phase delay syndrome, 161
sleep problems, 160–9
  as comorbidity, 164
  primary, 161–4
  screening, 167
  stimulant-related, 121, 161, 164–6, 178–9
  see also specific disorders
sleep-related breathing disorder, 161, 162
sleep–wake cycle, serotonin role, 38
Smith–Magennis syndrome, *208*
smoking
  ADHD and, 44
  parents of ADHD children, 15, 45

SNAP-25 gene
  animal models of ADHD, 37
  polymorphism, 43
snoring, 161–2
social factors, 162
  costs to society, 245
  influence on diagnosis, 11, 54
social skills training, 150–1
Sotos syndrome, 91, *208*
specific noradrenergic reuptake inhibitors (SNRIs), 238
  see also specific drugs
SPECT, *see* single-photon emission computed tomography (SPECT)
speech, self-directed internalized, 110
speech/language problems, 81–2
spelling disability, 206
spontaneously hypertensive rat, 37
STAR (Stop–Act–Review), 111
stereotypies, 95, 104
stimulant medication, *see* pharmacotherapy
Stop–Act–Review (STAR), 111
Stop–Think–Do, 111, 148
Strattera, *see* atomoxetine
Strengths and Difficulties Questionnaire (SDQ), 58, 213
stress, ADHD aetiology, 15
striatum, 27
  MRS studies, 34
substance abuse, 90, 101, 175, 242–3
  maternal, 15
  Tourette syndrome, 104
sucrose intake, 45
symptom domains, 9, *9*

T
talkativeness, assessment, 61–5
'talk down' technique, 198
teachers, 57–8
  see also school-based interventions
Teacher's Report Form (TRF), 129
television watching, assessment, 60–1, 213
temper tantrums
  autism spectrum disorder, 99–100
  preschool children, 196
Test of Everyday Attention for Children (TEA-Ch), 4, 80, 81
Test of Variables of Attention (TOVA), 3, 165
thalamocortical dysfunction, 27, *28*
Thames Valley Test Company, 80
thyroid abnormalities, 16, 88, 91, 216
tibialis anterior EMG, *163*
tic disorders, 95, 175, 222
  learning disability, 218
  pharmacotherapy, 104, 186–7
  Tourette syndrome, *see* Tourette syndrome

time out
  preschool children, 198
  school-based intervention, 110
tomoxetine, *see* atomoxetine
Tourette syndrome, 8, 91, 175, 222
  as comorbidity, 103–4, 127–8
  features associated, *185*, 186
  pharmacotherapy, 186
  substance abuse, 104
TOVA (Test of Variables of Attention), 3, 165
toxicological influences, 45
TPH2 (tryptophan hydroxylase-2) gene polymorphism, 42
treatment, *see* interventions
T2 relaxometry, 33
tricyclic antidepressants, 128, 186, 238
  see also specific drugs
tryptophan hydroxylase-2 (*TPH2*) gene polymorphism, 42
tuberous sclerosis, 90

V
validity
  animal models, 37
  diagnostic, 16–17, 18–19, 194
valproate, 182
variable number tandem repeats, *DAT1* gene, 41–2
velo–cardio–facial syndrome, 91, 208
venlafaxine, 124, 182

video
  family information, 24
  teacher information, 117
vigilance, noradrenergic systems and, 38
Vineland Adaptive Behavior Scales, 215
vision assessment, 90

W
websites, family information, 25–6
Wechsler Intelligence Scale for Children – 3rd edition (WISC-III), 78–9, 81
Wechsler Intelligence Scale for Children – 4th edition (WISC-IV), 78–9
weight measurement, 88, 90, 121
Wender–Utah Rating Scale (WURS), 235
Weschler Adult Intelligence Test – 3rd edition (WAIT-III), 79
Weschler Individual Achievement Test – 2nd edition (WIAT-II), 79–80
Weschler Preschool and Primary Scale of Intelligence – 3rd edition (WPPSI-III), 79
white matter, anatomical MRI studies, 29
Williams syndrome, 91, *208*, 210

X
X chromosome associations, 44

Z
zinc deficiency, 16